BIOAVAILABILITY OF NUTRIENTS FOR ANIMALS
Amino Acids, Minerals, and Vitamins

BIOAVAILABILITY OF NUTRIENTS FOR ANIMALS
Amino Acids, Minerals, and Vitamins

Edited by

Clarence B. Ammerman
Department of Animal Science
University of Florida
Gainesville, Florida

David H. Baker
Department of Animal Science
University of Illinois
Urbana, Illinois

Austin J. Lewis
Department of Animal Science
University of Nebraska
Lincoln, Nebraska

ACADEMIC PRESS
San Diego   New York   Boston   London   Sydney   Tokyo   Toronto

Find Us on the Web! http://www.apnet.com

This book is printed on acid-free paper.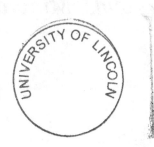

Copyright © 1995 by ACADEMIC PRESS

Academic Press
A Division of Harcourt Brace & Company
525 B Street, Suite 1900, San Diego, California 92101-4495

United Kingdom Edition published by
Academic Press Limited
24-28 Oval Road, London NW1 7DX

Library of Congress Cataloging-in-Publication Data

Bioavailability of nutrients for animals : amino acids, minerals, vitamins / edited
    by Clarence B. Ammerman, David H. Baker, Austin J. Lewis
        p.   cm.
    Includes index.
     ISBN 012-056250-2 (alk. paper)
      1. Animal nutrition.   2. Minerals—Bioavailability.   3. Amino
    acids—Bioavailability.   4. Vitamins—Bioavailability.
    I. Ammerman, Clarence B.   II. Baker, David H.   III. Lewis, Austin J.
    (David Hiram). date.
    SF95.B52   1995   95-10078
    636.08'52—dc20   CIP

Printed in the United States of America
98 99 IBT 7 5 4 3 2

CONTENTS

CONTRIBUTORS

Numbers in parentheses indicate the pages on which the authors' contributions begin.

Clarence B. Ammerman (83, 127, 157, 303, 349, 367), Department of Animal Science, University of Florida, Gainesville, Florida 32611

David H. Baker (67, 127, 367, 399), Department of Animal Sciences, University of Illinois, Urbana, Illinois 61801

Henry S. Bayley (35), Department of Nutritional Sciences, University of Guelph, Guelph, Ontario, Canada N1G 2W1

Sharon A. Benz (201), Food and Drug Administration, Center for Veterinary Medicine, Rockville, Maryland 20855

Pamela R. Henry (5, 119, 169, 201, 239, 303, 337, 349), Department of Animal Science, University of Florida, Gainesville, Florida 32611

Austin J. Lewis (5, 35, 67), Department of Animal Science, University of Nebraska, Lincoln, Nebraska 68583

Ramon C. Littell (5), Department of Statistics, University of Florida, Gainesville, Florida 32611

Elwyn R. Miller (157, 169, 295), Department of Animal Science, Michigan State University, East Lansing, Michigan 48824

Joseph H. Soares, Jr. (95, 257), Department of Animal Sciences, University of Maryland, College Park, Maryland 20740

FOREWORD

The formulation of animal diets that will assuredly and economically meet nutrient needs depends upon knowledge of (1) nutrient requirements, (2) nutrient concentrations in dietary ingredients, and (3) bioavailability of those nutrients. Information bases supporting the first two corners of this triad have been published by the Committee on Animal Nutrition of the National Research Council/National Academy of Sciences. The NRC series on nutrient requirements of domestic and laboratory animals includes current best estimates of minimum nutrient needs, often determined with purified diets. Also included are tables of feed composition in which average nutrient concentrations in individual ingredients are presented.

Until the publication of "Bioavailability of Nutrients for Animals: Amino Acids, Minerals, and Vitamins," there was no single source of information supporting the third corner of the diet-formulation triad. Now it is possible, with some assurance, to formulate diets that meet nutrient needs using ingredients in which some nutrients are bound and only partially available. "Bioavailability of Nutrients for Animals" includes information on the bioavailability of amino acids, minerals, and vitamins in natural feedstuffs plus useful data on the bioavailability of nutrients in a variety of supplements. Consideration is given to differences among species and to interacting factors that influence bioavailability, and methods for estimating and statistically evaluating bioavailability are described.

Those chapters on individual nutrients include a thorough but refined description of relevant literature plus a table summarizing the data in each reference. Where appropriate, the tabular data are organized by species, and nutrient bioavailability in an identified source has been given a relative value compared to that of a standard. The criteria used, methods of calculation, types of diets, and added nutrient levels are given for each citation. In most chapters, a second, shorter table has been prepared by summarizing all data on a single nutrient source and development of a single "best estimate" of bioavailability. The chapter on vitamins also considers issues of vitamin stability that influence amounts of nutrients that are available when diets are actually consumed.

This publication fills a serious void in the nutrition literature. It was written and edited by scientists who have been actively involved in bioavailability research. As is common for books with multiple authors, it has had a somewhat tortured evolutionary history. However, it is now in print, and those, like myself, who believed in this project and recognized the need for such a book will be pleased at what they find between its covers. I salute those who have labored so diligently to produce a truly useful document, and I am confident that you, the reader, will want to acknowledge and applaud this effort.

Duane E. Ullrey
Professor Emeritus
Michigan State University

PREFACE

This book represents a comprehensive effort to summarize research data relating to the bioavailability of amino acids, minerals, and vitamins in feeds, foods, and supplements for animals. This information can be used in conjunction with dietary requirement values in the formulation of diets in practical feeding situations. Factors that influence the bioavailability of these nutrients are discussed, and methodology for determining bioavailability is presented. Experimental data obtained for both ruminant and nonruminant species are summarized, and results with laboratory animals are included when considered appropriate. Experimental design and statistical evaluation of bioavailability assays are also discussed.

For amino acids, two general approaches to determining bioavailability are described in detail. The first approach is based on digestibility (usually true digestibility for poultry and apparent ileal digestibility for swine). Digestibility values have been widely adopted by the animal feed industry, and there have been several excellent reviews. Data from these reviews are summarized in tables. The second approach is the use of growth assays. Although the amount of data in this area is less abundant, bioavailability estimates from growth assays are needed to confirm the validity of the digestibility approach. A comprehensive table of data derived from growth assays with rats, chicks, and swine is provided. In a second chapter, the relative bioavailabilities of D-amino acids and amino acid analogs are reviewed.

Bioavailability information for seven macromineral and seven micromineral elements is presented. Extensive tables are included for each mineral wherein summaries of data from individual studies are provided together with references to the original publications. Data considered to be outside realistic experimental bounds were not included. Average bioavailability values for supplemental sources as well as the number of studies or individual samples contributing to the estimates are presented in abbreviated tables. Although these average bioavailability values serve as useful guides, consideration must be given to the limited number of determinations for certain estimates as well as the rather insensitive bioavailability assay procedures used for certain elements or classes of animals. This is especially true for values for calcium, phosphorus, and magnesium when determined with ruminants. Numerous references provide ready access to the literature for more detailed information. Grateful appreciation is expressed to Dr. Boyd L. O'Dell, Professor Emeritus, Biochemistry Department, University of Missouri—Columbia, for assistance in preparing the chapters on copper, selenium, and zinc.

Vitamins are discussed with reference to forms existing in foods and feeds, precursor compounds, enzymatic processes in the gut or body required to convert vitamins to their metabolically active form, and factors that affect the bioavailability of the vitamin per se or its bound cofactor or precursor form. A review of the pertinent literature is presented for 10 water-soluble vitamins and 4 fat-soluble vitamins.

Thanks are expressed to the contributors, who were willing to spend the time and effort necessary to make this book possible. Special appreciation is expressed to Ms. Cathy Brane for her assistance in preparation of the final manuscript.

Clarence B. Ammerman
David H. Baker
Austin J. Lewis

INTRODUCTION

Efficient production of livestock and poultry and the maintenance of normal health in animals require that essential nutrients be provided in appropriate amounts and in forms that are biologically utilizable. Deficiencies of certain nutrients occur frequently in diets consisting of common feed ingredients, and these nutrients must be provided in a supplemental form. Degree of bioavailability influences not only dietary requirement but also tolerance of a nutrient. Thus, it is important to know the bioavailability of nutrients in both common feed ingredients and dietary supplements that may be used in animal feeding. More research information exists on the utilization of nutrients in supplemental sources than on the nutrients present in feed ingredients. This book presents information on the bioavailability of amino acids, minerals, and vitamins in feeds and supplements used as dietary components.

Terms relating to nutrient utilization include "bioavailability," "availability," "biological availability," "bioactivity," "biopotency," and "bioefficiency." These terms are frequently used interchangably. The term "bioavailability" is defined as the degree to which an ingested nutrient in a particular source is absorbed in a form that can be utilized in metabolism by the animal. Similar definitions have been given by Forbes and Erdman (1983), Sauberlich (1987), and Southgate (1988). Other investigators (Fox *et al.*, 1981; O'Dell, 1984) have stressed that utilization of the nutrient within normal metabolic processes of the animal must be demonstrated to establish bioavailability. For some nutrients, measurement of actual utilization is extremely difficult, and researchers have often used estimates of utilization that do not fulfill the strictest definition of bioavailability.

In addition to identifying variables suitable as criteria in bioavailability studies the following quotation from Fairweather-Tait (1987) relating to research on iron bioavailability in foods seems both appropriate and instructive in emphasizing the variability associated with determination of nutrient bioavailability.

It is therefore apparent that the 'availability' of iron in any food is not an inherent property, characteristic of the material being assayed, but an experimentally determined value which reflects the absorption and utilization of the iron ingested under the conditions of the test.[1]

---

[1]Reprinted from *Nutrition Research* Vol. **7**, S.J. Fairweather-Tait, The concept of bioavailability as it relates to iron nutrition, pp. 319-325, 1987, with permission from Elsevier Science Ltd., The Boulevard, Langford Lane, Kidlington OX5 1GB, UK.

Values for bioavailability are frequently expressed in percentage units. In certain studies, such as those in which true absorption is obtained, the value represents the absolute proportion of a nutrient that is absorbed by the animal and presented to the tissues for utilization. Bioavailability values for nutrients are often expressed, however, in relation to a response obtained with a standard reference material. This approach results in a number referred to as the "relative bioavailability value". Relative values are useful in diet formulation, especially when applied to supplemental nutrient sources. Frequently, the nutrient source used as a standard reference material is the same as, or similar in bioavailability to, the source that was used to determine the animal's requirement for the nutrient. This adds validity to the use of relative bioavailability values with dietary supplements.

The reference standard used in bioavailability studies should be a highly available source, although reference standards that are less well utilized have been used for certain evaluations. For example, feed grade dicalcium phosphate rather than a highly soluble sodium phosphate has been used as a reference material. When feed grade dicalcium phosphate is used, the relative bioavailability values obtained for some phosphates tested may exceed 100%. With amino acids, the crystalline form of individual amino acids is generally the standard reference source, and true absorption in this instance is 100% (Chung and Baker, 1992). In contrast, $MnSO_4 \cdot H_2O$ is generally used as the standard reference for assessment of manganese bioavailability, but true absorption of the manganese in this compound is 2 to 8%, depending on the species and the diet to which manganese is added. This illustrates the vast difference between true absorption and relative bioavailability for standards such as crystalline amino acids and a micromineral that, even in its most bioavailable form, is poorly absorbed.

Bioavailability can be influenced by animal species and by nutrient demand of the animal in relation to dietary intake. Any physiological function or state that may increase nutrient demand (e.g., growth, bone development, pregnancy, lactation, or disease) can increase absolute nutrient utilization, especially when dietary intake of the nutrient is less than the animal's minimal requirement. The magnitude of the previous intake of a nutrient in relation to the animal's requirement can either reduce or enhance the utilization of that nutrient. Interactions with dietary nutrients and other factors or compounds within the diet, including certain medications, can affect bioavailability. This influence can occur both within the gastrointestinal tract before absorption or within the animal's tissues after absorption. The type of processing that the nutrient has undergone and particle size of the resulting feed ingredient or supplemental source may also be factors that influence utilization. With mineral elements in particular, chemical form and degree of solubility can have a profound effect on utilization of supplemental sources. Total measurable utilization of a nutrient in absolute terms may be influenced greatly by the factors just discussed, but the effect on relative bioavailability values for supplemental sources of the same nutrient may be minimal. In planning experimental approaches, interpreting results and implementing information from bioavailability assays, methods used in assessment and expression of bioavailability and factors that influence nutrient utilization must be taken into consideration.

REFERENCES

Chung T. K. and D. H.Baker. 1992. Apparent and true amino acid digestibility of a crystalline amino acid mixture and of casein: Comparison of values obtained with ileal-cannulated pigs and cecectomized cockerels. *J. Anim. Sci.* **70**:3781.

Fairweather-Tait, S. J. 1987. The concept of bioavailability as it relates to iron nutrition. *Nutr. Res.* **7**:319.

Forbes, R. M. and J. W. Erdman, Jr. 1983. Bioavailability of trace mineral elements. *Annu. Rev. Nutr.* **3**:213.

Fox, M. R. S., R. M. Jacobs, A. O. L. Jones, B. E. Fry, Jr., M. Rakowska, R. P. Hamilton, B. F. Harland, C. L. Stone and S. H.Tao. 1981. Animal models for assessing bioavailability of essential and toxic elements. *Cereal Chem.* **58**:6.

O'Dell, B. L. 1984. Bioavailabilty of trace elements. *Nutr. Rev.* **42**:301.

Sauberlich, H. E. 1987. Vitamins - How much is for keeps. *Nutr. Today* **22**(1):20.

Southgate, D. A. T. 1988. AFRC Institute of Food Research, Annual Report, Shinfield, Reading, U.K.

1

STATISTICAL EVALUATION OF BIOAVAILABILITY ASSAYS

Ramon C. Littell

Department of Statistics
University of Florida
Gainesville, Florida

Austin J. Lewis

Department of Animal Science
University of Nebraska
Lincoln, Nebraska

Pamela R. Henry

Department of Animal Science
University of Florida
Gainesville, Florida

I. INTRODUCTION

Bioavailability of a nutrient in a test substance relative to its bioavailabililty in a standard substance is usually defined to be the ratio of the amounts of the standard and test substances required to produce equivalent responses. Although the concept is simple, actual determination presents several problems. Some of these problems are statistical and involve modeling, experimental design, and estimation. This chapter describes some of the more common assays, and discusses some of the assumptions involved for assay validity, and strengths and weaknesses of each assay.

BIOAVAILABILITY OF NUTRIENTS FOR ANIMALS:
AMINO ACIDS, MINERALS, AND VITAMINS
Copyright © 1995 by Academic Press, Inc.
All rights of reproduction in any form reserved.

Methods described generally follow recommendations of Finney (1978). For brevity, bioavailability will be denoted RBV for relative bioavailability value.

Before discussing statistical aspects, two other issues must be addressed. First is the issue of what should constitute the "independent" variable. Two of the possibilities are the total amount of nutrient intake by the animal and the concentration of nutrient added to the diet. If dietary intakes are essentially identical among treatment groups, either approach is acceptable. If, however, dietary intakes differ among treatments, it is necessary to relate responses to total intake of the nutrient. This is especially important when the amount of a nutrient in the basal diet represents a major portion of the nutrient presented to the animal. Second is the question of the response to be measured, which in statistical terms would be called the "dependent" variable. Two examples of dependent variables are weight gain and bone ash. Choice of dependent variable depends on the nutrient to be assayed. Examples of independent and dependent variables specific for amino acids can be found in Chapter 2. In some cases the dependent variable must be transformed in order to obtain variance heterogeniety or other criteria for validity of the assay. Biological issues of what should be measured, both as dependent and independent variables, are better discussed in the subsequent chapters because they are nutrient specific.

Most statistical assays of bioavailability use regression methods, which require that independent and dependent variables be identified. In subsequent sections, x and y will denote the independent and dependent variables, respectively, following standard regression notation. Let x_s and x_t denote amounts of the standard and test substances required to produce a given value of the response y. It follows that RBV $= x_s/x_t$. It is possible that the ratio x_s/x_t depends on the value of y. In this case RBV would have different values corresponding to different values of y, and RBV would not be defined as a general entity. However, under conditions that hold at least approximately in many situations, the RBV is independent of the values of y, making it possible to define a single value for RBV. Two such conditions result in the so-called "slope ratio" and "parallel lines" assays.

Because assay methods are based on regression models, it is important to have an index of how well the model fits the data. The standard statistical index of goodness of fit of a regression model is R^2, and it is discussed in any textbook dealing with statistical regression analysis. The motivation for R^2 arises from the partitioning of total variation in a set of data into two parts according to the equation:

Total SS = regression SS + error SS,

where SS stands for "sum of squares," regression SS is the portion of total SS which is attributed to the relation between the dependent and the independent variables, and error SS is the portion of total SS that is not attributed to the relation between the dependent and independent variables. R^2 is calculated as the ratio of the regression sum of squares divided by the total sum of squares, and thereby measures the portion of the total variation in the dependent variable that is due to its relation with the independent variable. Clearly, R^2 is bounded between 0 and 1, and better fitting models have larger R^2 values than do poorer fitting models.

It is widely known that R^2 is not an infallible measure of goodness of fit. The value of R^2 can be artifically driven to 1 by adding unrelated variables to the model. Also, R^2 requires careful interpretation when several values of the dependent variable are taken at the same value of the independent variable. Nonetheless, R^2 is a useful statistic and it is informative to be reported in bioavailability studies.

There is no single value of R^2 that necessarily indicates a good fit of a model. It is possible, however, to recognize classes of response variables and types of experiments that tend to produce larger ranges of R^2 values than others. For example, R^2 in bioavailability studies for amino acids tend to be larger than for vitamins and R^2 for vitamin studies, in turn, tend to be greater than for minerals.

Basic experimental design issues for bioassays are discussed under Section II. Model validation and data analysis concepts for the slope ratio and the parallel lines assays will be presented under Sections III and IV. Other assay methods are variations of these two, and they will be discussed under Section V. Four examples illustrating model validation and data analysis are discussed under Section VI. An appendix to Section VI contains SAS computer programs for model validation and data analysis of some of the examples.

II. OVERVIEW OF EXPERIMENTAL DESIGN ISSUES

Bioavailability assays are based on experimental data, and properly designed experiments should be conducted to obtain valid and efficient assays. As in any experimental situation, the two basic components of treatment structure and assignment of treatments to experimental units must be addressed. Various levels of test and standard substances are mixed in diets and fed to animals. The diets, which usually include a zero supplemental level, or basal diet, constitute the treatments. The combinations of nutrient sources and dietary levels often can be considered factorial treatment combinations. The treatments can be assigned to experimental units according to any appropriate design, such as completely randomized, randomized blocks, etc. The experimental units might be individual animals, cages of animals, or even animals at a particular time in the case of crossover designs. Choices of treatment structure, treatment assignment, and experimental unit depend on the objectives of the study, prior knowledge of the statistical model, and the nature of experimental material. All principles of experimental design apply to bioavailability experiments. In addition, the design and statistical model must meet certain other requirements to make the assay valid, as will be discussed in subsequent sections.

III. SLOPE RATIO ASSAY

The slope ratio assay is the most common form of assay used in recent bioavailability experiments. Values of the independent and dependent variables, x and y, are determined from each experimental unit. It is assumed that there is a straight line relationship between y and x for both test and standard nutrient sources. Equations for regression lines are calculated, $y = a_s + b_s x$ for the standard nutrient and $y = a_t + b_t x$ for the test nutrient (Fig. 1a). It is assumed further that the responses of the two substances are the same at a zero value of x, making $a_s = a_t$. That is, the two lines intersect at $x = 0$, so that the common value of the intercepts can be denoted simply as a, giving regression equations $y = a + b_t x$ for the test substance and $y = a + b_s x$ for the standard. Then, again letting x_s and x_t denote amounts of the standard and test substances required to produce equivalent values of the response y, it follows that $a + b_s x_s = a + b_t x_t$. Solving gives RBV $= x_s/x_t = b_t/b_s$, the ratio of slopes of the regression lines. Hence the name "slope ratio" assay. Notice that RBV is a ratio estimate, and therefore it is more difficult to obtain an estimate of its standard error. This is illustrated under Section VI.

There may be several different test sources in an assay. In that event, the bioavailability of each test substance relative to the standard is computed in the same manner; the slope of a test source regression line is divided by the slope of the standard regression line.

For RBV estimates to be meaningful, the assumptions regarding linearity and intersection of the regression lines must hold. Statistical tests can be used to check the validity of the assumptions. These tests have been described by Finney (1978). Statistical regression computer programs can be used to perform the regression computations, although certain special features may be needed to perform the validity checks. Some programs, such as PROC GLM in the SAS system, contain these features and also can provide computations required to obtain standard error estimates for the RBV.

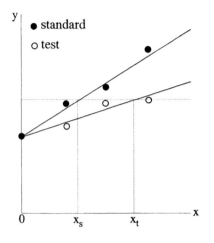

Fig. 1a. Slope-ratio assay

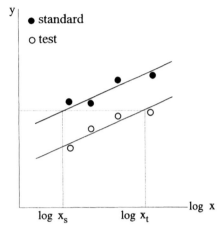

Fig. 1b. Parallel lines assay

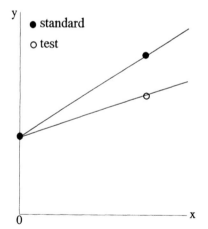

Fig. 1c. Three-point assay

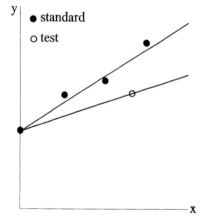

Fig. 1d. Standard curve assay

Fig 1. Four generalized assays to estimate biavailability of nutrients.

IV. PARALLEL LINES ASSAY

Some nutrient assays do not produce a linear relationship between y and x. Rather, a straight line relationship might be obtained by regressing y on the logarithm of x, giving $y = a_s + (b_s \cdot \log_{10} x)$ for the standard substance and $y = a_t + (b_t \cdot \log_{10} x)$ for the test substance (Fig.1b). If the slopes of the lines for standard and test are equal, then the equations become simply $y = a_s + (b \cdot \log_{10} x)$ for the standard and $y = a_t + (b \cdot \log_{10} x)$ for the test. Then $a_s + (b \cdot \log_{10} x_s) = a_t + (b \cdot \log_{10} x_t)$, and solving gives $\log_{10}(x_s/x_t) = (a_t - a_s)/b$. Thus, the bioavailability estimate is given by the equation RBV = antilog$((a_t - a_s)/b)$. Geometrically, RBV is the antilogarithm of the horizontal difference between two points on the lines of equal vertical height.

There is some controversy concerning which assay is better, the slope ratio or parallel lines. In fact, the best assay method is the one for which the corresponding model fits the data. If the regressions of y on x are linear and the intercepts are equal, then the model for the slope ratio assay fits the data, and the RBV should be estimated accordingly. On the other hand, if the regressions of y on $\log_{10} x$ are linear and have equal slopes, then the model for the parallel lines assay is appropriate, and the corresponding estimate of RBV should be used. In many cases, it will be known from experience which of the regressions is likely to be linear. Ordinarily, the study should be designed so that it is possible through preliminary statistical analysis to check the assumptions of the assay.

Note that parallelism of the lines implies that they never intersect. Mathematically, they can be considered to intersect at negative infinity, which is the logarithm of zero. Practically, data from the basal diet, with $x = 0$, are not usable in a parallel lines assay. This treatment is perhaps infeasible in a situation for which a parallel lines assay is appropriate. A basal diet resulting in excessive mortality due to a dietary deficiency would be an example.

V. OTHER ASSAY DESIGNS

If certain assumptions are known to be valid regarding the relationship between y and x, then simpler assay designs may be used to estimate RBV. These designs should be used, however, only in the presence of high confidence that the assumptions are valid, because data obtained from these designs provide little or no information to allow checks on the assumptions.

A. Three Point

The three point design, as the name implies, relies on only three design points to estimate RBV. It can be used in the case of either the assumption for the slope ratio or the parallel lines assays, but it must be known in advance which assumption is valid. If assumptions for the slope ratio assay are known to hold, that is, if regressions of y on x are known to be linear with equal intercepts, then the three point design ordinarily would include one point at $x = 0$ supplemental nutrient to define the intercept, and two other points obtained at a positive value for x for both standard and test sources. Then lines are struck by joining the intercept with each of the two points resulting from positive x (Fig.1c). The ratio of slopes of these two lines produces the RBV estimate as in the case of the slope ratio assay. In fact, the three point assay as just described is a special case of the slope ratio assay.

If assumptions for the parallel lines assay are known to hold, that is, if regressions of y on $\log_{10} x$ are linear for standard and test sources with equal slopes, then a version of the three point design can be used. Two points are obtained on the line for the standard source by taking relatively low and high values of $\log_{10} x$. The third point is obtained by taking $\log_{10} x$ for the test source somewhere between the values of $\log_{10} x$ used for the standard source, preferably near the larger value. Then a line is obtained by joining the points for the standard preparation. The horizontal distance from the test point to the standard line is computed, and the antilogarithm of this distance is the estimate of RBV, as in the case of the parallel lines assay.

Three point designs are highly efficient for estimating RBV, but they are also extremely dependent on validity of the assumptions for either the slope ratio or the parallel lines assays. They should be used only if one of these sets of assumptions is known to hold.

B. Standard Curve

The standard curve assay is a compromise between the three point assay and the slope ratio or parallel lines assays. It requires more than three data points, but usually not as many as the slope ratio or parallel lines assays. Basically, several points are obtained for the standard source to obtain the standard curve (Fig.1d). To provide a valid assay, the curve will be linear in either x or $\log_{10} x$. Usually, only one point is obtained for the test source, and RBV is estimated in the same manner as described above for the three point assay. If the curve is not linear in either x or $\log_{10} x$ over the entire range of x or $\log_{10} x$, then a portion of the curve might be suitably linear to justify estimation of RBV valid over the range of x or $\log_{10} x$ for which the curve is linear.

C. Mean Ratio

Some experiments have been conducted in which two or more sources of a nutrient were tested without a basal control group which is needed to make a three point comparison. In this case, the ratio of the test mean to the standard mean is calculated as an RBV estimate. Mean ratios as a test for comparing radioisotope techniques have compared the utilization of iodine sources (Aschbacher *et al.*, 1966). Both diiodosalicyclic acid ($D^{131}IS$) and ($^{125}I^-$) were given simultaneously as oral doses of iodine to cows. Mean ratio comparisons of radioiodine uptakes in the thyroid were appropriate and, in this case, were very sensitive because there was no residual isotope to dilute the supplemental effect of either isotope. Also, in experiments in which the basal portion of the diet is very low in the nutrient such that the response (y) would be minimal and supplemental concentrations of that nutrient from the standard and test sources represent by far the major percentage of the total amount in the diet, mean ratio comparisons of the response may be valid. On the contrary, when the standard and test sources constitute only a relatively small percentage of the total nutrient in the diet, mean ratio comparisons of responses become far less meaningful. As an example, assume numerical responses to some level of standard and test sources were 8 and 4, respectively. The RBV by mean ratio would equal 4/8 x 100 = 50%. If a control had been used in the design and a response value of 2 obtained, the RBV then becomes (4 - 2)/(8 - 2) x 100 = 33%. Under these conditions a mean ratio will bias an estimate upwards to some greater positive value. In another situation, if the test source were unavailable and would have produced a response identical to the control diet, the RBV would be a positive value, when it should actually be zero.

VI. EXAMPLES OF ASSAYS

In this section four examples of estimating bioavailability are shown. Each example illustrates a different type of statistical problem.

A. Bone Manganese in Poultry

This example using data from Henry *et al.* (1986) illustrates a slope ratio assay that was straightforward in design. The experiment had seven treatment groups consisting of a basal diet and diets supplemented with 40, 80, or 120 ppm of manganese from either manganese oxide or manganese sulfate. Sulfate was considered the standard source and oxide the test source. The response variable was bone manganese concentration. A plot of the means is shown in Fig. 2. The standard error of each of the means is approximately .4. There is essentially no difference between oxide and sulfate sources in diets that contain 40 ppm added manganese; however, means for sulfate are larger than means for oxide at 80 and 120 ppm added manganese. Results of a slope ratio assay will be presented. The methods used were described by Finney (1978, Chapter 7). Statistical computations were obtained using PROC GLM in the SAS system (Littell *et al.*, 1991). Critical portions of the SAS program are included in the Appendix.

Bone Mn ppm

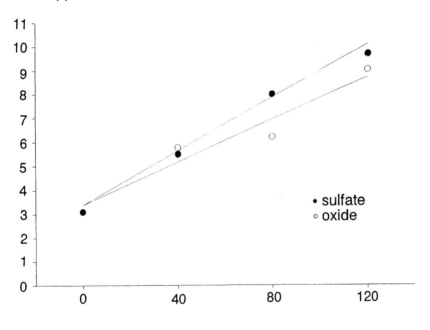

Supplemental Mn ppm

Fig. 2. Slope ratio assay of the effect of dietary manganese source and dietary manganese concentration on bone manganese concentration in poultry (Henry *et al.*, 1986).

Attention will focus first on checking validity of a slope ratio assay. Validity of the slope ratio assay requires that the response (bone Mn) is a linear function of the supplemented manganese for each source down to the zero supplemental level and that the regressions intersect at the zero supplemental level. Finney (1978) refers to linearity as a requirement for "statistical validity," and to intersection of the regression lines at the zero supplemental dose as "fundamental" validity. Finney (1978, Section 7.5) illustrates the use of a linear model and analysis of variance methods to test statistically for validity. Table I shows an analysis of variance for the bone manganese assay, which was extracted from SAS output shown in Table IVa. Details of the SAS program are under the Appendix. The methods in this example can be used to duplicate results by Finney (1978). Starting at the bottom line of the analysis of variance in Table I, the F-test labled "curvature" is statistically significant ($P = .018$). This indicates failure of linear regressions fitted to nonzero supplemental manganese levels to pass through the mean points plotted in Fig.2, evidently due to the nonlinearity of points for the test source (oxide). Thus, there is some doubt about the statistical validity of a slope ratio analysis of these data. Visual inspection of Fig. 2, however, shows that the trend is increasing over all levels of supplemental manganese, including the zero level, and that a linear fit captures the dominant aspect of the trend. Therefore, the analysis will proceed based on fitted linear regressions. It should be noted that the use of a standard curve assay design could have been highly misleading. If only one of the three points in Fig.2 had been obtained for the oxide source, the results would have depended greatly on which point was actually used. This reaffirms the desirability of several points to establish the test curve.

The F-test in Table I labeled "intersection" is a test of whether linear regressions fitted to data from the nonzero levels of supplemental manganese intersect at zero; that is, whether the lines have equal intercepts. The test outcome is nonsignificant ($P = .780$), consistent with the linear regressions having equal intercepts. Thus, fundamental validity is apparently satisfied. The F-test labeled "blanks" is a test of whether the common intercept of the regressions fitted to nonzero supplemental manganese levels coincides with the mean bone manganese for the basal diet. This test is also not significant ($P = .310$), consistent with the fitted regressions intersecting at the zero supplemental level mean point.

Failure of the means in Fig.2 to represent linear trends across added manganese could be due to true nonlinearity or to random variation. Although strict linearity is questionable, the overall trends are not severely nonlinear, so that two straight lines intersecting at 0 ppm supplemental manganese give a reasonably accurate representation of the general profiles.

The final step in this sequence of preliminary tests is to test for statistical significance of the difference between the slopes. This is the test, labeled "slope difference" in Table I, which is significant at the $P = .007$ level and leads to the conclusion that the slopes are different. It should be noted that the "average slope" in Table I provides a test of whether the average of the two slopes is different from zero. This test would not be of interest in this example because the slopes are significantly different. The sum of the sums of squares for average slope and slope difference would be the sum of squares called "regression" by Finney (1978).

Regression lines were refitted, forcing intersection at 0 ppm supplemental manganese. Details of the SAS program are shown under the Appendix. Output is shown in Table IVb. Slopes of the resulting lines are .0544 for the standard (sulfate) and .0452 for the test (oxide). Standard errors for both slopes are .0038. The common intercept is 3.333. In other words, the equations are

bone Mn = 3.333 + .0544 · (supplemental sulfate Mn)

and

bone Mn = 3.333 + .0452 · (supplemental oxide Mn).

Thus, the bioavailability estimate is RBV = .045/.054 = .83, which is usually expressed as 83%.

Finney (1978, pp. 155-156) describes how to obtain so-called "fiducial" limits for the RBV. Only essential parts of the process are outlined here. In practice, fiducial limits are used in the same manner as confidence limits, but are based on different theoretical principles. Computation of fiducial limits requires the matrix denoted V by Finney. This matrix is directly available as part of PROC GLM printout shown in Table IVb, and it is described in the appendix. For the bone manganese data the matrix is

$$V = 10^{-6} \begin{bmatrix} 35897 & -384.6 & -384.6 \\ -384.6 & 7.097 & 4.121 \\ -384.6 & 4.121 & 7.097 \end{bmatrix}$$

Multiplication of V by the error mean square (2.00 in Table IVb; denoted s^2 by Finney, 1978) produces the matrix of variances and covariances of the intercept and the two slope estimates. The quantity g in the fiducial limits (Finney, 1978) is $g = t^2 s^2 v_{11}/b_S^2$, where $t = 1.98$ (the tabled 95% two-tailed value for Student's t distribution with degrees of freedom = 102 from the error mean square), $v_{11} = 10^{-6} \times 7.097$ is the variance coefficient from V for the standard source (sulfate), and $b_S = .054$ is the slope of the regression line for the standard source. Thus, $g = (1.98)^2(2.00)(10^{-6} \times 7.097)/(.054)^2 = .019$. Considering this small value of g to be negligible, following Finney (1978, p. 156, Eq. 7.6.7), one may use the simplified approximate variance of RBV

$$\text{Var(RBV)} = (s^2/b_S^2) [v_{22} - 2 \cdot \text{RBV} \cdot v_{12} + \text{RBV}^2 \cdot v_{11}],$$

where v_{22}, v_{12}, and v_{11} are the elements in the lower right-hand 2 x 2 submatrix of V. Factoring 10^{-6} from each term in the brackets gives

$$Var(RBV) = (2.00/.054^2)10^{-6} [7.097 - 2 \cdot .83 \cdot 4.121 + .83^2 \cdot 7.097]$$
$$= (2.00/54^2) [5.145]$$
$$= .0035.$$

Thus, an approximate standard error of RBV is $.0035^{1/2} = .06$, and the resulting approximate 95% fiducial limits are $.83 - 1.98 \times .06 = .71$ and $.83 + 1.98 \times .06 = .95$. In terms of percentages, one concludes that manganese from the oxide source is between 71 and 95% as available as manganese from the sulfate source. Implicit in this conclusion is that RBV is significantly less than 100%. A test of whether the two regression lines have equal slopes should provide confirmation of this conclusion. Recall that the F-test for equality of slopes in Table I is significant at the $P = .007$ level, indicating that the slopes are different, which is in concert with the fiducial limits not containing the value 1.0.

As a cautionary note, the reader is reminded that the RBV estimate, fiducial limits, and conclusions for this example were computed despite failure in the validity check for linearity over the nonzero levels of supplemental manganese. As stated earlier, failure of the validity check could be due to true nonlinearity of the response to the oxide source, or it could be due to some unknown, random effect. If exhibited nonlinearity is due to random effect, then the standard error computed for the oxide slope estimate is biased downward, which propagates to the fiducial limits. On the other hand, true nonlinearity of the response to the oxide source indicates that the true bioavailability of the manganese in oxide, relative to sulfate, varies with the level of supplementation. The RBV of .83 would then represent an intermediate value of the true RBV values over the range of supplemental manganese levels, 0 to 120 ppm.

B. Hemoglobin Repletion as an Assay for Iron in Rats

Fritz et al. (1974) reported results from eight laboratories that conducted bioavailability assays of four iron sources. Each laboratory evaluated aliquots of each of the original four substances. Source 1 was reagent grade ferrous sulfate, which was considered the standard source of iron. Source 2 (7 to 10 μm) and source 3 (27 to 40 μm) were different particle sizes from the same lot of electrolytically reduced iron. Source 4 was ferric orthophosphate. Fritz et al. (1974) combined results across laboratories and used the parallel lines method to estimate RBV. Plots of hemoglobin vs level of supplemental iron in Fig. 3 suggest that the slope ratio method would be appropriate. In this section, slope ratio estimates are computed and compared with results reported by Fritz et al. (1974).

Hemoglobin g/dL

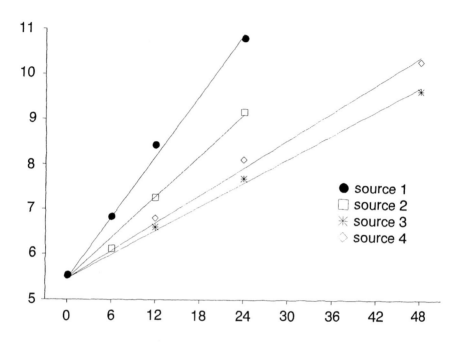

Supplemental Fe ppm

Fig. 3. Slope ratio assay of the effect of dietary iron source and dietary iron concentration on hemoglobin concentration in rats (Fritz *et al.*, 1974).

Table II contains an analysis of variance for the hemoglobin data. This analysis treats data in Table 2 of Fritz *et al.* (1974) as resulting from a randomized blocks experimental design with laboratories as blocks and combinations of iron sources and levels of supplemental iron as treatments. Proceeding as in the previous example to check the validity assumptions, the value $F = .51$ labeled "curvature" is not significant ($P = .729$). Thus, nonlinearity evidently is not a problem. Next, $F = 1.06$ for intersection also is nonsignificant ($P = .371$), so the lines can be assumed to intersect at the zero supplemental level of iron. The test labeled "blanks" for whether the linearity holds down to the zero supplemental level of iron has $F = 1.85$ with $P = .177$ and is nonsignificant. Having passed all validity checks, slope ratio RBV estimates can be computed.

Linear equations intersecting at the origin have equations

Hemoglobin = 5.45 + .227· (source 1 iron)
Hemoglobin = 5.45 + .152· (source 2 iron)
Hemoglobin = 5.45 + .089· (source 3 iron)
Hemoglobin = 5.45 + .103· (source 4 iron).

Slopes of these lines yield bioavailability values relative to source 1 of .668, .392, and .454 for sources 2, 3, and 4, respectively.

The V matrix needed to compute standard errors for RBV is:

$$
V = 10^{-4}
\begin{bmatrix}
340.9 & -18.93 & -18.93 & -9.470 & -9.470 \\
-18.93 & 2.706 & 1.052 & .526 & .526 \\
-18.93 & 1.052 & 2.706 & .526 & .526 \\
-9.470 & .526 & .526 & .676 & .263 \\
-9.470 & .526 & .526 & .263 & .676
\end{bmatrix}
$$

The g value is $(2.0)^2(.308)(.00027)/(.227)^2 = .0065$, which is sufficiently small to justify using the simpler variance formula, Eq. [7.6.7] of Finney (1978). Resulting fiducial limits are $.668 \pm .077$ for source 2, $.392 \pm .040$ for source 3, and $.454 \pm .042$ for source 4.

It is noteworthy to compare the slope ratio RBV computed here with those computed by Fritz *et al.* (1974) using the parallel lines method. Using RBV and standard deviations from Fritz *et al.* (1974, Table 3) to obtain standard errors, one obtains confidence intervals of $.635 \pm .088$ for source 2, $.379 \pm .099$ for source 3, and $.445 \pm .039$ for source 4. Intervals from the preceeding analysis using slope ratio estimates are shorter for two of the three test sources. This is possibly because the slope ratio estimates utilize data from the zero level of iron, and the parallel lines estimates do not.

C. Toe Ash Phosphorus in Poultry

Phosphorus from three different sources was added to poultry diets at four concentrations creating 12 diets (Miles *et al.*, 1993). Four birds were fed each of the 12 diets. No basal control diet was fed in this experiment as the low phosphorus concentration would have resulted in considerable mortality. Feed intake for each bird was measured and supplemental phosphorus intake was calculated as (feed intake) · (concentration added phosphorus). Therefore, values of the independent variable, supplemental phosphorus intake, differ from bird to bird in the same treatment group. The response criterion was toe ash percentage, which is plotted *vs* supplemental phosphorus intake in Fig. 4a. Source 1 (reagent grade dicalcium

Toe Ash %

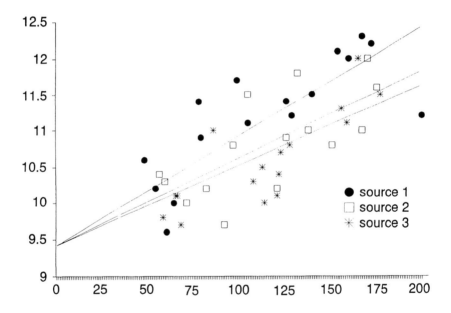

Supplemental P Intake mg

Fig 4a. Slope ratio assay of the effect of dietary phosphorus source and supplemental phosphorus intake on toe ash percentage in poultry (Miles *et al.*, 1993).

phosphate) was the standard, source 2 was a feed grade monocalcium/dicalcium phosphate, and source 3 was a feed grade defluorinated phosphate. Toe ash percentage is plotted *vs* $\log_{10}$ supplemental phosphorus intake in Fig. 4b. Because of the small number of birds assigned to each of the diets and the relatively large variation within diets, statistical tests are unable to reveal definitively whether the model appropriate for slope ratio or parallel lines assays is best. Both models were fitted and corresponding RBV estimates were calculated. The slope ratio model had $R^2 = .63$ and the parallel lines model had $R^2 = .65$.

Toe Ash %

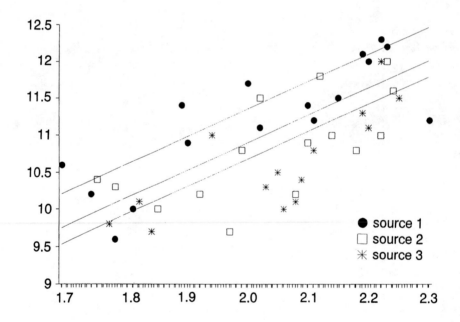

Log Supplemental P Intake mg

Fig 4b. Parallel lines assay of the effect of dietary phosphorus source and $\log_{10}$ supplemental phosphorus intake on toe ash percentage in poultry (Miles *et al.*, 1993)

Regressions of toe ash on added phosphorus intake were tested for equality of intercepts to check the assumption for slope ratio assays. The result showed no significant evidence of different intercepts ($P = .34$), so models were refitted with equal intercepts. Parameter estimates with standard errors were: intercept = 9.417 ±.204, slope 1 = .015 ±.0018, slope 2 = .012 ±.0019, and slope 3 = .011 ±.0019. Slope ratio bioavailablity estimates are: RBV2 = .012/.015 = .8 and RBV3 = .011/.015 = .733.

Regressions of toe ash on $\log_{10}$ supplemental phosphorus were tested for equality of slopes to check the assumption for parallel lines assays. The result showed no significant evidence of different slopes ($P = .97$). Models were refitted with equal slopes, producing the following parameter estimates with standard errors: slope = 3.234 ±.397, intercept 1 = 4.705 ±.812, intercept 2 = 4.250 ±.813, and intercept 3 = 4.027 ±.818. From these parameter estimates bioavailability estimates were computed: RBV2 = antilog((4.250-4.705)/3.234) = .723 and RBV3 = antilog((4.027-4.705)/3.234) = .617.

Comparisons of RBV from slope ratio and parallel lines assays show larger values from slope ratio assays by approximately 10 to 18%. The discrepancies are within the margin of error of estimation. In cases such as this in which one model does not emerge as distinctly superior to the other, either by graphical or statistical investigations, both models should be fitted and estimates derived from both to check general agreement. If greatly different bioavailability estimates are obtained, then neither should be used with confidence.

D. Liver Copper in Poultry

It is often necessary to transform data in order to meet mathematical requirements for valid statistical analyses. This is sometimes the case in bioavailability studies. Variance homogeneity (equality of variances) is a requirement for valid ordinary least squares regression analysis. Pott *et al.* (1994) used a logarithmic transformation to remove heterogeneity of variances in a bioavailability assessment of copper. Chicks were fed a basal diet containing 11 ppm copper or the basal diet supplemented with 150, 300, or 450 ppm copper from either a sulfate or lysine source. Copper intake for each chick was used as the independent variable. The response variable was liver copper, which is plotted in Fig. 5a. Liver copper is clearly more variable at high levels of copper intake than at low levels of copper intake. Also, the response trend appears more exponential in form than linear. $\log_{10}$ liver copper is plotted versus copper intake in Fig. 5b, in which variation appears stabilized over levels of copper intake. Also, the trends in $\log_{10}$ liver copper appear linear over the nonzero levels of copper intake and projected regression lines appear reasonably to intersect at the zero level, i.e., to have equal intercepts. The logarithmic transformation, therefore, has accomplished two objectives, linearity and variance homogeniety. But the response to the basal diet appears to be larger than the common intercept of regression lines fitted to nonzero levels of the two sources. Statistical tests in Table III support the visual assessments. Curvature is not significant ($P = .204$), intercepts are not significantly different ($P = .125$), and the common value of the intercepts is significantly different from the mean $\log_{10}$ liver copper of the basal diet ($P = .001$). Thus, a condition for statistical validity (linearity holding near the zero level of the independent variable) is not met. This is a situation

Liver Cu ppm

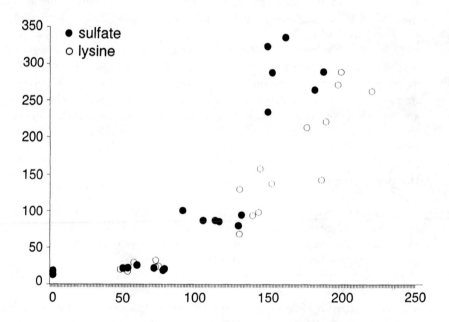

Supplemental Cu Intake mg

Fig 5a. Effect of dietary copper source and supplemental copper intake on liver copper concentration in poultry (Pott *et al.*, 1994).

similar to the one addressed by Finney (1978, p. 154), but will not be discussed further here. Instead, regression lines are fitted to data for nonzero levels of supplemental copper intake, with equal intercepts. The slope ratio estimate of bioavailability is computed: $b_t/b_s = .00798/.00936 = .85$, where b_s and b_t are slopes of regression lines over the nonzero levels of supplemental copper. Details of SAS programs to produce the validity tests and the regression lines are discussed in the Appendix. Since each animal has its individual copper intake value, curvature should be tested differently than illustrated with the bone manganese data of Example A.

Log Liver Cu ppm

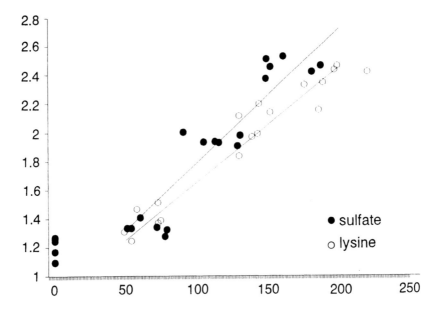

Supplemental Cu Intake mg

Fig 5b. Slope ratio assay of the effect of dietary copper source and supplemental copper intake on $\log_{10}$ transformed liver copper concentration in poultry (Pott *et al.*, 1994).

Now the question arises of how to interpret the RBV of 85% which has been calculated using logarithms of the response for the dependent variable. If one regards the logarithm as the response, then the RBV estimate has the usual interpretation. That is, if a certain value of $\log_{10}$ liver copper is obtained using a given level x_t of copper intake from the test source, then the same value of $\log_{10}$ liver copper would be expected from using a level $x_s = .85x_t$ of copper intake from the standard source. Using logarithms as the response is a common practice in some scientific areas, for example, pH values in chemistry and Richter scale values in seismology, and may have direct interpretive value. But if interpretations must be made in terms of the original response, then the meaning of RBV must be deciphered in terms of the original response. It will now be shown that RBV may be interpreted in the same manner, regardless of the transformation that was used for the statistical analysis.

Let y denote the original response and let $f(y)$ denote the transformed responses through the function f. If the transformed response $f(y)$ is a linear function of the independent variable for each nutrient source, that is, if $f(y_t) = a + bx$ for each source, then the bioavailability of a test source relative to the standard source is equal to b_t/b_s. In other words, bioavailability is measured in the same manner using the transformed data as it would be using original data. To see that this is true, return to the definition of the RBV: If x_s and x_t are amounts of the standard and test nutrient, respectively, which produce equal expected values of the response, then RBV $= x_s/x_t$. The key to the argument is the fact that if x_s and x_t produce the same amounts of y, then they also produce the same amounts of $f(y)$. Thus, since $f(y) = a + b_s x_s$ and $f(y) = a + b_t x_t$, it follows that $a + b_s x_s = a + b_t x_t$. As in the original definition of RBV, solution of this equation results in RBV $= x_s/x_t = b_t/b_s$, which is the desired result.

APPENDIX

Following are SAS programs which produce output for the bone manganese and liver copper examples described under Sections VI, A and IV, D. This is not intended to be a complete explanation of the programs and outputs. Rather, it is material which persons familiar with linear statistical models and PROC GLM in SAS might follow and modify for their particular needs.

A. Bone Manganese

Create a SAS data set named BONEMN which has variables SOURCE, LEVEL, and MNPPM. The variable SOURCE has values 1 and 2 for those respective sources of manganese, and SOURCE may be arbitrarily assigned the value 1 when LEVEL

= 0. The variable LEVEL has values 0, 40, 80, and 120 corresponding to those levels of supplemental manganese. Next create a variable named X0, with X0 = 1 when LEVEL = 0 and X0 = 0 otherwise. Also, create a variable named CLEVEL whose values are the same as LEVEL, i.e., CLEVEL = LEVEL. Following are SAS statements which create the SAS data set, and one example data line :

```
OPTIONS PS=60 NODATE;
DATA BONEMN;
INPUT ROW SOURCE LEVEL REPS BIRD MNPPM;
IF LEVEL=0 THEN X0=1;
ELSE X0=0;
CLEVEL=LEVEL;
CARDS;
1    1    40    1    1   4.7745;
RUN;
```

To obtain the validity tests, execute the SAS statements

```
PROC GLM DATA=BONEMN;
CLASS SOURCE CLEVEL;
MODEL MNPPM = LEVEL SOURCE*LEVEL X0 SOURCE
    CLEVEL(SOURCE) /SS1;
RUN;
```

Output, which has been edited, is shown in Table IVa from which computations in Table I are obtained. The following relations hold between labels in Tables I and IVa:

average slope = level
slope differences = level*source
blanks = x0
intersection = source
curvature = clevel(source).

Notice that the GLM Type I sums of squares are used. Equations for regression lines in Fig. 2 are obtained from the statements:

```
PROC GLM DATA=BONEMN;
CLASS SOURCE;
MODEL MNPPM = SOURCE*LEVEL / SOLUTION I;
RUN;
```

Output appears in Table IVb. Intercept and slopes for the lines are obtained directly from parameter estimates on the printout. Also, coefficients for the V matrix are printed in the X'X inverse matrix.

Placing SOURCE in the CLASS statement causes GLM to create "dummy" variables named DUMMY001 and DUMMY002 corresponding to the values 1 and 2 of SOURCE. DUMMY001 is equal to 1 if SOURCE = 1 and DUMMY001 is equal to 0 otherwise. DUMMY002 is defined similarly with regard to SOURCE 2. The linear model is

MNPPM = $a + b_1$(DUMMY001)(LEVEL) + b_2(DUMMY002)(LEVEL).

When SOURCE = 1 the equation becomes

MNPPM = $a + b_1$(LEVEL)

and when SOURCE = 2 the equation is

MNPPM = $a + b_2$(LEVEL).

Thus, regression equations are obtained which have equal intercepts.

A multiple regression model is often used which has equivalent results. Define variables LEVEL1 and LEVEL2 to be the respective levels of supplemental manganese from sources 1 and 2. Then the multiple regression model is

MNPPM = $a + b_1$(LEVEL1) + b_2(LEVEL2).

Equivalence of the multiple regression model and the dummy variable model is apparent upon recognition that LEVEL1 = (DUMMY001)(LEVEL) and LEVEL2 = (DUMMY002)(LEVEL).

Two remaining points should be made regarding the manner in which the zero level of the independent variable is accomodated in the model. First, if the condition for fundamental validity is met, that is, if intercepts of regression lines fitted to nonzero levels of the independent variable do not differ significantly, then the model should be refitted with intercepts forced to be equal. Slopes of regression lines with common intercepts are more stable than slopes of regression lines which have different intercepts, and the former will produce more stable RBV estimates. Second, it sometimes happens that data from the basal treatment are included multiple times in the data set, once for each nutrient source. In other words, the basal data are included once with SOURCE = 1 and LEVEL = 0; they are included again with SOURCE = 2 and LEVEL = 0, and so on. This is erroneous. The basal data should be included only once in the data set, with LEVEL = 0 and SOURCE set equal to a single value for all the basal data. The value of SOURCE may be one of the other values of SOURCE, or it may be some other value, typically zero. For the SAS programs illustrated in this Appendix, all of these choices will lead to the same computations, although labeling on the output will differ slightly.

D. Liver Copper

Details of this example differ from those of the bone manganese data in two ways. First, the independent variable, supplemental copper intake (CUINT), has different values for every animal. Curvature should be assessed by testing polynomial effects of CUINT. This is in contrast to creating the alias variable CLEVEL and using it in the CLASS statement of the SAS GLM program, as was done with the bone manganese data. Using the variable CLEVEL in a CLASS statement with the copper intake data would have the effect of treating each intake value as a separate "treatment," and would absorb all (or nearly all) degrees of freedom from error.

A quadratic polynomial is used to check for significance of curvature. Choice of a quadratic was based on visual inspection of the data plots in Fig.5b. SAS statements for the validity checks are

```
PROC GLM DATA=LIVCU; CLASS SOURCE;
   MODEL LOGLIVCU=CUINT CUINT*SOURCE X0 SOURCE
         CUINT*CUINT(SOURCE)/SS1;
RUN;
```

Results appear in Table Va.

Second, because the common intercept of the regression lines differs significantly from the mean for the basal diet, the slopes should be obtained from regressions using data points with nonzero copper intake. This can be done by leaving the variable X0 in the MODEL statement. Appropriate SAS statements are

```
PROC GLM DATA=LIVCU; CLASS SOURCE;
   MODEL LOGLIVCU=CUINT(SOURCE) X0/SOLUTION;
RUN;
```

Results appear in Table Vb.

In other applications it might be desirable to use a higher degree polynomial than quadratic. The objective is to account for the dominant aspects of nonlinearity, rather than to weave a curve through all the localized twists and turns of the data. Usually, this can be accomplished with a quadratic or cubic polynomial. SAS statements to include cubic terms are

```
PROC GLM DATA=LIVCU; CLASS SOURCE;
   MODEL LOGLIVCU=CUINT CUINT*SOURCE X0 SOURCE
      CUINT*CUINT(SOURCE)  CUINT*CUINT*CUINT(SOURCE) /SS1;
RUN;
```

Ramon C. Littell, Austin J. Lewis, and Pamela R. Henry

Output from these statements is not shown. It would have the same appearance as that in Table Va, except that there would be another line under Type I SS for the cubic term. The cubic term should be tested first, then the quadratic term. Statistical significance of either of these terms indicates nonlinearity.

Table I. Analysis of variance for slope ratio validity tests on poultry bone manganese data

Source of variation	df	Sum of squares	Mean square	F value	Pr>F
Average slope	1	442.13	442.13	232.37	.001
Slope difference	1	14.29	14.29	7.51	.007
Blanks	1	1.90	1.90	1.00	.310
Intersection	1	.15	.15	.08	.780
Curvature	2	15.92	7.96	4.18	.018
Error	98	186.46	1.90		

Table II. Analysis of variance for slope ratio validity tests on rat hemoglobin data

Source of variation	df	Sum of squares	Mean square	F Value	Pr > F
Laboratories	7	156.05	22.29	72.40	.001
Regression	4	268.28	67.07	217.83	.001
Blanks	1	.57	.57	1.85	.177
Intersection	3	.98	.33	1.06	.371
Curvature	4	.63	.16	.51	.729
Error	84	25.86	.31		

Table III. Analysis of variance for slope ratio validity tests on poultry liver copper data

Source of variation	df	Sum of squares	Mean square	F Value	Pr>F
Average slope	1	8.245	8.245	443.03	.001
Slope difference	1	.193	.193	10.35	.003
Blanks	1	.356	.356	19.15	.001
Intersection	1	.046	.046	2.47	.125
Curvature	2	.062	.031	1.67	.204
Error	35	.651	.019		

Table IVa. General linear models procedure output for poultry bone manganese data validity tests

Source	df	Sum of squares	Mean square	F Value	Pr > F
Model	6	474.390892	79.065148	41.55	.0001
Error	98	186.461735	1.902671		
Total	104	660.852627			
		Type I SS			
LEVEL	1	442.129523	442.129523	232.37	.0001
LEVEL*SOURCE	1	14.288124	14.288124	7.51	.0073
X0	1	1.901790	1.901790	1.00	.3100
SOURCE	1	.148743	.148743	.08	.7804
CLEVEL(SOURCE)	2	15.922729	7.961364	4.18	.0180

Table IVb. General linear models procedure output for bone manganese regression coefficients

General Linear Models Procedure

Dependent Variable: MNPPM

Source	DF	Sum of Squares	Mean Square	F Value	Pr > F
Model	2	456.417647	228.208823	113.86	0.0001
Error	102	204.434980	2.004265		
Total	104	660.852627			

R-Square	C.V.	Root MSE	MNPPM Mean
0.690650	20.98007	1.41572	6.7479314

Parameter		Estimate	Std Error of Estimate
INTERCEPT		3.333175385	0.26823116
LEVEL*SOURCE	1	0.045187442 B	0.00377153
	2	0.054409609 B	0.00377153

Matrix Element Representation

Effect		Representation
INTERCEPT		INTERCEPT
LEVEL*SOURCE	1	DUMMY001
	2	DUMMY002

X'X Generalized Inverse (g2)

	INTERCEPT	DUMMY001	DUMMY002
INTERCEPT	0.0358974359	-0.000384615	-0.000384615
DUMMY001	-0.000384615	7.0970696E-6	4.1208791E-6
DUMMY002	-0.000384615	4.1208791E-6	7.0970696E-6

Table Va. General linear models output for liver copper data validity tests

General Linear Models Procedure

Dependent Variable: LOGLIVCU

Source	DF	Sum of Squares	Mean Square	F Value	Pr > F
Model	6	8.90164295	1.48360716	79.72	0.0001
Error	35	0.65134089	0.01860974		
Corrected Total	41	9.55298384			

R-Square	C.V.	Root MSE	LOGLIVCU Mean
0.931818	7.494185	0.13642	1.82031

Source	DF	Type I SS	Mean Square	F Value	Pr > F
CUINT	1	8.24475150	8.24475150	443.03	0.0001
CUINT*SOURCE	1	0.19262315	0.19262315	10.35	0.0028
X0	1	0.35630881	0.35630881	19.15	0.0001
SOURCE	1	0.04594566	0.04594566	2.47	0.1251
CUINT*CUINT(SOURCE)	2	0.06201383	0.03100691	1.67	0.2036

Table Vb. General linear models output for liver copper regression coefficients

General Linear Models Procedure

Dependent Variable: LOGLIVCU

Source	DF	Sum of Squares	Mean Square	F Value	Pr > F
Model	3	8.79368346	2.93122782	146.70	0.0001
Error	38	0.75930038	0.01998159		
Total	41	9.55298384			

R-Square	C.V.	Root MSE	LOGLIVCU Mean
0.920517	7.765498	0.14136	1.82031

Parameter	Estimate	Std Error of Estimate
INTERCEPT	0.8513348937	13.12
CUINT(SOURCE) 1	0.0079864002	16.75
2	0.0093647616	16.50
X0	0.3667012983	4.22

REFERENCES

Aschbacher, P. W., R. G. Cragle, E. W. Swanson and J. K. Miller. 1966. Metabolism of oral iodide and 3,5-diiodosalicylic acid in the pregnant cow. *J. Dairy Sci.* **49**:1042.

Finney, D. J. 1978. "Statistical Method in Biological Assay," 3rd ed. Griffen, London, UK.

Fritz, J. C., G. W. Pla, B. N. Harrison and G. A. Clark. 1974. Collaborative study of the rat hemoglobin repletion test for bioavailability of iron . *J. Assoc. Off. Anal. Chem.* **57**:513.

Henry, P. R., C. B. Ammerman and R. D. Miles. 1986. Bioavailability of manganese sulfate and manganese monoxide in chicks as measured by tissue uptake of manganese from conventional dietary levels. *Poult. Sci.* **65**:983.

Littell, R. C., R. J. Freund and P. C. Spector. 1991. "SAS System for Linear Models," 3rd. ed., p. 329. SAS Institute, Cary, NC.

Miles, R. D., C. W. Comer and P. R. Henry. 1993. Relative phosphorus bioavailability of two feed-grade phosphate sources for chicks. *Poult. Sci.* **72** (Suppl.1):182 [Abstract].

Pott, E. B., P. R. Henry, C. B. Ammerman, A. M. Merritt, J. B. Madison and R. D. Miles. 1994. Relative bioavailability of copper in a copper-lysine complex for chicks and lambs. *Anim. Feed Sci. Technol.* **45**:193.

Florida Agricultural Experiment Station Journal Series No. R-04363.

2

AMINO ACID BIOAVAILABILITY

Austin J. Lewis

Department of Animal Science
University of Nebraska
Lincoln, Nebraska

Henry S. Bayley

Department of Nutritional Sciences
University of Guelph
Guelph, Ontario

I. INTRODUCTION

The amino acid composition of a feedstuff or a diet can be determined by chemical procedures, usually acid hydrolysis followed by ion-exchange chromatography with colorimetric or fluorimetric detection of the amino acids. Chemical procedures do not, however, determine the amounts of amino acids that are available to an animal. To be "bioavailable," an amino acid must be absorbed and presented to the tissues in a form that can be used for normal metabolic functions.

Various methods have been developed to determine the availability of amino acids in feedstuffs, and no single procedure has emerged as universally applicable. It is convenient to divide the methods into three major groups: *in vitro*, indirect *in vivo*, and direct *in vivo*.

II. *IN VITRO* METHODS

The goal of *in vitro* procedures is to predict from laboratory tests of feedstuffs the amounts of amino acids that will be available to animals. The *in vitro* procedures are of three types: chemical, enzymic, and microbiological.

BIOAVAILABILITY OF NUTRIENTS FOR ANIMALS:
AMINO ACIDS, MINERALS, AND VITAMINS
Copyright © 1995 by Academic Press, Inc.

35

A. Chemical Tests

Most chemical tests of availability are specific for lysine. They are based on the premise that the ε-amino group of lysine must be free (not bound to another molecule) for the lysine to be biologically available. The original procedures used the reaction of lysine with 1-fluoro-2,4-dinitrobenzene (FDNB; Carpenter et al., 1957; Carpenter, 1960). A modification was developed by Roach et al. (1967). Other procedures using different reagents, such as 2,4,6-trinitrobenzene sulfonic acid (TNBS; Kakade and Liener, 1969), have also been published. Simplified methods based on the adsorption of dyes, such as acid orange 12, by proteins have been described (Hurrell and Carpenter, 1975; Goh et al., 1979a,b).

Although chemical procedures can differentiate among samples of the same feedstuff and may have a role to play in quality control, comparisons between chemical procedures and direct determinations of availability in animals have not always been encouraging. In a series of experiments in which lysine availability was evaluated in the same feedstuff by chemical procedures and growth experiments with pigs (Batterham et al., 1978, 1979, 1981, 1984, 1986a,b), there was little relationship between the chemical estimates and those obtained with pigs. A similar comparison of lysine availability in cereal grains by Taverner and Farrell (1981) also revealed a poor relationship between chemical and biological estimates. Nordheim and Coon (1984) measured the lysine availability in several fish meals, meat and bone meals, feather meals, and hair meals using the FDNB and TNBS methods and also using a chick growth assay. The correlation coefficients (r) of the chick growth assay results vs FDNB–lysine and TNBS–lysine were .83 and .90, respectively. An r of .96 between FDNB–lysine and chick assay available methionine was reported by Miller et al. (1965).

B. Enzymic Procedures

In vitro tests using enzymic digestion to simulate digestion within the intestine have been proposed. Several enzymes including pepsin, pronase, pancreatin, and papain have been tested. The primary difficulty with this approach has been to identify an enzyme or mixture of enzymes that truly imitates the action of the mixed enzymes in vivo and is effective for a wide variety of feedstuffs. The end products of in vitro enzymic digestion consist of amino acids, peptides of various lengths, and undigested proteins.

C. Microbiological Assays

Microbiological assays, which were once the primary method of determining the amino acid content of feedstuffs, have been used to estimate biological availability. The method is based on growth of a microorganism that has a specific requirement for the amino acid being studied. Organisms that have been used are the bacterium *Streptococcus zymogenes* (Ford, 1960) and the protozoan *Tetrahymena pyriformis* (Stott and Smith, 1966). There are numerous theoretical and practical difficulties with microbiological assays of amino acid availability, and these assays are little used today.

In general, the *in vitro* methods provide useful information about the effects of processing on amino acid availability, particularly any damage caused to lysine by heating. Data obtained from *in vitro* methods have not, however, found acceptance as a basis for diet formulation. More details about *in vitro* methods are found in the reviews of Carpenter (1973) and Sibbald (1987).

III. INDIRECT *IN VIVO* METHODS

Measurement of amino acid bioavailability in the target species is obviously more desirable than tests performed solely in the laboratory, but direct measurements with animals are both time consuming and expensive. Consequently, there have been efforts to establish indirect *in vivo* methods of determining amino acid availability. Two such methods are the use of plasma amino acid concentrations and the measurement of nitrogen digestibility.

It has been known since the experiments of Richardson *et al.* (1953) and Denton and Elvehjem (1954) that the concentrations of amino acids in the blood of animals are affected by dietary levels, and that use of the plasma concentration of the limiting amino acid to estimate amino acid requirements of poultry and swine is well established (Zimmerman and Scott, 1965; Lewis and Speer, 1975; Lewis *et al.*, 1977). There have been proposals that changes in plasma amino acid concentrations can also be used to estimate the availabilities of amino acids in feedstuffs (Morrison and McLaughlan, 1972). The method has never been fully developed, primarily because of the wide range of factors that can influence plasma amino acid concentrations, and because of the difficulties and expense involved in plasma amino acid analysis (Perry and Hansen, 1969).

Prediction of amino acid availabilities from measurements of nitrogen digestibility would offer a convenient indirect *in vivo* method if there were close relationships between the digestibilities of individual amino acids and overall protein digestibility.

In some experiments, reasonable relationships between the availabilities of specific amino acids and nitrogen digestibility have been reported (Uhlemann and Poppe, 1970; Borggreve and Veen, 1984), but the general consensus (Darcy *et al.*, 1982; Tanksley and Knabe, 1984) is that this method is of limited value.

IV. DIRECT *IN VIVO* METHODS

A. Amino Acid Digestibility

The digestibility of feeds and their proximate components is an important determinant of their relative worth as components of mixed diets for animals (Schneider and Flatt, 1975). A logical extension of the measurement of the digestibility of proximate components was to measure the digestibility of the individual amino acids in feedstuffs (Dammers, 1964). Since then there has been a vigorous research effort to use the digestible amino acid levels in feeds as a basis for diet formulation. The progress in this area during the 30 years since Dammers applied the classical concept of digestibility to the modern knowledge of amino acids has been reviewed extensively by Low (1982), Tanksley and Knabe (1984), Sauer and Ozimek (1986), Sibbald (1987), and den Hartog *et al.* (1989).

Microbial fermentation in the hindgut changes amino acid flux to the feces, leading to amino acid disappearances (or appearances) from the digestive tract that do not contribute to the amino acid nutrition of the animal. Thus, digestibility values measured by comparing dietary intakes and fecal outputs do not give credible estimates of the fraction of the amino acid in the feed that is useful to the animal (Cho and Bayley, 1971). This led to measurements of amino acid flow at the distal ileum on the assumption that the disappearance to this point in the digestive tract was the result of enzymic digestion and absorption, with microbial degradation accounting for a substantial fraction of the amino acid disappearances from the hindgut (Zebrowska, 1982). These studies measured ileal digestibilities, in contrast to fecal digestibilities, and in the majority of cases the ileal values were lower than the fecal values, indicating that fecal digestibilities overestimated the value of feeds as sources of amino acids (Low, 1979).

Digestibilities based on direct comparisons of feed intake and ileal or fecal output are affected by the contributions of endogenously derived material to the ileal or fecal output. For nitrogen compounds, including the amino acids, these contributions can be substantial because of the proteinaceous nature of the digestive enzymes and the mucosal cells added to the digesta. To minimize the effects of these residues of endogenous materials on the digestibility data, estimates of the amounts of endogenous nitrogen in the feces are made to allow calculation of "true" (or "corrected") digestibility values; these are distinguished from the "apparent" digestibilities (Taverner *et al.*, 1981).

One method of estimating the contribution of endogenous amino acids is to measure the fecal amino acid loss when a protein-free diet is consumed. However, endogenous losses are influenced by the amount and nature of dietary intakes. For example, Craig and Broderick (1981) found that in rats 1.84 g of nitrogen was excreted for each kilogram of dry matter consumed. An alternative approach is to regress fecal nitrogen (or amino acid) loss on protein (or amino acid) intake (Carlson and Bayley, 1970). Both methods fail to account for the effect of dietary protein intake on endogenous protein secretions into the digestive tract.

Souffrant *et al.* (1986) compared amino acid intake and portal blood uptake and found more amino acid in the portal blood flux than in the diet because of recycling of endogenous amino acids. They calculated that in pigs given a semipurified, casein-based diet at least 85% of the endogenous amino acids was absorbed. Siriwan *et al.* (1989) showed that the amounts of endogenous amino acids in ileal digesta of broiler chickens were influenced by both dietary fiber and dietary protein levels. It thus seems that all attempts to determine corrected or true digestibilities incur the uncertainty of the endogenous fraction, which can account for up to a quarter of the total amino acid input to the small intestine.

An alternative approach was developed by Krawielitzki *et al.* (1977), who used the flux of ^{15}N-labeled amino acids to quantify directly the residues of dietary amino acids in the feces and termed the digestibility values determined in this way "real." Thus, for each amino acid in a feedstuff, there are six possible values to describe the digestibility: apparent, true, and real for both fecal and ileal digestibilities. Not surprisingly, there has been some confusion surrounding the utility of these measures to characterize feeds.

An ingenious application of the ^{15}N label was made by de Lange *et al.* (1990), who labeled the endogenous protein by providing a continuous intravenous infusion of ^{15}N-labeled leucine. This approach coupled with data on the amino acid composition of the endogenous protein in the terminal ileum (de Lange *et al.*, 1989) allowed determination of the real ileal digestibilities of the amino acids in feedstuffs. The great differences between the apparent, true, and real ileal digestibility values illustrate the problem of ascribing a single number to this nutritional parameter. As an example, the apparent, true, and real ileal digestibilities of lysine in wheat were 71, 85, and 102%, respectively. However, the possibilities of using a wider range of feed ingredients, and the widespread use of crystalline amino acids in diets, have increased the importance of evaluating feedstuffs in a biologically consistent way and of quantifying their differences. Thus, establishment of the utility of the different measures of digestibility has become of both theoretically interesting and of pressing practical importance.

1. Determination of Ileal Digestibilities of Amino Acids in Pigs

On the assumption that amino acids that disappear from the digestive tract in the hindgut are of no value to the animal (Rerat, 1978), the flux of amino acids from the ileum must be measured. This requires surgical intervention to allow either collection of all the digesta or sampling of the digesta as it passes into the colon. The method adopted is to cut through the terminal ileum and attach a canula which is exteriorized; a second canula is attached to the distal end of the ileum to allow the return of the digesta once it has been measured and sampled. Sauer *et al.* (1989) have described the surgical procedures for pigs. Huisman *et al.* (1985) examined the effect of reentrant cannulation on digestion in the pig and found that it did not influence overall (fecal) digestibilities of the proximate components of the diet.

The use of reentrant cannulas allows unequivocal quantification of digesta flux, but disruption of the gastrointestinal tract may influence the functioning of the small intestine. An alternate procedure, the use of a simple T-cannula, permits the sampling of digesta as it leaves the ileum without complete disruption of the gut. However, T-cannulas require the use of a "marker" to quantify the flux, with all the assumptions inherently involved in the use of markers.

Cannulated animals are restricted in cages and the collections are made over a 24-hr period. Successive samples of digesta are collected for periods of 30 to 120 min and the total amount is measured, a sample removed, and the remainder returned to the pig through the distal cannula. Comparison of the ileal amino acid flux with the dietary intake allows calculation of apparent ileal digestibility. Low (1982) concluded that this measure is useful because it indicates the minimal net amount of amino acids, irrespective of origin, that is lost to the animal.

Apparent digestibilities are increased by correction for endogenous losses and depend on the dietary intake of the amino acids. But Buraczewski and Horaczynski (1983) found that increasing the protein level from 10 to 20% had no effect on apparent ileal digestibilities. In practice, most investigations have determined apparent ileal digestibilities as an index of amino acid availability in feedstuffs.

Sauer and Ozimek (1986) reviewed the apparent ileal digestibilities for pigs for three cereals and eight protein supplements. These values are from data reported since 1976, and the mean values are widely used to compare feeds (NRC, 1988). Unfortunately, mean values provide no indications of the wide ranges that they represent. For example, the lysine values ranged from 62.3 to 81.0% for 15 samples of wheat; the use of a mean of 74.5% is a poor indication of the value of any one sample of wheat as a source of lysine. Taverner *et al.* (1981) measured both apparent and true ileal digestibilities of amino acids in cereals. For lysine, the apparent values for three samples of wheat ranged from 70 to 81% and the true values from 79 to 89%, so "correction" for endogenous lysine did little to reduce the range.

2. Determination of Amino Acid Digestibility in Birds

Measurements of digestibility in birds are complicated by their voiding feces and urine together, and because urine contains amino acids (Gruhn and Raue, 1974) it is necessary to ensure separation of the feces and urine by surgical intervention (Shannon and McNab, 1973). Summers and Robblee (1985) sampled digesta from the terminal ileum of birds and used these samples to calculate apparent ileal digestibilities.

Likuski and Dorrell (1978) compared intake and output of amino acids by previously fasted, precision-fed roosters and used their observations to calculate "true metabolizability of amino acids." Papadopoulos (1985) concluded that this method, despite its shortcomings, was currently the most practical way of comparing feedstuffs as amino acid sources for poultry.

Data from precision-fed, cecectomized roosters for the true digestibility of amino acids are being used to evaluate feeds for poultry; but there is wide variation in these results. The true digestibilities of lysine in wheat ranged from 62 to 93% (Parsons, 1990) making it just as imprecise to use these values for poultry as it is to use the corresponding ileal digestibilities for swine.

3. Utility of Amino Acid Digestibilities in Feed Evaluation

The purpose of determining amino acid digestibilities is to optimize the use of feed resources for animal production. Tanskley and Knabe (1984) formulated the question: "Can ileal digestibility values help in formulating diets more precisely?" The investigators carried out the crucial experiments to answer this question by formulating pig diets based upon either total amino acid levels or upon the levels of digestible (ileal) amino acids. There was no advantage to using the ileal digestibility values for diets based on corn and soybean meal. They used cottonseed meal as a substitute for soybean meal and found apparent ileal digestibilities of lysine were 86 and 70% for the soybean and cottonseed meals, respectively. Formulating diets to equal levels of ileal digestible lysine resulted in slower growth for the pigs given cottonseed meal in their diets, indicating that the ileal digestibility was not precise in predicting equivalence of the nutritional values of the soybean and cottonseed meals.

Batterham et al. (1990) measured both the apparent ileal digestibility of lysine and lysine availability by slope ratio growth assay in cottonseed and soybean meals. They found that the availability of the lysine in the cottonseed meal was much lower than its apparent ileal digestibility. However, both values were similar for soybean meal. Growth studies with cottonseed meal confirmed the utility of the growth assay value for lysine in cottonseed meal. Ileal digestibility of lysine was of limited use as a basis for formulation of diets containing cottonseed meal. Unfortunately, few other investigations have shown the utility of ileal digestibilities in formulating diets.

4. Summaries of Amino Acid Digestibilities in Poultry and Swine

Comprehensive reviews of digestibility data in poultry (Parsons, 1991) and swine (Southern, 1991) have been published by Nutri-Quest, Inc. (a subsidiary of BioKyowa, Inc.). Data from these reviews are summarized in Tables I and II.

B. Growth Assays

Assays of bioavailability that involve some measurement of animal growth are usually considered the ultimate standards against which other methods are judged. Growth assays of amino acid bioavailability measure the capacity of a protein to provide a specific limiting amino acid and promote growth. This ability is normally compared to the response obtained with a crystalline amino acid, which is assumed to be fully available.

Growth assays have at least two very attractive features. First, they measure a response (growth) that has important practical and economic consequences. Second, they indicate the net effect of all the components that can affect bioavailability (digestion, absorption, and utilization). On the other hand, growth assays of amino acid availability have serious limitations. Growth assays are expensive and time consuming and they yield data for one amino acid only. Furthermore, growth assays are subject to many sources of interference, and they often contain a large amount of inherent animal variation.

Because they are so laborious, growth assays cannot serve as a routine method of feedstuff evaluation. They are important, however, because they "remain the only direct means to check the validity of claims for the nutritional relevance of values obtained by other procedures" (Carpenter, 1973). The design and conduct of a growth assay can have a large effect on the result obtained. Because they tend to serve as the "absolute" standard, it is particularly crucial that growth assays be conducted well. Previous reviews of various aspects of the methodology of growth assay of amino acid availability include those of Meade (1972), Carpenter (1973), Baker (1978), McNab (1979), Parsons (1985), and Sibbald (1987).

1. Principles of Growth Assays

Although many variants of growth assays of amino acid availability have been proposed, most are based on the same principles. A dose–response relationship between the crystalline form of the amino acid of interest and some measure of growth is established. This serves as the standard. The standard response relationship is then compared with the dose–response relationship of a test protein (or other amino acid source). To simplify both the statistical analysis and the interpretation of the results, linear dose–response relationships are normally assumed. Linear methods are not adequate, however, to describe the full biological relationship in most situations. Thus, both linear and nonlinear methods merit consideration. Chapter 1 of this book describes the statistical principles of growth assays of bioavailability.

2. Technical Aspects

a. Basal Diets.' Basal diets used in growth assays need to be deficient in the amino acid under investigation but adequate in all other nutrients, including other amino acids. Two approaches have been used to accomplish this. The first consists of using purified diets in which the amino acid requirements (except the test amino acid) are provided by crystalline amino acids. This approach has been adopted in experiments with rats (Tsien et al., 1957; Calhoun et al., 1960) and particularly with chicks (Netke and Scott, 1970; Sasse and Baker, 1973; Baker et al., 1979). It has the advantage that the available amino acid content of the basal diet is known (assuming that crystalline amino acids are 100% available). The obvious disadvantage is the high cost of these diets, which precludes their use in large animals.

The second approach is to use a basal diet containing protein sources relatively low in the amino acid of interest together with supplementary amino acids. This has invariably been the approach chosen for experiments with pigs (Batterham et al., 1979; Parsons et al., 1985; Sato et al., 1987). The use of intact proteins allows less control over the levels of other amino acids. These can become very high, with the potential to lead to the adverse effects of amino acid disproportion. Both types of diets seem to be valid if formulated correctly. An advantage of the purified diet is that it allows partition of the response between that due to the basal diet and that due to the supplemental protein, as described by Netke and Scott (1970) and Parsons (1986).

b. Bioavailability of Crystalline Amino Acids. In most growth assays of amino acid bioavailability, the dose–response relationship for a crystalline amino acid serves as the standard of reference. It is assumed that crystalline amino acids are completely absorbed and are therefore 100% bioavailable. In a digestibility study with adult cockerels, Sibbald and Wolynetz (1985) indicated that only 92% of L-lysine·HCl was "bioavailable." Most other reports, however, in both poultry (Nelson et al., 1986; Han et al., 1990; Izquierdo et al., 1988) and swine (Buraczewska, 1981; Leibholz et al., 1986; Chung and Baker, 1991) have indicated that crystalline amino acids are fully absorbed from the lumen of the gut. Disappearance from the gut, however, is not evidence of complete bioavailability. Heat-damaged proteins may contain amino acid derivatives that are absorbed, but which are excreted in the urine rather than being metabolized (Carpenter, 1973).

Crystalline amino acids may be absorbed more rapidly than amino acids from proteins, and this may influence bioavailability. Early research (Cannon *et al.*, 1947; Geiger, 1947) indicated that the timing of an amino acid supplement may affect its efficiency of utilization. Subsequent studies (Yang *et al.*, 1963, 1968; Baker and Izquierdo, 1985) have revealed that this may vary among amino acids and may depend on the level of amino acid supplementation. Experiments with swine (Batterham, 1984; Partridge *et al.*, 1985), however, have shown clearly that the efficiency of crystalline lysine utilization is lower when pigs are fed once daily than when they are fed more frequently. The overall question regarding the utilization of crystalline amino acids remains unanswered, but it is evident that there are situations when crystalline amino acids may be completely absorbed but not completely bioavailable. The extent to which they are less than fully utilized may depend on the individual amino acid and the experimental procedure.

c. Interfering Substances. A persistent problem with growth assays is the issue of interfering substances present in the feedstuff to be assayed. Although the assay is based on the premise that any growth response is caused solely by the provision of the limiting amino acid, there may be other substances present that can either stimulate or depress growth. These problems can be particularly acute in low-protein feedstuffs, such as cereal grains, in which the contribution of the limiting amino acid is small relative to the amount of feedstuff added.

i. Amino acids. All proteins contribute amino acids in addition to the one being assayed. Because of the complex interrelationships among amino acids (Harper *et al.*, 1970), these additional amino acids have the potential to modify the growth response and thus affect the estimate of bioavailability. The issue has been recognized for some time, but no completely satisfactory solution has been found.

There is clear evidence (Netke *et al.*, 1969) that the addition of a mixture of crystalline amino acids lacking the first limiting amino acid can reduce feed intake and weight gain. The efficiency of feed utilization and, therefore, the efficiency with which the first limiting amino acid is used, may or may not be affected. This indicates that whether the presence of excess amino acids in a test feedstuff affects the bioavailability estimate may depend on the independent variable of the assay. If the independent variable is dietary amino acid *concentration*, there will probably be an effect on the bioassay, but if the independent variable is amino acid *intake*, there is less likelihood that the pattern of excess amino acids will affect the outcome of the bioavailability growth assay.

Experiments that have included designs to address the problem of excess amino acids have yielded conflicting results. The general approach has been to include in the assay a mixture of crystalline amino acids that simulates the test protein. In some experiments this "simulated protein" has been added at one level, whereas in others graded levels have been included.

Smith and Scott (1965a) in a comprehensive series of experiments determined the available amino acid content of fish meal by growth assay. Diets that included simulated fish meal were used as a reference standard. The independent variable was dietary amino acid concentration. Their estimates of bioavailability were very high (most were greater than 100%). In a subsequent report (Smith and Scott, 1965b), they established that their simulated fish meal reduced performance relative to fish meal itself, and that this was at least partially responsible for their high estimates of bioavailability.

A somewhat different approach was taken by Uwaegbute and Lewis (1966a,b). These researchers attempted to account for what they termed the "protein effect" in bioassays of amino acid availability. They equalized the essential amino acid content (except lysine, which was the test amino acid) in all diets by additions of crystalline amino acids. Their estimates of the available lysine contents of a series of feedstuffs were reasonably similar to estimates obtained by the FDNB procedure.

A third approach, developed by Robel and Frobish (1977), has been used by subsequent researchers. Robel and Frobish (1977) measured the bioavailability of sulfur amino acids in soybean meal with a chick bioassay. They used as their standard of reference either graded levels of crystalline sulfur amino acids or graded levels of all amino acids (essential and nonessential) in a pattern designed to simulate soybean meal. They found that the "excess" amino acids in simulated soybean meal did not affect the estimate of bioavailability. The independent variable in their experiment was the amount of sulfur amino acids consumed.

In contrast, Baker (1978) and Hirakawa and Baker (1986) in the measurement of lysine availability in chick bioassays found that the addition of a crystalline amino acid mixture simulating the test protein (soybean meal or a corn gluten meal–sesame meal–meat and bone meal mixture, respectively) reduced the efficiency of lysine utilization. Relative to the utilization of crystalline lysine alone, the utilization of lysine in a simulated protein was 80% for soybean meal and 60% for the corn gluten meal–sesame meal–meat and bone meal mixture.

Sato et al. (1987), in experiments with swine, reported that the excess amino acids in soybean meal affected the estimate of tryptophan bioavailability. They found that the efficiency of tryptophan utilization in a mixture of crystalline amino acids that simulated soybean meal was 82% of that of crystalline tryptophan alone.

In recent experiments concerning the availability of threonine in soybean meal, Radke and co-workers found that the excess amino acids in simulated soybean meal were without effect in experiments with rats and chicks (Radke *et al.*, 1988) or swine (Radke *et al.*, unpublished). The efficiency of utilization of threonine in simulated soybean meal was 98 to 102% of that of crystalline threonine alone. Similarly, Izquierdo *et al.* (1988) evaluated the bioavailability of lysine in simulated casein using a chick assay. The availability was 99% relative to crystalline lysine.

Thus, it remains unclear how the excess amino acids in proteins may affect the results. Perhaps there are differences among amino acids. It is important to keep in mind that a mixture of crystalline amino acids that simulates a protein is not the same as an intact protein itself. Intact proteins must undergo hydrolysis and can also impart chemical and physical features to diets that are different than mixtures of crystalline amino acids. Furthermore, the excess amino acids present in a protein are an inherent feature of that protein and perhaps no special adjustments should be made for them.

ii. Other substances. There may be other substances present in the feedstuff to be assayed that can affect the response. Plant protein sources often have a low digestible energy content because they contain relatively large amounts of fiber. This may either increase or decrease feed intake and influence estimates of availability even when adjustments for differences in intake are made. Other growth inhibitors can also have large effects. Batterham *et al.* (1981) reported a negative value (-23%) for the availability of lysine in linseed meal for pigs. This estimate implies that the available lysine contribution from linseed meal decreased as the amount of linseed meal in the diet was increased. Apparently, some other factor present in the linseed meal interfered with pig performance, although the authors could not identify what it was. Particularly surprising was that in a similar experiment using rats instead of pigs the estimate of lysine bioavailability in the same source of linseed meal was 82%.

Even more difficult to deal with is the possibility of growth-enhancing factors that may be present in some feedstuffs. In some experiments, addition of the test protein seems to increase feed intake. This may influence the estimate of bioavailability even when attempts are made to adjust for the differences in intake. Relatively high values for the availability of amino acids in fish meal have been reported in several experiments (Carpenter *et al.*, 1963; Smith and Scott, 1965a; Uwaegbute and Lewis 1966b; Carpenter *et al.*, 1972; Major and Batterham, 1981).

d. Length of the Assay. Experiments with chicks have demonstrated that the length of the assay can affect the estimate of bioavailability. Carpenter *et al.* (1963) compared estimates of lysine bioavailability based on assays of 3, 6, or 10 days.

There was a tendency for the estimate of bioavailability to decrease as the assay period increased. The fiducial limits of the estimate also decreased as the time period increased. Similarly, Hill *et al.* (1966) reported that a 9-day assay produced an estimate of lysine availability in soybean meal that was about 10% lower than that of a 5-day assay. In contrast, Robel and Frobish (1977) found that 8-day assays of sulfur amino acids, lysine, and tryptophan in soybean meal yielded estimates that were higher than 4- or 6-day estimates. The reasons for the differences among experiments are not clear, but they could be related to the time after hatching that the experiments were started. Most chick assays now consist of a 7- to 10-day growth period that is begun approximately 1 week posthatching.

3. Statistical Aspects

a. Independent Variable. The independent variable in most growth assays of amino acid availability has been either amino acid concentration in the diet or amino acid intake (usually supplemental amino acid intake). Although the choice may be influenced by the choice of dependent variable, amino acid intake has been preferred by most investigators.

When weight gain is the dependent variable, analyses based on amino acid intake result in more valid assays than analyses based on dietary amino acid level. This has been established in experiments with both rats (Gupta *et al.*, 1958; de Muelenaere *et al.*, 1967) and chicks (Carpenter *et al.*, 1963; Campbell, 1966; Smith, 1968; Guo *et al.*, 1971, Oh *et al.*, 1972; Cave and Williams, 1980). When the basal diet contains the test amino acid (i.e., the concentration of the test amino acid in the basal diet is greater than zero), the independent variable should be intake of amino acid from supplemental sources rather than total amino acid intake (Netke and Scott, 1970).

In cases in which the dependent variable includes adjustments for differences in feed intake (e.g., feed conversion efficiency), the choice of either amino acid concentration or amino acid intake has little effect on the precision of the estimate (Carpenter *et al.*, 1963). Batterham and co-workers (Batterham *et al.*, 1979, 1981) used feed conversion efficiency on a carcass basis *vs* dietary lysine concentration in experiments with pigs, but feed intake was equalized in these studies. The merits and demerits of equalized feeding have been reviewed by Baker (1984).

b. Dependent Variable. Most assays have used body weight gain as the dependent variable. This has the advantage of being easy to measure. In rats, the use of empty body weight gain eliminates inaccuracies caused by differences in gastrointestinal contents, but estimates of lysine bioavailability are affected little (de Muelenaere *et al.*, 1967). Major and Batterham (1981) reported that estimates of lysine bioavailability in chicks that were fasted at the end of an experiment were similar to those that were allowed access to feed throughout the experiment.

Bioavailability estimates based on feed conversion efficiencies of chicks are usually higher than those based on weight gain (Miller *et al.*, 1965; Uwaegbute and Lewis, 1966b; Carpenter *et al.*, 1972; Oh *et al.*, 1972; Njike *et al.*, 1975; Major and Batterham, 1981). There is, however, little or no improvement in the precision of the estimates. Results with rats (Batterham *et al.*, 1979, 1981) also indicate that estimates based on feed conversion efficiency tend to be higher than those based on weight gain. Data from the same group with swine, however, indicate that estimates based on feed conversion efficiency and weight gain are similar, but that the use of feed conversion efficiency tends to improve precision. Feed intake was equalized in these swine experiments. Feed conversion efficiency on a carcass basis was judged to be the most appropriate criterion for both rats and swine.

Several groups have suggested that the deposition of protein in rats and chicks, as measured by either carcass nitrogen (Calhoun *et al.*, 1960; de Muelenaere *et al.*, 1967) or nitrogen balance (Uwaegbute and Lewis, 1966b), is the most appropriate and reliable criterion for assessment of amino acid bioavailability. The results of Radke *et al.* (1988) support the contention that carcass nitrogen gain is superior to weight gain, but this finding has not been universal (Cave and Williams, 1980). Sibbald (1987) concluded that although some measure of nitrogen retention is preferable, "weight gain appears to give comparable results and is much easier to measure."

c. Tests of Validity. Procedures to determine whether a particular slope ratio assay of amino acid bioavailability is valid are the same as for other bioassays using slope ratio procedures. Unfortunately, with few exceptions (e.g., Campbell, 1966; Oh *et al.*, 1972; Cave and Williams, 1980; Parsons, 1986) tests of validity are rarely described or even mentioned. Statistical procedures are outlined by Finney (1978) and a specific example dealing with lysine bioavailability in a chick assay is provided by Campbell (1966).

Tests for *statistical validity* determine whether the responses to increasing amounts of standards and test substances are linear and whether there is curvature at low amino acid levels (intakes). Failure to achieve statistical validity does not invalidate the assay procedure *per se*, but does cast doubts on the model being tested. A change in the model may result in a valid assay. In contrast, *fundamental validity* refers to whether the regression lines for the individual substances intersect at the point of the basal diet. A lack of fundamental validity indicates that the test substances cannot be assayed against each other, and that an expression of ratios of slopes is inappropriate. Although some authors (Carpenter *et al.*, 1972; Cave and Williams, 1980) have rejected certain of their assays or components of assays because of lack of validity, others (Netke and Scott, 1970; Robel and Frobish, 1977; Hirakawa and Baker, 1986; Leibholz, 1986) have identified fundamental invalidity and/or have based estimates of bioavailability on the ratios of slopes of independent regression equations with different intercepts.

d. Partitioning the Response. In slope ratio assays of amino acid availability, there is usually an increase in feed intake when the dietary concentration of the test amino acid is increased. Unless the basal diet is completely devoid of the test amino acid, this means that part of the increase in weight gain will be due to the consumption of more of the test amino acid from the basal diet. This issue was discussed by Netke and Scott (1970) who proposed a method of "partitioning" weight gain between that due to the basal diet and that due to the test ingredient. The partitioning is relatively simple if crystalline amino acid basal diets are used. This is because the source of amino acid in the basal diet and the reference source is the same and therefore has the same bioavailability. When the basal diet contains intact proteins, assumptions have to be made about the bioavailability of the test amino acid in these proteins (Oh *et al.*, 1972; Parsons, 1986). With crystalline amino acid diets, partitioning seems to yield higher values than nonpartitioning (Hirakawa and Baker, 1986; Parsons, 1986). With a basal diet containing feather meal, Oh *et al.* (1972) found that partitioning tended to yield somewhat lower estimates of bioavailability.

4. Summaries of Growth Assays of Amino Acid Bioavailability

A list of studies in which relative bioavailabilities of amino acids have been measured in experiments with rats, chicks, and swine is provided in Table III. Summary values derived from Table III are presented in Table IV for poultry and Table V for swine.

Table I. True digestibilities of amino acids in poultry[a]

Feedstuff	n	Arg	Cys	Lys	Met	Thr	Val
Alfalfa	8	82	40	59	73	71	75
Animal protein blend	17	88	65	84	91	84	87
Bakery meal	8	83	81	61	84	71	80
Barley	24	85	81	78	79	77	81
Blood meal	18	84	73	82	88	85	84
Canola	26	90	71	78	90	78	82
Casein	1	97	84	97	99	98	98
Corn	19	95	86	78	91	84	88
Corn gluten feed	14	88	65	71	84	75	83
Corn gluten meal	11	96	87	88	97	93	95
Distillers grains with solubles	5	63	77	65	84	72	81
Feather meal	24	83	56	65	75	72	81
Field peas	1	89	78	87	89	88	80
Fish meal	30	92	75	88	92	90	91
Gelatin	1	96	68	94	93	95	97
Groundnut meal	2	92	78	73	87	85	90
Lupin	2	96	88	92	86	91	91
Meat meal	43	85	59	79	85	79	82
Oats	15	94	84	87	86	85	88
Oat groats	4	92	84	80	90	83	88
Poultry by-product	23	87	62	80	86	80	83
Rice bran	7	87	68	75	78	70	77
Soybeans, raw	3	79	57	78	68	68	69
Soybean meal	35	92	83	90	92	89	91
Sesame meal	2	92	82	88	94	87	91
Sorghum	16	77	83	76	88	81	86

Sunflower meal	8	95	80	85	93	85	86
Wheat	23	88	88	81	87	83	86
Wheat shorts	15	86	69	81	80	79	82

[a]Adapted from Parsons (1991) with permission.

Table II. Apparent ileal digestibilities of amino acids in swine[a]

Feedstuff	n	Arg	His	Ile	Leu	Lys	Met	Cys	Phe	Tyr	Thr	Trp	Val
Barley	19	79	77	76	79	70	79	75	80	76	67	68	73
Blood meal	3	94	94	70	93	93	-	-	92	-	87	89	92
Bone meal	1	79	74	76	79	77	81	38	78	72	75	-	77
Canola meal	5	84	80	77	79	76	84	84	76	72	69	77	70
Casein	2	94	95	92	96	95	96	66	96	96	88	91	94
Corn	13	82	82	79	88	64	86	76	84	83	66	62	79
Corn gluten feed	3	-	-	59	-	41	-	-	-	-	47	-	-
Corn gluten meal	2	86	80	84	90	74	86	73	88	81	80	72	81
Cottonseed meal	7	90	80	72	74	65	75	-	84	80	66	75	75
Feather meal	2	79	45	78	77	45	64	72	81	74	70	60	78
Fish meal	8	88	80	83	85	83	83	63	81	83	78	74	81
Groundnut meal	6	92	79	81	82	75	87	74	88	91	67	71	81
Meat meal	1	91	82	84	84	85	85	58	84	81	81	-	81
Meat and bone meal	25	81	70	70	73	70	78	49	76	72	65	54	72
Milk, dried, skim	3	88	92	86	91	91	86	79	89	93	81	-	85
Oats	1	-	-	-	-	70	79	64	-	-	55	-	-
Oat groats	1	90	86	86	85	82	89	-	90	82	78	81	86
Rapeseed meal	8	84	81	75	79	73	86	76	79	73	68	-	70
Rye	2	71	70	66	70	65	75	72	74	63	57	-	65
Sorghum	5	84	-	89	91	58	86	-	-	-	64	72	87
Soybeans, extruded	1	81	79	70	69	78	78	64	77	69	67	69	69
Soybeans, raw	3	56	48	43	37	57	47	35	45	40	48	25	35
Soybean meal, 48.5%	12	89	85	83	82	85	86	79	83	83	76	79	79
Soybean meal, 44%	17	90	86	83	83	85	87	76	84	83	76	80	80
Soy flour	1	91	88	83	81	88	91	78	87	83	76	79	81

Soy protein isolate	1	91	88	90	92	88	-	-	88	89	85	-	86
Sunflower meal	9	89	79	78	77	74	87	74	80	77	71	76	75
Triticale	5	80	78	78	80	72	83	81	80	77	61	70	76
Wheat	23	84	85	84	85	73	85	82	88	84	72	79	80
Wheat bran	1	-	-	-	-	74	78	67	-	-	55	-	-
Wheat middlings	6	84	79	70	72	72	79	-	82	74	60	78	73

[a]Adapted from Southern (1991) with permission.

Table III. Relative bioavailabilities of amino acids based on growth assays[a]

Source	Amino acid	RV	Standard	Response criterion	Method of calc	Diet	Age /wt	Reference
Chickens								
Blood meal	Lys	60	Cryst Lys	Gain	TP	N	7 d	Kratzer and Green (1957)
Blood meal	Lys	70	Cryst Lys	Gain	SR	SP	7 d	Guo et al. (1971)
Blood meal	Lys	105	Cryst Lys	Gain/feed	SR	N	8 d	Batterham et al. (1986a)
Blood meal	Met	66	Cryst Met	Partitioned gain	SR	SP	7 d	Oh et al. (1972)
Casein	Lys	99	Cryst Lys	Gain	SR	AA	8 d	Izquierdo et al. (1988)
Corn	Lys	73	Cryst Lys	Gain	SR	AA	9 d	Costa et al. (1977)
Corn	SAA	97	Cryst SAA	Gain	SR	AA	5 d	Sasse and Baker (1973a)
Corn, high moisture	Lys	72	Cryst Lys	Gain	SR	AA	9 d	Costa et al. (1977)
Corn gluten meal	SAA	99	Cryst SAA	Gain	SR	AA	5 d	Sasse and Baker (1973a)
Cottonseed meal	Lys	83	Cryst Lys	Gain	SR	N	8 d	Major and Batterham (1981)
Feather meal	Lys	5	Cryst Lys	Gain	SC	AA	8 d	Smith (1968)
Feather meal	Lys	68	Cryst Lys	Gain	SC	N	10 d	Nordheim and Coon (1984)
Feather meal	Met	75	Cryst Met	Gain	SC	AA	8 d	Smith (1968)
Feather meal	Met	35	Cryst Met	Partitioned gain	SR	SP	7 d	Oh et al. (1972)
Feather meal	Thr	63	Cryst Thr	Gain	SC	AA	8 d	Smith (1968)
Feather meal	Trp	46	Cryst Trp	Gain	SC	AA	8 d	Smith (1968)
Fish meal	Lys	90	Cryst Lys	Gain	SR	N	10 d	Carpenter et al. (1963)
Fish meal	Lys	113	Cryst Lys	Gain	SR	N	10 d	Carpenter et al. (1963)
Fish meal	Lys	90	Cryst Lys	Gain	SR	SP	7 d	Guo et al. (1971)
Fish meal	Lys	90	Cryst Lys	Gain	TP	AA	12 d	Ousterhout et al. (1959)
Fish meal	Lys	122	Cryst Lys	Gain	PL	N	7 d	Uwaegbute and Lewis (1966b)
Fish meal	Lys	90	Cryst Lys	Gain	SC	N	10 d	Nordheim and Coon (1984)
Fish meal	Lys	100	Cryst Lys	Gain/feed	SR	N	8 d	Major and Batterham (1981)
Fish meal	Lys	125	Cryst Lys	Gain	SC	AA	8 d	Smith and Scott (1965a)

Feedstuff	AA	Value	Supplement	Response				Reference
Fish meal	Lys	85	Cryst Lys	Gain	SC	AA	8 d	Smith (1968)
Fish meal	Met	93	Cryst Met	Gain	SC	AA	8 d	Smith (1968)
Fish meal	Met	98	Cryst Met	Gain	TP	AA	12 d	Ousterhout et al. (1959)
Fish meal	Met	92	Cryst Met	Gain	SR	SP	10 d	Carpenter et al. (1972)
Fish meal	Met	108	Cryst Met	Gain	SC	AA	8 d	Smith and Scott (1965a)
Fish meal	Met	90	Cryst Met	Partitioned gain	SR	SP	7 d	Oh et al. (1972)
Fish meal	Met	100	Cryst Met	Gain/feed	SR	SP	10 d	Miller et al. (1965)
Fish meal	Thr	85	Cryst Thr	Gain	SC	AA	8 d	Smith (1968)
Fish meal	Trp	115	Cryst Trp	Gain	TP	AA	12 d	Ousterhout et al. (1959)
Fish meal	Trp	100	Cryst Trp	Gain	SC	AA	8 d	Smith (1968)
Hair meal	Lys	57	Cryst Lys	Gain	SC	N	10 d	Nordheim and Coon (1984)
Meat meal	Cys	56	Cryst Cys	Partitioned gain	SR	AA	8 d	Parsons (1986)
Meat meal	Lys	52	Cryst Lys	Gain	SR	SP	7 d	Guo et al. (1971)
Meat meal	Lys	72	Cryst Lys	Gain/feed	SR	N	8 d	Batterham et al. (1986a)
Meat meal	Lys	75	Cryst Lys	Partitioned gain	SR	AA	8 d	Parsons (1986)
Meat meal	Lys	83	Cryst Lys	Gain	PL	N	7 d	Uwaegbute and Lewis (1966b)
Meat meal	Met	106	Cryst Met	Gain	SR	SP	10 d	Carpenter et al. (1972)
Meat meal	Met	48	Cryst Met	Gain/feed	SR	SP	10 d	Miller et al. (1965)
Meat meal	Met	81	Cryst Met	Partitioned gain	SR	N	8 d	Parsons (1986)
Meat meal	Met	91	Cryst Met	Partitioned gain	SR	SP	7 d	Oh et al. (1972)
Meat and bone meal	Lys	83	Cryst Lys	Gain/feed	SR	N	8 d	Batterham et al. (1986a)
Meat and bone meal	Lys	91	Cryst Lys	Gain	SC	N	10 d	Nordheim and Coon (1984)
Meat and bone meal	Lys	31–93	Cryst Lys	Carcass gain/feed	SR	N	8 d	Batterham et al. (1986b)
Meat and bone meal	Lys	86	Cryst Lys	Gain/feed	SR	N	8 d	Major and Batterham (1981)
Peanut meal	Lys	92	Cryst Lys	Gain	PL	N	7 d	Uwaegbute and Lewis (1966b)
Peanut meal	Met	76	Cryst Met	Gain	SR	SP	10 d	Carpenter et al. (1972)
Rapeseed meal	Lys	90	Cryst Lys	Gain	SR	SP	7 d	Guo et al. (1971)
Rapeseed meal	Met	87	Cryst Met	Partitioned gain	SR	SP	7 d	Oh et al. (1972)
Soybean meal	Lys	93	Cryst Lys	Gain/feed	SR	N	8 d	Major and Batterham (1981)
Soybean meal	Lys	90	Cryst Lys	Gain	SR	SP	14 d	Hill et al. (1966)

Table III. (continued)

Source	Amino acid	RV	Standard	Response criterion	Method of calc	Diet	Age/wt	Reference
Soybean meal	Lys	98	Cryst Lys	Gain	SC	AA	8 d	Smith (1968)
Soybean meal	Lys	83	Cryst Lys	Gain	PL	N	7 d	Uwaegbute and Lewis (1966b)
Soybean meal	Lys	77	Cryst Lys	Partitioned gain	SR	AA	7 d	Netke and Scott (1970)
Soybean meal	Lys	90	Cryst Lys	Gain	SR	AA	8 d	Robel and Frobish (1977)
Soybean meal	Met	95	Cryst Met	Partitioned gain	SR	SP	7 d	Oh et al. (1972)
Soybean meal	Met	93	Cryst Met	Gain	SC	AA	8 d	Smith (1968)
Soybean meal	SAA	88	Cryst SAA	Gain	SR	AA	8 d	Robel and Frobish (1977)
Soybean meal	Thr	104	Cryst Thr	Gain	SC	AA	8 d	Smith (1968)
Soybean meal	Trp	100	Cryst Trp	Gain	SC	AA	8 d	Smith (1968)
Soybean meal	Trp	83	Cryst Trp	Gain	SR	AA	8 d	Robel and Frobish (1977)
Sunflower meal	Lys	101	Cryst Lys	Gain/feed	SR	N	8 d	Major and Batterham (1981)
Sunflower meal	Met	101	Cryst Met	Gain	SR	SP	10 d	Carpenter et al. (1972)
Whale meal	Met	67	Cryst Met	Gain/feed	SR	SP	10 d	Miller et al. (1965)
Wheat	Lys	78	Cryst Lys	Gain	SR	SP	8 d	Cave and Williams (1980)
Swine								
Alfalfa, freeze dried	Trp	80	Cryst Trp	Gain/feed	SC	SP	5 kg	Rivera et al. (1976)
Blood meal	Lys	108	Cryst Lys	Carcass gain/feed	SR	N	20 kg	Batterham et al. (1986a)
Blood meal	Lys	74	Cryst Lys	Gain	SC	N	5 wk	Parsons et al. (1985)
Corn	Trp	77	Cryst Trp	Gain/feed	SC	SP	5 kg	Rivera et al. (1976)
Corn	Trp	94	Sim corn	Gain	SR	SP	10 kg	Sato et al. (1987)
Corn, opaque 2	Trp	65	Cryst Trp	Gain/feed	SC	SP	5 kg	Rivera et al. (1976)
Cottonseed meal	Lys	39	Cryst Lys	Carcass gain	SR	N	20 kg	Batterham et al. (1984)
Cottonseed meal	Lys	39	Cryst Lys	Carcass gain	SR	N	20 kg	Batterham et al. (1979)
Cottonseed meal	Lys	72	Cryst Lys	Gain	SR	N	21 d	Leibholz (1986)
Cottonseed meal	Met	87	Cryst Met	Gain	SR	N	28 d	Leibholz and Kirby (1985)
Cottonseed meal	Trp	81	Sim CSM	Gain	SR	SP	10 kg	Sato et al. (1987)

Ingredient	Amino acid	Value	Source	Criterion	Assay	N/SP	Weight/Duration	Reference
Field peas	Lys	93	Cryst Lys	Carcass gain	SR	N	20 kg	Batterham et al. (1984)
Fish meal	Lys	89	Cryst Lys	Carcass gain	SR	N	20 kg	Batterham et al. (1979)
Linseed meal	Lys	-23	Cryst Lys	Carcass gain/feed	SR	N	20 kg	Batterham et al. (1981)
Lupins	Lys	90	Cryst Lys	Gain	SR	N	21 d	Leibholz (1986)
Lupin seed meal	Lys	53	Cryst Lys	Carcass gain/feed	SR	N	20 kg	Batterham et al. (1984)
Lupin seed meal	Lys	51	Cryst Lys	Carcass gain/feed	SR	N	20 kg	Batterham et al. (1986c)
Lupin seed meal	Lys	74	Cryst Lys	Carcass gain/feed	SR	N	20 kg	Batterham et al. (1981)
Meat meal	Lys	87	Cryst Lys	Gain	SR	N	21 d	Leibholz (1986)
Meat meal	Lys	71	Cryst Lys	Carcass gain/feed	SR	N	20 kg	Batterham et al. (1986a)
Meat meal	Met	93	Cryst Met	Gain	SR	N	28 d	Leibholz and Kirby (1985)
Meat and bone meal	Lys	38–97	Cryst Lys	Carcass gain/feed	SR	N	20 kg	Batterham et al. (1986b)
Meat and bone meal	Lys	50	Cryst Lys	Carcass gain	SR	N	20 kg	Batterham et al. (1979)
Meat and bone meal	Lys	42	Cryst Lys	Carcass gain/feed	SR	N	20 kg	Batterham et al. (1986c)
Meat and bone meal	Lys	70	Cryst Lys	Carcass gain/feed	SR	N	20 kg	Batterham et al. (1986a)
Meat and bone meal	Trp	82	Sim MBM	Gain	SR	SP	10 kg	Sato et al. (1987)
Milk	Lys	99	Cryst Lys	Gain	SR	N	21 d	Leibholz (1986)
Milk, dried skim	Lys	88	Cryst Lys	Carcass gain	SR	N	20 kg	Batterham et al. (1979)
Milk, dried skim	Met	104	Cryst Met	Gain	SR	N	28 d	Leibholz and Kirby (1985)
Peanut meal	Lys	57	Cryst Lys	Carcass gain/feed	SR	N	20 kg	Batterham et al. (1984)
Rapeseed meal	Lys	87	Cryst Lys	Carcass gain/feed	SR	N	20 kg	Batterham et al. (1981)
Sorghum	Lys	63	Casein	Gain	SC	SP	8 kg	Copelin et al. (1978)
Sorghum	Thr	89	Casein	Gain	SC	SP	8 kg	Copelin et al. (1978)
Sorghum	Trp	93	Casein	Gain	SC	SP	13 kg	Copelin et al. (1978)
Sorghum	Trp	86	Sim sorgh	Gain	SR	SP	10 kg	Sato et al. (1987)
Sorghum	Trp	85	Cryst Trp	Gain/feed	SC	SP	5 kg	Rivera et al. (1976)
Soybean meal	Lys	80	Cryst Lys	Carcass gain/feed	SR	N	20 kg	Batterham et al. (1986c)
Soybean meal	Lys	94	Cryst Lys	Carcass gain/feed	SR	N	20 kg	Batterham et al. (1984)
Soybean meal	Lys	87	Cryst Lys	Carcass gain	SR	N	20 kg	Batterham et al. (1979)
Soybean meal	Lys	97	Cryst Lys	Gain	SR	N	21 d	Leibholz (1986)
Soybean meal	Met	102	Cryst Met	Gain	SR	N	28 d	Leibholz and Kirby (1985)

Table III. (continued)

Source	Amino acid	RV	Standard	Response criterion	Method of calc	Diet	Age /wt	Reference
Soybean meal	Trp	95	Sim SBM	Gain	SR	SP	10 kg	Sato et al. (1987)
Sunflower meal	Lys	60	Cryst Lys	Carcass gain/feed	SR	N	20 kg	Batterham et al. (1981)
Rats								
Blood meal	Lys	81	Cryst Lys	Carcass gain/feed	SR	N	25 d	Batterham et al. (1986a)
Cottonseed meal	Lys	35	Cryst Lys	Carcass gain/feed	SR	N	25 d	Batterham et al. (1984)
Cottonseed meal	Lys	58	Cryst Lys	Gain/feed	SR	N	25 d	Batterham et al. (1979)
Field peas	Lys	76	Cryst Lys	Carcass gain/feed	SR	N	25 d	Batterham et al. (1984)
Fish meal	Lys	104	Cryst Lys	Gain/feed	SR	N	25 d	Batterham et al. (1979)
Linseed meal	Lys	82	Cryst Lys	Carcass gain/feed	SR	N	25 d	Batterham et al. (1981)
Lupin seed meal	Lys	81	Cryst Lys	Carcass gain/feed	SR	N	25 d	Batterham et al. (1984)
Lupin seed meal	Lys	86	Cryst Lys	Carcass gain/feed	SR	N	25 d	Batterham et al. (1981)
Meat meal	Lys	63	Cryst Lys	Carcass gain/feed	SR	N	25 d	Batterham et al. (1986a)
Meat and bone meal	Lys	21–88	Cryst Lys	Carcass gain/feed	SR	N	25 d	Batterham et al. (1986b)
Meat and bone meal	Lys	64	Cryst Lys	Gain/feed	SR	N	25 d	Batterham et al. (1979)
Meat and bone meal	Lys	77	Cryst Lys	Carcass gain/feed	SR	N	25 d	Batterham et al. (1986a)
Milk, dried skim	Lys	94	Cryst Lys	Gain/feed	SR	N	25 d	Batterham et al. (1979)
Peanut meal	Lys	76	Cryst Lys	Carcass gain/feed	SR	N	25 d	Batterham et al. (1984)
Soybean meal	Lys	90	Cryst Lys	Carcass gain/feed	SR	N	25 d	Batterham et al. (1984)
Soybean meal	Lys	89	Cryst Lys	Gain/feed	SR	N	25 d	Batterham et al. (1979)
Sunflower meal	Lys	60	Cryst Lys	Carcass gain/feed	SR	N	25 d	Batterham et al. (1981)
Wheat	Lys	75	Cryst Lys	Carcass N gain	SC	N	44 g	Calhoun et al. (1960)

[a]Abbreviations can be found in Appendix I.

Table IV. Summary of bioavailabilities of amino acids for poultry based on growth assays

Feedstuff	Arg	Lys	Met	Thr	Trp
Blood meal	-	78	66	-	-
Canola meal	-	90	87	-	-
Corn	-	73	97	-	-
Meat meal	-	71	93	-	-
Soybean meal	-	90	94	100	92
Wheat	-	78	-	-	-
Arginine·HCl	83	-	-	-	-
Lysine·HCl	-	79	-	-	-
DL-Methionine	-	-	98	-	-
Methionine hydroxy analog–Ca	-	-	65	-	-
Methionine hydroxy analog–liquid	-	-	66	-	-
Threonine	-	-	-	100	-
Tryptophan	-	-	-	-	100

Table V. Summary of bioavailabilities of amino acids for swine based on growth assays

Feedstuff	Arg	Lys	Met	Thr	Trp
Blood meal	-	91	-	-	-
Canola meal	-	87	-	-	-
Corn	-	-	-	-	86
Dried skimmed milk	-	99	-	-	-
Meat meal	-	79	93	-	-
Sorghum grain	-	63	-	89	88
Soybean meal	-	90	100	-	95
Arginine·HCl	83	-	-	-	-
Lysine·HCl	-	79	-	-	-
DL-Methionine	-	-	100	-	-
Methionine hydroxy analog–liquid	-	-	100	-	-
Threonine	-	-	-	100	-
Tryptophan	-	-	-	-	100

V. REFERENCES

Baker, D. H. 1978. Nutrient bioavailability in feedstuffs: Methodology for determining amino acid and B-vitamin availability in cereal grains and soybean meal. In "Proceedings of the Georgia Nutrition Conference," p. 1. University of Georgia, Athens, GA.

Baker, D. H. 1984. Equalized versus ad libitum feeding. Nutr. Rev. 42:269.

Baker, D. H. and O. A. Izquierdo. 1985. Effect of meal frequency and spaced crystalline lysine ingestion on the utilization of dietary lysine by chickens. Nutr. Res. 5:1103.

Baker, D. H., K. R. Robbins and J. S. Buck. 1979. Modification of the level of histidine and sodium bicarbonate in the Illinois crystalline amino acid diet. Poult. Sci. 58:749.

Batterham, E. S. 1984. Utilization of free lysine by pigs. Pig News Info. 5:85.

Batterham, E. S., L. M. Anderson, D. R. Baigent, R. E. Darnell and M. R. Taverner. 1990. A comparison of the availability and ileal digestibility of lysine in cottonseed and soyabean meals for grower/finisher pigs. Br. J. Nutr. 64:663.

Batterham, E. S., L. M. Anderson, R. F. Lowe and R. E. Darnell. 1986c. Nutritional value of lupin (Lupinus albus)–seed meal for growing pigs: Availability of lysine, effect of autoclaving and net energy content. Br. J. Nutr. 56:645.

Batterham, E. S., R. E. Darnell, L. S. Herbert and E. J. Major. 1986b. Effect of pressure and temperature on the availability of lysine in meat and bone meal as determined by slope-ratio assays with growing pigs, rats and chicks and by chemical techniques. Br. J. Nutr. 55:441.

Batterham, E. S., R. F. Lowe, R. E. Darnell and E. J. Major. 1986a. Availability of lysine in meat meal, meat and bone meal and blood meal as determined by the slope-ratio assay with growing pigs, rats and chicks and by chemical techniques. Br. J. Nutr. 55:427.

Batterham, E. S., R. D. Murison and L. M. Anderson. 1984. Availability of lysine in vegetable protein concentrates as determined by the slope-ratio assay with growing pigs and rats and by chemical techniques. Br. J. Nutr. 51:85.

Batterham, E. S., R. D. Murison and C. E. Lewis. 1978. An evaluation of total lysine as a predictor of lysine status in protein concentrates for growing pigs. Br. J. Nutr. 40:23.

Batterham, E. S., R. D. Murison and C. E. Lewis. 1979. Availability of lysine in protein concentrates as determined by the slope-ratio assay with growing pigs and rats and by chemical techniques. Br. J. Nutr. 41:383.

Batterham, E. S., R. D. Murison and R. F. Lowe. 1981. Availability of lysine in vegetable protein concentrates as determined by the slope-ratio assay with growing pigs and rats and by chemical techniques. Br. J. Nutr. 45:401.

Borggreve, G. J. and W. A. G. Veen. 1984. Requirement of fattening pigs for gross and digestible lysine in feeds with easily digested protein. Neth. J. Agric. Sci. 32:23.

Buraczewska, L. 1981. Absorption of amino acids in different parts of the small intestine in growing pigs. I. Absorption of free amino acids and water. Acta Physiol. Pol. 32:419.

Buraczewska, L. and H. Horaczynski. 1983. Influence of dry matter intake on ileal nitrogen output and of protein intake on digestibility of amino acids in pigs. In "Protein Metabolism and Nutrition" (R. Pion, M. Arnal and D. Bonin, Eds.), Vol. II, p. 381. Paris, France: Les Colloques de l'INRA, 16, EAPP Publication 31.

Calhoun, W. K., F. N. Hepburn and W. B. Bradley. 1960. The availability of lysine in wheat, flour, bread and gluten. J. Nutr. 70:337.

Campbell, R. C. 1966. The chick assay of lysine. Biometrics 22:58.

Cannon, P. R., C. H. Steffee, L. J. Frazier, D. A. Rowley and R. C. Stepto. 1947. The influence of time of ingestion of essential amino acids upon utilization in tissue synthesis. *Fed. Proc.* 6:390. [Abstract]

Carlson, K. H. and H. S. Bayley. 1970. Nitrogen and amino acids in the feces of young pigs receiving a protein-free diet and diets containing graded levels of soybean oil meal or casein. *J. Nutr.* 100:1353.

Carpenter, K. J. 1960. The estimation of the available lysine in animal-protein foods. *Biochem. J.* 77:604.

Carpenter, K. J. 1973. Damage to lysine in food processing: Its measurement and its significance. *Nutr. Abstr. Rev.* 43:423.

Carpenter, K. J., G. M. Ellinger, M. I. Munro and E. J. Rolfe. 1957. Fish products as protein supplements to cereals. *Br. J. Nutr.* 11:162.

Carpenter, K. J., B. E. March, C. K. Milner and R. C. Campbell. 1963. A growth assay with chicks for the lysine content of protein concentrates. *Br. J. Nutr.* 17:309.

Carpenter, K. J., I. McDonald and W. S. Miller. 1972. Protein quality of feedingstuffs. 5. Collaborative studies on the biological assay of available methionine using chicks. *Br. J. Nutr.* 27:7.

Cave, N. A. and C. J. Williams. 1980. A chick assay for availability of lysine in wheat. *Poult. Sci.* 59:799.

Cho, C. Y. and H. S. Bayley. 1971. Amino acid composition of digesta taken from swine receiving diets containing rapeseed meals as sole source of protein. *Can. J. Physiol. Pharmacol.* 50:513.

Chung, T. K. and D. H. Baker. 1991. Apparent and true digestibility of amino acids in casein and in a complete amino acid mixture: Comparison of ileal digestibility in pigs with the cecectomized cockerel assay. *J. Anim. Sci.* 69(Suppl. 1):381. [Abstract]

Copelin, J. L., C. T. Gaskins and L. F. Tribble. 1978. Availability of tryptophan, lysine and threonine in sorghum for swine. *J. Anim. Sci.* 46:133.

Costa, P. M. A., A. H. Jensen, D. H. Baker and H. W. Norton. 1977. Lysine availability of roasted dried and high-moisture corns as determined by the chick growth assay. *J. Anim. Sci.* 46:457.

Craig, W. M. and G. A. Broderick. 1981. Effect of the treatment on true digestibility in the rat, *in vitro* proteolysis and available lysine content of cottonseed meal protein. *J. Anim. Sci.* 52:292.

Dammers, J. 1964. Verteringsstudies bij het varken. Factoren van invloed op de vertering der voedercomponenten en de verteerbaarheid der aminozuren. Ph.D. thesis, University of Leuven, Belgium.

Darcy, B., J. P. Laplace and P. H. Duee. 1982. Protein digestion in the small intestine of the pig. 1. Amino acid digestibility according to the dietary protein source of a maize starch based diet. *Ann. Zootech.* 31:279.

de Lange, C. F. M., W. C. Sauer and W. Souffrant. 1989. The effect of protein status of the pig on the recovery and amino acid composition of endogenous protein in digesta collected from the distal ileum. *J. Anim. Sci.* 67:755.

de Lange, C. F. M., W. B. Souffrant and W. C. Sauer. 1990. Real ileal protein and amino acid digestibilities in feedstuffs for growing pigs as determined with the ^{15}N-isotope dilution technique. *J. Anim. Sci.* 68:409.

de Muelenaere, H. J. H., M-L Chen and A. E. Harper. 1967. Assessment of factors influencing estimation of lysine availability in cereal products. *J. Agric. Food Chem.* 15:310.

den Hartog, L. A., M. W. A. Verstegen and J. Huisman. 1989. Amino acid digestibility in pigs as affected by diet composition. *In* "Absorption and Utilization of Amino Acids. Volume III" (M. Friedman, Ed.), p. 201. CRC Press, Boca Raton, FL.

Denton, A. E. and C. A. Elvehjem. 1954. Availability of amino acids *in vivo*. *J. Biol. Chem.* 206:449.

Finney, D. J. 1978. "Statistical Method in Biological Assay," 3rd ed. Hafner, New York.

Ford, J. E. 1960. A microbiological method for assessing the nutritional value of proteins. *Br. J. Nutr.* 14:485.

Geiger, E. 1947. Experiments with delayed supplementation of incomplete amino acid mixtures. *J. Nutr.* 34:97.

Goh, Y. K., D. R. Clandinin and A. R. Robblee. 1979a. The application of the dye-binding method for measuring protein denaturation of rapeseed meals caused by autoclave or oven heat treatments for varying periods of time. *Can. J. Anim. Sci.* 59:189.

Goh, Y. K., D. R. Clandinin and A. R. Robblee. 1979b. Application of the dye-binding technique for quantitative and qualitative estimation of rapeseed meal protein. *Can. J. Anim. Sci.* 59:181.

Gruhn, K. and B. Raue. 1974. Ausscheidungen der Amino Sauren mid dem Harn und Kot von kolostomierten und nicht operierten Hennen-Beitrag zur Methode de Amino sauren resorbierbarkeit. 1. Mitteilung Abhangigkeit der Exkretion der Harnaminosauren von Aminosaurebverzehr. *Arch. Tierernahr.* 24:67.

Guo, L. S., J. D. Summers and E. T. Moran, Jr. 1971. Assaying feedstuffs for available lysine content using a feather meal basal diet. *Can. J. Anim. Sci.* 51:161.

Gupta, J. D., A. M. Dakroury, A. E. Harper and C. A. Elvehjem. 1958. Biological availability of lysine. *J. Nutr.* 64:259.

Han Y., F. Castanon, C. M. Parsons and D. H. Baker. 1990. Absorption and bioavailability of DL-methionine hydroxy analog compared to DL-methionine. *Poult. Sci.* 69:281.

Harper, A. E., N. J. Benevenga and R. M. Wohlueter. 1970. Effects of ingestion of disproportionate amounts of amino acids. *Physiol. Rev.* 50:428.

Hill, D. C., J. Singh and G. C. Ashton. 1966. A chick bioassay for lysine. *Poult. Sci.* 45:554.

Hirakawa, D. A. and D. H. Baker. 1986. Assessment of lysine bioavailability in an intact protein mixture: Comparison of chick growth and precision-fed rooster assays. *Nutr. Res.* 6:815.

Huisman, J., E. J. Van Weerden, G. Hof, K. K. Van Hellemond and P. Van Leeuwen. 1985. The effect of insertion of re-entrant cannulae on digestive processes. *In* "Proceedings of the 3rd International Seminar on Digestive Physiology in the Pig" (A. Just, H. Jorgensen and J. A. Fernandez. Eds.), p. 341. Copenhagen, Denmark.

Hurrell, R. F. and K. J. Carpenter. 1975. The use of three dye-binding procedures for the assessment of heat damage to food proteins. *Br. J. Nutr.* 33:101.

Izquierdo, O. A., C. M. Parsons and D. H. Baker. 1988. Bioavailability of lysine in L-lysine·HCl. *J. Anim. Sci.* 66:2590.

Kakade, M. L. and I. E. Liener. 1969. Determination of available lysine in proteins. *Anal. Biochem.* 27:273.

Kratzer, F. H. and N. Green. 1957. The availability of lysine in blood meal for chicks and popults. *Poult. Sci.* 36:562.

Krawielitzki, K., T. Volker, S. Smulikowska, H. D. Bock and J. Wunsche. 1977. Weitere Untersuchungen zum Multikompartment-Modell des Protienstoffwechsels. *Arch. Tierernahr.* 27:609.

Leibholz, J. 1986. The utilization of lysine by young pigs from nine protein concentrates compared with free lysine in young pigs fed *ad lib. Br. J. Nutr.* 55:179.

Leibholz, J. and A. C. Kirby. 1985. The utilization of methionine from five protein concentrates compared with synthetic methionine. *Br. J. Nutr.* 53:391.

Leibholz, J., R. J. Love, Y. Mollah and R. R. Carter. 1986. The absorption of dietary L-lysine and extruded L-lysine in pigs. *Anim. Feed Sci. Technol.* 15:141.

Lewis, A. J., E. R. Peo, Jr., P. J. Cunningham and B. D. Moser. 1977. Determination of the optimum dietary proportions of lysine and tryptophan for growing rats based on growth, food intake and plasma metabolites. *J. Nutr.* **107**:1361.

Lewis, A. J. and V. C. Speer. 1975. A multiple parameter approach to the estimation of amino acid requirements of lactating sows. *In* "Protein Nutritional Quality of Foods and Feeds" (M. Friedman, Ed.), Part 1, p. 51. Dekker, New York.

Likuski, H. J. A. and H. G. Dorrell. 1978. A bioassay for rapid determinations of amino acid availabilities. *Poult. Sci.* **57**:1658.

Low, A. G. 1979. Studies on digestion and absorption in the intestines of growing pigs. 6. Measurements of the flow of amino acids. *Br. J. Nutr.* **41**:147.

Low, A. G. 1982. Digestibility and availability of amino acids from feedstuffs for pigs: A review. *Livest. Prod. Sci.* **9**:511.

Major, E. J. and E. S. Batterham. 1981. Availability of lysine in protein concentrates as determined by the slope-ratio assay with chicks and comparisons with rat, pig and chemical assays. *Br. J. Nutr.* **46**:513.

McNab, J. M. 1979. Growth tests for the determination of available amino acids. *In* "Proceedings of the 2nd European Symposium on Poultry Nutrition" (C. A. Kan and P. C. M. Simons, Eds.), p. 102. Beekbergen, The Netherlands.

Meade, R. J. 1972. Biological availability of amino acids. *J. Anim. Sci.* **35**:713.

Miller, E. L., K. J. Carpenter and C. B. Morgan. 1965. Availability of sulphur amino acids in protein foods. 2. Assessment of available methionine by chick and microbiological assays. *Br. J. Nutr.* **19**:249.

Morrison, A. B. and J. M. McLaughlan. 1972. Availability of amino acids in foods. *In* "Protein and Amino Acid Functions" (E. J. Bigwood, Ed.), p. 389. Pergamon Press, New York.

National Research Council. 1988. "Nutrient Requirements of Swine," 9th ed. National Academy Press, Washington DC.

Nelson, T. S., L. K. Kirby and J. T. Halley. 1986. Digestibility of crystalline amino acids and the amino acids in corn and poultry blend. *Nutr. Rep. Int.* **34**:903.

Netke, S. P. and H. M. Scott. 1970. Estimates on the availability of amino acids in soybean oil meal as determined by chick growth assay: Methodology as applied to lysine. *J. Nutr.* **100**:281.

Netke, S. P., H. M. Scott and G. L. Allee. 1969. Effect of excess amino acids on the utilization of the first limiting amino acid in chick diets. *J. Nutr.* **99**:75.

Njike, M. C., A. U. Mba and V. A. Oyenuga. 1975. Chick bioassay of available methionine and methionine plus cystine. Development of assay procedure. *J. Sci. Food Agric.* **26**:175.

Nordheim, J. P. and C. N. Coon. 1984. A comparison of four methods for determining available lysine in animal protein meals. *Poult. Sci.* **63**:1040.

Oh, S., J. D. Summers and A. S. Wood. 1972. Availability of methionine in various protein supplements as determined by chick bioassay. *Can. J. Anim. Sci.* **52**:171.

Ousterhout, L. E., C. R. Grau and B. D. Lundholm. 1959. Biological availability of amino acids in fish meals and other protein sources. *J. Nutr.* **69**:65.

Papadopoulos, M. C. 1985. Estimations of amino acid digestibility and availability in feedstuffs for poultry. *World's Poult. Sci. J.* **41**:64.

Parsons, C. M. 1985. Amino acid availability in feedstuffs for poultry and swine. *In* "Recent Advances in Amino Acid Nutrition" (D. H. Baker and C. M. Parsons, Eds.), p. 35. Ajinomoto, Tokyo, Japan.

Parsons, C. M. 1986. Determination of digestible and available amino acids in meat meal using conventional and caecetomized cockerels or chick growth assays. *Br. J. Nutr.* **56**:227.

Parsons, C. M. 1990. Digestibility of amino acids in feedstuffs for poultry. *In* "Proceedings of the Maryland Nutrition Conference," p. 22. University of Maryland, Baltimore, MD.

Parsons, C. M. 1991. Amino acid digestibilities for poultry: Feedstuff evaluation and requirements. *In* "BioKyowa Technical Review—1." Nutri-Quest, Inc., Chesterfield, MO.

Parsons, M. J., P. K. Ku and E. R. Miller. 1985. Lysine availability in flash-dried blood meals for swine. *J. Anim. Sci.* **60**:1447.

Partridge, I. G., A. G. Low and H. D. Keal. 1985. A note on the effect of feeding frequency on nitrogen use in growing boars given diets with varying levels of free lysine. *Anim. Prod.* **40**:375.

Perry, T. L. and S. Hansen. 1969. Technical pitfalls leading to errors in the quantitation of plasma amino acids. *Clin. Chim. Acta* **25**:53.

Radke, T. R., A. J. Lewis, E. R. Peo, Jr., J. D. Hancock and W. W. Stroup. 1988. Determination of the bioavailability of threonine in soybean meal using rats and broiler chicks. *J. Anim. Sci.* **66**(Suppl. 1):94. [Abstract]

Rerat, A. 1978. Digestion and absorption of carbohydrates and nitrogenous matters in the hindgut of the omnivorous nonruminant animal. *J. Anim. Sci.* **46**:1808.

Richardson, L. R., L. G. Blaylock and C. M. Lyman. 1953. Influence of dietary amino acid supplements on the free amino acids in the blood plasma of chicks. *J. Nutr.* **51**:515.

Rivera L., P. H., E. R. Peo, Jr., T. Stahly, B. D. Moser and P. J. Cunningham. 1976. Availability of tryptophan in some feedstuffs for swine. *J. Anim. Sci.* **43**:432.

Roach, A. G., P. Sanderson and D. Williams. 1967. Comparison of methods for the determination of available lysine value in animal and vegetable protein sources. *J. Sci. Food Agric.* **18**:274.

Robel, E. J. and L. T. Frobish. 1977. Evaluation of the chick bio-assay for estimating sulfur amino acid, lysine, and tryptophan availability in soybean meal. *Poult. Sci.* **56**:1399.

Sasse, C. E. and D. H. Baker. 1973. Modification of the Illinois reference standard amino acid mixture. *Poult. Sci.* **52**:1970.

Sato, H., T. Kobayashi, R. W. Jones and R. A. Easter. 1987. Tryptophan availability of some feedstuffs determined by pig growth assay. *J. Anim. Sci.* **64**:191.

Sauer, W., M. Dugan, K. de Lange, M. Imbeah and R. Mosenthim. 1989. Considerations in methodology for the determination of amino acid digestibilities in feedstuffs for pigs. *In* "Absorption and Utilization of Amino Acids. Vol. III" (M. Friedman, Ed.), p. 217. CRC Press, Boca Raton, FL.

Sauer, W. C. and L. Ozimek. 1986. Digestibility of amino acids in swine: results and their practical applications. A review. *Livest. Prod. Sci.* **15**:367.

Schneider, B. H. and W. P. Flatt. 1975. "The Evaluation of Feeds through Digestibility Experiments." University of Georgia Press, Athens, GA.

Shannon, D. W. F. and J. M. McNab. 1973. The digestibility of the nitrogen, amino acids, lipid, carbohydrates, ribonudeic acid and phosphorus of an n-paraffin grown yeast when given to colostomised laying hens. *J. Sci. Food Agric.* **24**:27.

Sibbald, I. R. 1987. Estimation of bioavailable amino acids in feedingstuffs for poultry and pigs: A review with emphasis on balance experiments. *Can. J. Anim. Sci.* **67**:221.

Sibbald, I. R. and M. S. Wolynetz. 1985. The bioavailability of supplementary lysine and its effect on the energy and nitrogen excretion of adult cockerels fed diets diluted with cellulose. *Poult. Sci.* **64**:1972.

Siriwan, P., W. L. Bryden and E. F. Annison. 1989. Effects of dietary fiber and protein levels on endogenous protein secretions in chickens. *Proc. Nutr. Soc. Aust.* **14**:143.

Smith, R. E. 1968. Assessment of the availability of amino acids in fish meal, soybean meal and feather meal by chick growth assay. *Poult. Sci.* **47**:1624.

Smith, R. E. and H. M. Scott. 1965a Measurement of the amino acid content of fish meal proteins by chick growth assay. 1. Estimation of amino acid availability in fish meal proteins before and after heat treatment. *Poult. Sci.* **44**:401.

Smith, R. E. and H. M. Scott. 1965b. Measurement of the amino acid content of fish meal proteins by chick growth assay. 2. The effects of amino acid imbalances upon estimations of amino acid availability by chick growth assay. *Poult. Sci.* **44**:408.

Souffrant, W. B., B. Darcy-Vrillon, T. Corring, J. P. Leplace, R. Kohler, G. Gebhardt and A. Rerat. 1986. Recycling of endogenous nitrogen in the pig. *Arch. Tierernahr.* **36**:269.

Southern, L. L. 1991. Digestible amino acids and digestible amino acid requirements for swine. *In* "BioKyowa Technical Review—2." Nutri-Quest, Inc. Chesterfield, MO.

Stott, J. A. and H. Smith. 1966. Microbiological assay of protein quality with Tetrahymena pyriformis W. 4. Measurement of available lysine, methionine, arginine and histidine. *Br. J. Nutr.* **20**:663.

Summers, D. J. and A. R. Robblee. 1985. Comparison of apparent amino acid digestibilities in anaesthetized versus sacrificed chickens using diets containing soybean meal and canola meal. *Poult. Sci.* **64**:536.

Tanksley T. D. and D. A. Knabe. 1984. Ileal digestibilities of amino acids in pig feeds and their use in formulating diets. *In* "Recent Advances in Animal Nutrition – 1984" (D. J. A. Cole and W. Haresign, Ed.), p. 75. Butterworths, London.

Taverner, M. R. and D. J. Farrell. 1981. Availability to pigs of amino acids in cereal grains. 3. A comparison of ileal availability values with faecal, chemical and enzymic estimates. *Br. J. Nutr.* **46**:173.

Taverner, M. R., I. D. Hume and D. J. Farrell. 1981. Availability to pigs of amino acids in cereal grains. 2. Apparent and true ileal availability. *Br. J. Nutr.* **46**:159.

Tsien, W. S., E. L. Johnson and I. E. Liener. 1957. The availability of lysine from Torula yeast. *Arch. Biochem. Biophys.* **71**:414.

Uhlemann, H. and S. Poppe. 1970. Zur Verdaulichkeit des Proteins und der Resorbierbarkeit van Lysin, Methionin un Zystin aus verschiedenen Proteintragern bei wachsenden Albinoratten. *Arch. Tierernahr.* **20**:165.

Uwaegbute, H. O. and D. Lewis. 1966a. Chick bioassay of lysine. I. Development of assay procedure. *Br. Poult. Sci.* **7**:249.

Uwaegbute, H. O. and D. Lewis. 1966b. Chick bioassay of lysine. II. Assay of fishmeals, meat meals, soyabean meals and groundnut meals. *Br. Poult. Sci.* **7**:261.

Yang, S. P., J. E. Steinhauer and J. E. Masterson. 1963. Utilization of a delayed lysine supplement by young rats. *J. Nutr.* **79**:257.

Yang, S. P., K. S. Tilton and L. L. Ryland. 1968. Utilization of a delayed lysine or tryptophan supplement for protein repletion of rats. *J. Nutr.* **94**:178.

Zebrowska, T. 1982. Nitrogen digestion in the large intestine. *In* "Physiologie digestive chez le porc." INRA, Paris.

Zimmerman, R. A. and H. M. Scott. 1965. Interrelationship of plasma amino acid levels and weight gain as influenced by suboptimal and superoptimal dietary concentrations of single amino acids. *J. Nutr.* **87**:13.

3

BIOAVAILABILITY OF D-AMINO ACIDS
AND DL-HYDROXY-METHIONINE

Austin J. Lewis

Department of Animal Science
University of Nebraska
Lincoln, Nebraska

David H. Baker

Department of Animal Sciences
University of Illinois
Urbana, Illinois

I. BIOAVAILABILITY OF D-AMINO ACIDS

The tissues of animals do not normally contain D-amino acids, and before an animal can utilize an ingested D-amino acid it must convert the amino acid to the L form. This conversion, known as inversion, consists of two steps: (1) oxidative deamination to the α-keto analog and (2) transamination of an amino group from glutamate.

Amino acids differ greatly in the extent to which they can be inverted by animals and consequently in the degree to which the D forms are bioavailable. Some amino acids (e.g., methionine) are readily inverted and may be completely bioavailable, others (e.g., lysine) do not undergo inversion and therefore cannot be utilized by animals. In general, with the exception of tryptophan, avian species invert D-amino acids more efficiently than do mammalian species (Baker, 1986).

The experiments that form the basis for the following summary are identified in Table I. Bioavailabilities relative to the L-isomer are listed in the table. Previous reviews of the bioavailabilities of amino acid isomers and analogs include those of Berg (1953, 1959), Meister (1965), Sunde (1972), Baker (1986), and Baker (1994).

A. Arginine

Although an early experiment suggested some utilization of D-arginine by rats, later research with both rats and chicks has indicated that this amino acid is not utilized by either species.

BIOAVAILABILITY OF NUTRIENTS FOR ANIMALS:
AMINO ACIDS, MINERALS, AND VITAMINS

67

B. Cystine

D-Cystine is not utilized by any species in which it has been tested (rats, chicks, and dogs).

C. Histidine

D-Histidine is relatively poorly utilized in mice, rats, and chicks. Early experiments indicated moderate utilization by mice and rats, but this has not been confirmed in recent, more extensive studies. It is possible the D-histidine used in some of the early experiments was contaminated with the L-isomer.

D. Isoleucine

Of the four isomers of isoleucine (L- and D-isoleucine and L- and D-alloisoleucine), only L-isoleucine and D-alloisoleucine are utilized. Recent experiments with chicks suggest that D-alloisoleucine has a 60% bioefficacy relative to L-isoleucine. DL-Isoleucine as sold commercially generally contains 25% of each of the four isomers. Thus, DL-isoleucine would be expected to have a bioefficacy value of 40%.

E. Leucine

Mammals are able to use some D-leucine but the bioavailability is less than 50% and may be zero in some species (e.g., humans). In contrast, the bioavailability of D-leucine is high in chicks, with most experiments indicating that it is almost as bioavailable as the L form.

F. Lysine

Lysine is not metabolized at a significant rate by D-amino acid oxidase, and furthermore lysine does not undergo transamination. Consequently, D-lysine cannot substitute for the natural isomer. Experiments have confirmed that D-lysine is not utilized by mice, rats, chicks, poults, or humans.

G. Methionine

There have been more investigations of the bioavailability of D-methionine than other D-amino acids, undoubtedly because of the importance of methionine in practical diets and the commercial production of DL-methionine. D-Methionine is well utilized in all animals except primates. Bioavailability is usually equal to the L-isomer when relatively small amounts of D-methionine are fed in practical diets.

In purified diets, particularly those containing other D-amino acids, the utilization of D-methionine is lower than that of L-methionine. In primates (humans and monkeys) D-methionine is less well utilized.

H. Phenylalanine

D-Phenylalanine is readily inverted, and the bioavailability of D-phenylalanine is high in most species. Estimates vary, but in general the bioavailability of D-phenylalanine approaches that of the L form in mice, rats, chicks, and humans. The one determination with poults indicated a lower bioavailability.

I. Threonine

Threonine, like lysine, is metabolized only slowly by D-amino acid oxidase and does not undergo transamination. Consequently, of the four isomers of threonine, only the naturally occurring L-threonine is utilized.

J. Tryptophan

There is a large difference among animal species in their ability to use D-tryptophan. In rats and pigs the bioavailability of the D-isomer is high and has been reported as almost equal to the L-isomer. In other species, such as chicks, rabbits, and dogs, the bioavailability of D-tryptophan seems to be much lower, and in humans the bioavailability is considered to be zero.

K. Tyrosine

The limited data that are available indicate that D-tyrosine has a high bioavailability in rats but is of no nutritional value in humans.

L. Valine

D-Valine is of little biological value to mammals, and initial experiments with chicks indicated that the same thing was true in poultry. More recent experiments with chicks, however, have indicated that the bioavailability of D-valine is higher than was originally thought and may be as high as 70% relative to the L-isomer.

II. BIOAVAILABILITY OF DL-HYDROXY-METHIONINE

Most research on 2-hydroxy-4-methylthiobutyric acid often referred to as methionine hydroxy analog (OH-M), has involved poultry, for which this methionine analog is an important commercial product. It is sold as either free OH-M, a liquid, or OH-M (Ca), a solid consisting of 2 mol of OH-M bound to calcium by the two carboxyl carbons. As marketed, liquid OH-M contains 88% OH-M; OH-M (Ca) contains 86% OH-M. Liquid OH-M contains monomers, dimers, trimers, and a small amount of OH-M oligomers (Boebel and Baker, 1982a). In all cases, OH-M products are 50% L-OH-M and 50% D-OH-M.

Considerable controversy has surrounded the biological availability of DL-OH-M relative to DL-methionine. The primary questions are: on a weight or concentration basis, does DL-OH-M free acid contain 88% DL-methionine activity, and does DL-OH-M (Ca) contain 86% DL-methionine activity? A "yes" answer to these questions would suggest that on a molar basis (or isosulfurous basis), these OH-M products are 100% efficacious relative to DL-methionine. Research has yielded various efficacy values for DL-OH-M (Ca) and for liquid DL-OH-M, relative to DL-methionine (Bird, 1952; Gordon and Sizer, 1955; Sullivan and Bird, 1957; Machlin and Gordon, 1959; Marrett and Sunde, 1965; Tipton et al., 1965, 1966; Scott et al., 1966; Smith, 1966; Creger et al., 1968; Featherston and Horn, 1974; Katz and Baker, 1975a; Romoser et al., 1976; Harter and Baker, 1977; Bishop and Halloran, 1977; Baker and Boebel, 1980; Christensen and Anderson, 1980; Christensen et al., 1980; Waldroup et al., 1981; Boebel and Baker, 1982a; Reid et al., 1982; van Weerden et al., 1982; Harms and Miles, 1983; van Weerden et al., 1983; Elkin and Hester, 1983; Muramatsu et al., 1984; Noll et al., 1984; Garlich, 1985; Harms and Buresh, 1987; Summers et al., 1987; Thomas et al., 1991; Huyghebaert, 1993).

In reviews by Potter (1984) and Potter et al. (1984) molar biopotency values of DL-OH-M free acid (relative to DL-methionine) for poultry were 76, 75, and 74% based on a summary of literature values using crystalline amino acid, semipurified, and practical-type diets, respectively. Assuming an average molar efficacy value of 75%, the bioequivalency value of DL-OH-M free acid calculates to be 66% (75 × 88%) on a weight basis.

In both rats (Boebel and Baker, 1983) and mice (Friedman and Gumbmann, 1988), DL-OH-M has been estimated as having a lower bioavailability than an isosulfurous level of DL-methionine. Recent research (Chung and Baker, 1991) has indicated that young pigs utilize DL-OH-M with the same free molar efficiency as L-methionine.

Table I. Relative bioavailability of D-amino acids[a]

Amino acid	Bioavailability	Reference
D-Arginine		
Rat	50[b]	Winitz et al. (1957)
Rat	0	Baker and Boebel (1981)
Chick	0	Sugahara et al. (1967)
Chick	0	Baker and Boebel (1981)
D-Cystine		
Rat	0	du Vigneaud et al. (1932a)
Rat	0	Loring et al. (1933)
Chick	0	Baker and Harter (1978)
Dog	0	Stekol (1934a,b)
D-Histidine		
Mouse	46[b]	Totter and Berg (1939)
Mouse	0	Celander and Berg (1953a)
Mouse	9	Friedman and Gumbmann (1982)
Rat	64[b]	Cox and Berg (1934)
Rat	83[b]	Celander and Berg (1953b)
Rat	22[b]	Kamath and Berg (1964a,b)
Rat	0	Baker and Boebel (1981)
Adult rat	100	Nasset and Gatewood (1954)
Chick	0	Fell et al. (1959)
Chick	9[b]	Sugahara et al. (1967)
Chick	19	Baker and Boebel (1981)
D-Isoleucine (2R, 3R)		
Mouse	0	Bauer and Berg (1943)
Mouse	1	Friedman and Gumbmann (1982)
Rat	0	Rose (1938)
Rat	0	Albanese (1945a)
Rat	0	Greenstein et al. (1951)
Rat	16[c]	Boebel and Baker (1982b)
Chick	0	Grau and Peterson (1946)
Chick	25[b]	Sugahara et al. (1967)
Chick	0	Funk and Baker (1989)
Adult rooster	0[c]	Leveille and Fisher (1960)
Human	0	Rose (1949)
Human	0	Rose et al. (1955c)
D-Alloisoleucine (2R, 3S)		
Chick	70[c]	Boebel and Baker (1982b)
Chick	60	Funk and Baker (1989)
D-Leucine		
Mouse	0	Bauer and Berg (1943)

Table I. (continued)

Amino acid	Bioavailability	Reference
Mouse	12	Friedman and Gumbmann (1982)
Rat	0	Rose (1938)
Rat	16[b,c]	Rechcigl et al. (1958)
Rat	48	Boebel and Baker (1982b)
Adult rat	83[b]	Anderson and Nasset (1950)
Chick	100	Grau and Peterson (1946)
Chick	84[b]	Sugahara et al. (1967)
Chick	100	Robbins and Baker (1977)
Human	0	Rose et al. (1955c)
D-Lysine		
Mouse	0	Totter and Berg (1939)
Mouse	-4	Friedman and Gumbmann (1982)
Rat	0[c]	McGinty et al. (1924–25)
Rat	0[c]	Berg and Dalton (1934)
Rat	0	Berg (1936)
Rat	0	Rose (1938)
Chick	0[c]	Fell et al. (1959)
Chick	0	Sugahara et al. (1967)
Poult	0	Kratzer (1950)
Human	0	Rose et al. (1955a)
D-Methionine		
Mouse	100	Bauer and Berg (1943)
Mouse	76	Friedman and Gumbmann (1984)
Rat	100	Jackson and Block (1932–33, 1937–38)
Rat	100	Rose (1938)
Rat	84	Wretlind (1950)
Rat	100	Wretlind and Rose (1950)
Rat	100	Sauberlich (1961)
Rat	88	Funk et al. (1990)
Adult rat	100	Nasset and Anderson (1951)
Chick	100	Grau and Almquist (1943)
Chick	100	Fell et al. (1959)
Chick	82	Bruggemann et al. (1962)
Chick	100	Bauriedel (1963)
Chick	100[c]	Gutteridge and Lewis (1964)
Chick	100[c]	Smith (1966)
Chick	100	Tipton et al. (1966)
Chick	89[b]	Sugahara et al. (1967)
Chick	100	Marrett et al. (1964)
Chick	100	Marrett and Sunde (1965)

Table I. (continued)

Amino acid	Bioavailability	Reference
Chick	92[b]	Bhargava et al. (1970)
Chick	74[b]	Bhargava et al. (1971)
Chick	100[d]	Katz and Baker (1975b)
Chick	100[c]	Baker and Boebel (1980)
Rabbit	100[c]	Cho et al. (1980)
Dog	100	Stekol (1935)
Dog	100	Cho et al. (1980)
Miniature pig	100[c]	Cho et al. (1980)
Pig (very young)	50	Kim and Bayley (1983)
Pig	100[c]	Reifsnyder et al. (1984)
Monkey	< 73	Stegink et al. (1980)
Human	100	Rose (1949)
Human	100	Rose et al. (1955b)
Human	14[b]	Kies et al. (1975)
Human	45[b]	Zezulka and Calloway (1976)
D-Phenylalanine		
Mouse	100	Bauer and Berg (1943)
Mouse	20	Friedman and Gumbmann (1982)
Rat	100	Rose (1938)
Rat	100	Rose and Womack (1946)
Rat	100	Wretlind (1952)
Rat	52[b]	Armstrong (1953)
Rat	68	Boebel and Baker (1982c)
Chick	100	Grau (1947)
Chick	30[b,c]	Fisher et al. (1957)
Chick	100	Fell et al. (1959)
Chick	89[b]	Sugahara et al. (1967)
Chick	75	Boebel and Baker (1982c)
Poult	28	Snetsinger et al. (1964)
Human	< 100	Rose (1949)
Human	100[c]	Rose et al. (1955d)
D-Threonine (D-allothreonine; 2R, 3R)		
Mouse	0	Bauer and Berg (1943)
Mouse	3	Friedman and Gumbmann (1982)
Rat	0	West and Carter (1938)
Chick	0	Grau (1949)
Chick	0	Sugahara et al. (1967)
Adult rooster	0[c]	Leveille and Fisher (1960)
Human	0	Rose (1949)
Human	0	Rose et al. (1955b)

Table I. (continued)

Amino acid	Bioavailability	Reference
D-Tryptophan		
Mouse	31[b]	Totter and Berg (1939)
Mouse	0	Celender and Berg (1953a)
Mouse	27	Friedman and Gumbmann (1982)
Rat	100[c]	Berg and Potgieter (1931–32)
Rat	100	du Vigneaud et al. (1932b)
Rat	100	Berg (1934)
Rat	75	Oesterling and Rose (1952)
Rat	50	Sauberlich (1961)
Rat	100	Ohara et al. (1980)
Chick	0	Grau and Almquist (1944)
Chick	< 40[c]	Wilkening and Schweigert (1947)
Chick	50[c]	Anderson et al. (1950)
Chick	100[c]	West et al. (1952)
Chick	7[b]	Morrison et al. (1956)
Chick	15[b]	Sugahara et al. (1967)
Chick	21	Ohara et al. (1980)
Rabbit	0	Schayer (1950)
Rabbit	< 75[b]	Loh and Berg (1971)
Dog	> 30	Triebwasser et al. (1976)
Dog	36	Czarnecki and Baker (1982)
Pig	60	Baker et al. (1971)
Pig	70	Arentson and Zimmerman (1985)
Pig	100[c]	Kirchgessner and Roth (1985)
Pig	100[c]	Schutte et al. (1988)
Human	0[c]	Albanese et al. (1948)
Human	0	Baldwin and Berg (1949)
Human	0	Rose (1949)
Human	0[c]	Rose et al. (1954)
D-Tyrosine		
Rat	100	Bubl and Butts (1948)
Human	0	Albanese et al. (1946)
D-Valine		
Mouse	0	Bauer and Berg (1943)
Mouse	5	Friedman and Gumbmann (1982)
Rat	0	Rose (1938)
Rat	50	White et al. (1952)
Rat	8[b]	Womack et al. (1957)
Rat	< 33	Sauberlich (1961)
Rat	16	Boebel and Baker (1982b)

Table I. (continued)

Amino acid	Bioavailability	Reference
Chick	0	Grau and Peterson (1946)
Poult	25	Snetsinger et al. (1964)
Chick	43[b]	Sugahara et al. (1967)
Chick	72	Boebel and Baker (1982b)
Adult rooster	100[c]	Leveille and Fisher (1960)
Human	0	Rose (1949)
Human	0	Rose et al. (1955e)

[a]Values represent bioavailability (or bioefficacy) relative to the L-isomer.

[b]Values estimated from data given by the authors.

[c]Values were derived from experiments in which DL- (racemic) mixtures were compared with L-isomers.

[d]When fed at levels close to the requirement.

[e]100% in a semipurified (soy protein diet); estimated to be 80% in a purified (amino acid) diet.

REFERENCES

Albanese, A. A. 1945. Studies on human blood proteins. I. The isoleucine deficiency of hemoglobin. J. Biol. Chem. 157:613.

Albanese, A. A., V. I. Davis and M. Lein. 1948. The utilization of D-amino acids by man. VIII. Tryptophan and acetyltryptophan. J. Biol. Chem. 172:39.

Albanese, A. A., V. Irby and M. Lein. 1946. The utilization of d-amino acids by man. VI. Tyrosine. J. Biol. Chem. 166:513.

Anderson, J. O., G. F. Combs and G. M. Briggs. 1950. Niacin-replacing value of L- and DL-tryptophan in chick diets as influenced by carbohydrate source. J. Nutr. 42:463.

Anderson J. T. and E. S. Nasset. 1950. The utilization by the adult rat of amino acid mixtures low in leucine. J. Nutr. 40:625.

Arentson, B. E. and D. R. Zimmerman. 1985. Nutritive value of D-tryptophan for the growing pig. J. Anim. Sci. 60:474.

Armstrong, M. D. 1953. The utilization of L- and D-phenylalanine by the rat. J. Biol. Chem. 205:839.

Baker, D. H. 1986. Utilization of isomers and analogs of amino acids and other sulfur-containing compounds. Prog. Food Nutr. Sci. 10:133.

Baker, D. H. 1994. Utilization of precursors for L-amino acids. In "Amino Acids in Farm Animal Nutrition" (J. P. F. D'Mello, Ed.), Chap. 3, pp. 37–61. CAB International, Wallingford, U.K.

Baker, D. H., N. K. Allen, J. Boomgaardt, G. Graber and H. W. Norton. 1971. Quantitative aspects of D- and L-tryptophan utilization by the young pig. J. Anim. Sci. 33:42.

Baker, D. H. and K. P. Boebel. 1980. Utilization of the D- and L-isomers of methionine and methionine hydroxy analogue as determined by chick bioassay. *J. Nutr.* **110**:959.

Baker, D. H. and K. P. Boebel. 1981. Utilization of the D-isomers of arginine and histidine by chicks and rats. *J. Anim. Sci.* **53**:125.

Baker, D. H. and J. M. Harter. 1978. D-cystine utilization by the chick. *Poult. Sci.* **57**:562.

Baldwin, H. R. and C. P. Berg. 1949. The influence of optical isomerism and acetylation upon the availability of tryptophan for maintenance in man. *J. Nutr.* **39**:203.

Bauer, C. D. and C. P. Berg. 1943. The amino acids required for growth in mice and the availability of their optical isomers. *J. Nutr.* **26**:51.

Bauriedel, W. R. 1963. The effect of feeding D-methionine on the D-amino acid oxidase activity of chick tissues. *Poult. Sci.* **42**:214.

Berg, C. P. 1934. Tryptophane metabolism. IV. The influence of the optical activity on the utilization of tryptophane for growth and for kynurenic acid production. *J. Biol. Chem.* **104**:373.

Berg, C. P. 1936. The availability of d(-)-lysine for growing rats. *J. Nutr.* **12**:671.

Berg, C. P. 1953. Physiology of the amino acids. *Physiol. Rev.* **33**:145.

Berg, C. P. 1959. Utilization of the D-amino acids. *In* "Protein and Amino Acid Nutrition" (A. A. Albanese, Ed.), Chap 4, pp. 57–66. Academic Press, New York.

Berg, C. P. and J. L. Dalton. 1934. Influence of optical activity on the utilization of lysine for growth. *Proc. Soc. Exp. Biol. Med.* **31**:709.

Berg, C. P. and M. Potgieter. 1931–32. Tryptophan metabolism. II. The growth-promoting ability of dl-tryptophan. *J. Biol. Chem.* **94**:661.

Bhargava, K. K., R. P. Hanson and M. L. Sunde. 1970. Effects of methionine and valine on antibody production in chicks infected with Newcastle disease virus. *J. Nutr.* **100**:241.

Bhargava, K. K., R. P. Hanson and M. L. Sunde. 1971. Effects of methionine and valine on antibody production in chicks infected with live or killed Newcastle disease virus. *Poult. Sci.* **50**:614.

Bird, F. H. 1952. A comparison of methionine and two of its analogues in the nutrition of the chick. *Poult. Sci.* **31**:1095.

Bishop, R. B. and H. R. Halloran. 1977. The effect of methionine or methionine hydroxy analogue supplementation on chick response to total sulfur amino acid intake. *Poult. Sci.* **56**:383.

Boebel, K. P. and D. H. Baker. 1982a. Efficacy of calcium salt and free acid forms of methionine hydroxy analog for chicks. *Poult. Sci.* **61**:1167.

Boebel, K. P. and D. H. Baker. 1982b. Comparative utilization of the α-keto and D- and L-α-hydroxy analogs of leucine, isoleucine and valine by chicks and rats. *J. Nutr.* **112**:1929.

Boebel, K. P. and D. H. Baker. 1982c. Comparative utilization of the isomers of phenylalanine and phenyllactic acid by chicks and rats. *J. Nutr.* **112**:367.

Boebel, K. P. and D. H. Baker. 1983. Utilization of the D- and L-isomers of methionine and 2-hydroxy-4-(methylthiobutyrate)Ca by rats. *Fed. Proc.* **42**:543. [Abstract]

Bruggemann, J., K. Drepper and H. Zucker. 1962. Quantitative determination of the utilization of D-, L- and DL-methionine and DL-2-hydroxy-4- methylthiobutyric acid-Ca by the chick. *Die Naturwissenschaften* **49**:334.

Bubl, E. C. and J. S. Butts. 1948. The utilization of D-tyrosine for growth in the rat. *J. Biol. Chem.* **174**:637.

Celander, D. R. and C. P. Berg. 1953a. The availability of D-histidine, related imidazoles, and D-tryptophan in the mouse. *J. Biol. Chem.* **202**:339.

Celander, D. R. and C. P. Berg. 1953b. The metabolism of urocanic acid, imadazoleacetic acid and D-histidine in the intact rat. *J. Biol. Chem.* **202**:351.

Cho, E. S., D. W. Anderson, L. J. Filer, Jr. and L. D. Stegink. 1980. D-methionine utilization in young miniature pigs, adult rabbits, and adult dogs. *J. Parenter. Enteral Nutr.* **4**:544.

Christensen, A. C. and J. O. Anderson. 1980. Factors affecting efficacy of methionine hydroxy analogue for chicks fed practical diets. *Poult. Sci.* **59**:2485.

Christensen, A. C., J. O. Anderson and D. C. Dobson. 1980. Factors affecting efficacy of methionine hydroxy analogue for chicks fed amino acid diets. *Poult. Sci.* **59**:2480.

Chung, T. K. and D. H. Baker. 1991. Sulfur amino acid nutrition of the young pig: Cystine replacement value and utilization of methionine isomers and analogs. *J. Anim. Sci.* **69** (Suppl. 1):113. [Abstract]

Cox, G. J. and C. P. Berg. 1934. The comparative availability of d and l- histidine for growth. *J. Biol. Chem.* **107**:497.

Creger, C. R., J. R. Couch and H. L. Ernst. 1968. Methionine hydroxy analogue and L-methionine in broiler diets. *Poult. Sci.* **47**:229.

Czarnecki, G. L. and D. H. Baker. 1982. Utilization of D- and L-tryptophan by the growing dog. *J. Anim. Sci.* **55**:1405.

du Vigneaud, V., R. Dorfmann and H. S. Loring. 1932a. A comparison of the growth-promoting properties of d- and l-cystine. *J. Biol. Chem.* **98**:577.

du Vigneaud, V., R. R. Sealock and C. Van Etten. 1932b. The availability of d-tryptophan and its acetyl derivative to the animal body. *J. Biol. Chem.* **98**:565.

Elkin, R. G. and P. Y. Hester. 1983. A comparison of methionine sources for broiler chickens fed corn-soybean meal diets under simulated commercial grow-out conditions. *Poult. Sci.* **62**:2030.

Featherston, W. R. and G. W. Horn. 1974. Studies on the utilization of the α-hydroxy acid of methionine by chicks fed crystalline amino acid diets. *Poult. Sci.* **53**:680.

Fell, R. V., W. S. Wilkinson and A. B. Watts. 1959. The utilization by the chick of D and L amino acids in liquid and dry diets. *Poult. Sci.* **38**:1203. [Abstract]

Fisher, H., D. Johnson, Jr. and G. A. Leveille. 1957. The phenylalanine and tyrosine requirement of the growing chick with special reference to the utilization of the D-isomer of phenylalanine. *J. Nutr.* **62**:349.

Friedman, M. and M. R. Gumbmann. 1982. Bioavailability of D-amino acids in mice. *Fed. Proc.* **41**:392. [Abstract]

Friedman, M. and M. R. Gumbmann. 1984. The utilization and safety of isomeric sulfur-containing amino acids in mice. *J. Nutr.* **114**:2301.

Friedman, M. and M. R. Gumbmann. 1988. Nutritional value and safety of methionine derivatives, isomeric dipeptides and hydroxy analogs in mice. *J. Nutr.* **118**:388.

Funk, M. A. and D. H. Baker. 1989. Utilization of isoleucine isomers and analogs by chicks. *Nutr. Res.* **9**:523.

Funk, M. A., A. E. Hortin and D. H. Baker. 1990. Utilization of D-methionine by rats. *Nutr. Res.* **10**:1029.

Garlich, J. D. 1985. Response of broilers to DL-methionine hydroxy analog free acid, DL-methionine, and L-methionine. *Poult. Sci.* **64**:1541.

Gordon, R. S. and I. W. Sizer. 1955. The biological equivalence of methionine hydroxy analogue. *Poult. Sci.* **34**:1198. [Abstract]

Grau, C. R. 1947. Interrelationships of phenylalanine and tyrosine in the chick. *J. Biol. Chem.* **170**:661.

Grau, C. R. 1949. The threonine requirement of the chick. *J. Nutr.* **37**:105.

Grau, C. R. and H. J. Almquist. 1943. The utilization of the sulfur amino acids by the chick. *J. Nutr.* **26**:631.

Grau, C. R. and H. J. Almquist. 1944. Requirement of tryptophane by the chick. *J. Nutr.* **28**:263.

Grau, C. R. and D. W. Peterson. 1946. The isoleucine, leucine and valine requirements of the chick. *J. Nutr.* **32**:181.

Greenstein, J. P., L. Levintow, C. G. Baker and J. White. 1951. Preparation of the four stereoisomers of isoleucine. *J. Biol. Chem.* **188**:647.

Gutteridge, D. G. A. and D. Lewis. 1964. Chick bioassay of methionine and cystine. II. Assay of soyabean meals, groundnut meals, meat meals, methionine isomers and methionine analogue. *Br. Poult. Sci.* **5**:193.

Harms, R. H. and R. E. Buresh. 1987. Influence of three levels of copper on the performance of turkey poults with diets containing two sources of methionine. *Poult. Sci.* **66**:721.

Harms, R. H. and R. D. Miles. 1983. A comparison of DL-methionine and Liquimeth® as a source of supplemental methionine for the turkey poult. *Poult. Sci.* **62**:1025.

Harter, J. M. and D. H. Baker. 1977. Sulfur amino acid activity of glutathione, DL-α-hydroxy-methionine, and α-keto-methionine in chicks. *Proc. Soc. Exp. Biol. Med.* **156**:201.

Huyghebaert, G. 1993. Comparison of DL-methionine and methionine hydroxy analogue-free acid in broilers by using multi-exponential regression models. *Br. Poult. Sci.* **34**:351.

Jackson, R. W. and R. J. Block. 1932–33. Metabolism of d and l-methionine. *Proc. Soc. Exp. Biol. Med.* **30**:587.

Jackson, R. W. and R. J. Block. 1937–38. Metabolism of cystine and methionine II. The availability of d- and l-methionine and their formyl derivatives in the promotion of growth. *J. Biol. Chem.* **122**:425.

Kamath, S. H. and C. P. Berg. 1964a. Antagonism of poorly invertable D-amino acids toward growth promotion by readily invertable D-amino acids. *J. Nutr.* **82**:237.

Kamath, S. H. and C. P. Berg. 1964b. Antagonism of the D-forms of the essential amino acids toward the promotion of growth by D-histidine. *J. Nutr.* **82**:243.

Katz, R. S. and D. H. Baker. 1975a. Factors associated with utilization of the calcium salt of methionine hydroxy analogue by the young chick. *Poult. Sci.* **54**:584.

Katz, R. S. and D. H. Baker. 1975b. Efficacy of D-, L- and DL-methionine for growth of chicks fed crystalline amino acid diets. *Poult. Sci.* **54**:1667.

Kies, C., H. Fox and S. Aprahamian. 1975. Comparative value of L- DL- and D-methionine supplementation of an oat-based diet for humans. *J. Nutr.* **105**:809.

Kim, K. I. and H. S. Bayley. 1983. Amino acid oxidation by young pigs receiving diets with varying levels of sulphur amino acids. *Br. J. Nutr.* **50**:383.

Kirchgessner, V. M. and F. X. Roth. 1985. Biologische wirksamkeit von DL-tryptophan bei mastschweinen. *Z. Tierphysiol. Tierernähr. Futtermittelkd.* **54**:135.

Kratzer, F. H. 1950. The activities of D and L lysine for turkey poults. *J. Nutr.* **41**:153.

Leveille, G. A. and H. Fisher. 1960. Amino acid requirement for maintenance in the adult rooster. III. The requirements for leucine, isoleucine, valine and threonine, with reference also to the utilization of the D- isomers of valine, threonine and isoleucine. *J. Nutr.* **70**:135.

Loh, H. H. and C. P. Berg. 1971. Production of D-kynurenine and other metabolites from D-tryptophan by the intact rabbit and rabbit tissue. *J. Nutr.* **101**:465.

Loring, H. S., R. Dorfmann and V. du Vigneaud. 1933. The availability of mesocystine for promotion of growth in connection with cystine-deficient diets. *J. Biol. Chem.* **103**:399.

Machlin, L. J. and R. S. Gordon. 1959. Equivalence of methionine hydroxy analog and methionine for chickens fed low-protein diets. *Poult. Sci.* **38**:650.

Marrett, L., H. R. Bird and M. L. Sunde. 1964. The effects of different isomers of methionine on the growth of chicks fed amino acid diets. *Poult. Sci.* **43**:1113.

Marrett, L. E. and M. L. Sunde. 1965. The effect of other D-amino acids on the utilization of the isomers of methionine and its hydroxy analogue. *Poult. Sci.* **44**:957.

McGinty, D. A., H. B. Lewis and C. S. Marvel. 1924–25. Amino acid synthesis in the animal organism. The availability of some caproic acid derivatives for the synthesis of lysine. *J. Biol. Chem.* **62**:75.

Meister, A. 1965. "Biochemistry of the Amino Acids," Vol. I, Chap. II. Academic Press, New York.

Morrison, W. D., T. S. Hamilton and H. M. Scott. 1956. Utilization of D-tryptophan by the chick. *J. Nutr.* **60**:47.

Muramatsu, T., H. Yokota, J. Okumura and I. Tasaki. 1984. Biological efficacy of liquid methionine and methionine hydroxy analogue-free acid in chicks. *Poult. Sci.* **63**:1453.

Nasset, E. S. and J. T. Anderson. 1951. Nitrogen balance index in the adult rat as affected by diets low in L- and DL-methionine. *J. Nutr.* **44**:237.

Nasset, E. S. and V. H. Gatewood. 1954. Nitrogen balance and hemoglobin of adult rats fed amino acid diets low in L- and D-histidine. *J. Nutr.* **53**:163.

Noll, S. L., P. E. Waibel, R. D. Cook and J. A. Witmer. 1984. Biopotency of methionine sources for young turkeys. *Poult. Sci.* **63**:2458.

Oesterling, M. J. and W. C. Rose. 1952. Tryptophan requirement for growth and utilization of its optical isomers. *J. Biol. Chem.* **196**:33.

Ohara, I., S. Otsuka, Y. Yugari and S. Ariyoshi. 1980. Comparison of the nutritive values of L-, DL- and D-tryptophan in the rat and chick. *J. Nutr.* **110**:634.

Potter, L. M. 1984. Limiting amino acids in poultry diets. *In* "Proceedings of the Degussa Technical Symposium," p. 4. Charlotte, North Carolina.

Potter, L. M., G. P. Schmidt, M. E. Blair, J. R. Shelton and B. A. Bliss. 1984. MHAC versus DL-methionine. *Anim. Nutr. Health* (March–April, 1984), p. 14.

Rechcigl, M., Jr., J. K. Loosli and H. H. Williams. 1958. The utilization of D-leucine for growth by the rat. *J. Biol. Chem.* **231**:829.

Reid, B. L., A. Madrid and P. M. Maiorino. 1982. Relative biopotency of three methionine sources for laying hens. *Poult. Sci.* **61**:726.

Reifsnyder, D. H., C. T. Young and E. E. Jones. 1984. The use of low protein liquid diets to determine the methionine requirement and the efficacy of methionine hydroxy analogue for the three-week-old pig. *J. Nutr.* **114**:1705.

Robbins, K. R. and D. H. Baker. 1977. Comparative utilization of L-leucine, D-leucine and DL-hydroxy-leucine by the chick. *Nutr. Rep. Int.* **16**:611.

Romoser, G. L., P. L. Wright and R. B. Grainger. 1976. An evaluation of the L-methionine activity of the hydroxy analogue of methionine. *Poult. Sci.* **55**:1099.

Rose, W. C. 1938. The nutritive significance of the amino acids. *Physiol. Rev.* 18:109.

Rose, W. C. 1949. Amino acid requirements of man. *Fed. Proc.* **8**:546.

Rose, W. C., A. Borman, M. J. Coon and G. F. Lambert. 1955a. The amino acid requirements of man. X. The lysine requirement. *J. Biol. Chem.* **214**:579.

Rose, W. C., M. J. Coon, H. B. Lockhart and G. F. Lambert. 1955b. The amino acid requirements of man XI. The threonine and methionine requirements. *J. Biol. Chem.* **215**:101.

Rose, W. C., C. H. Eades, Jr. and M. J. Coon. 1955c. The amino acid requirements of man. XII. The leucine and isoleucine requirements. *J. Biol. Chem.* **216**:225.

Rose, W. C., G. F. Lambert and M. J. Coon. 1954. The amino acid requirements of man. VII. General procedures; The tryptophan requirement. *J. Biol. Chem.* **211**:815.

Rose, W. C., B. E. Leach, M. J. Coon and G. F. Lambert. 1955d. The amino acid requirements of man. IX. The phenylalanine requirement. *J. Biol. Chem.* **213**:913.

Rose, W. C., R. L. Wixom, H. B. Lockhart and G. F. Lambert. 1955e. The amino acid requirements of man. XV. The valine requirement; summary and final observations. *J. Biol. Chem.* **217**:987.

Rose, W. C. and M. Womack. 1946. The utilization of the optical isomers of phenylalanine, and the phenylalanine requirement for growth. *J. Biol. Chem.* **166**:103.

Sauberlich, H. E. 1961. Effect of vitamin B_6 on the growth of rats fed diets limiting in an essential amino acid and on the utilization of the isomers of tryptophan, methionine and valine. *J. Nutr.* **74**:289.

Schayer, R. W. 1950. Studies of the metabolism of tryptophan labeled with ^{15}N in the indole ring. *J. Biol. Chem.* **187**:777.

Schutte, J. B., E. J. Van Weerden and F. Koch. 1988. Utilization of DL- and L-tryptophan in young pigs. *Anim. Prod.* **46**:447.

Scott, H. M., M. Kelly and R. L. Huston. 1966. L-methionine *versus* methionine hydroxy analogue in basal diets containing either isolated soybean protein or crystalline amino acids. *Poult. Sci.* **45**:1123.

Smith, R. E. 1966. The utilization of L-methionine, DL-methionine and methionine hydroxy analogue by the growing chick. *Poult. Sci.* **45**:571.

Snetsinger, D. C., D. G. Britzman, R. C. Fitzsimmons and P. E. Waibel. 1964. The L-phenylalanine and L-valine requirement of the turkey poult and the utilization of their D-isomers. *Poult. Sci.* **43**:675.

Steginck, L. D., J. Moss, K. J. Printen and E. S. Cho. 1980. D-methionine utilization in adult monkeys fed diets containing DL-methionine. *J. Nutr.* **110**:1240.

Stekol, J. 1934a. Metabolism of l-cystine and dl-cystine in adult dogs maintained on a protein-free diet. *J. Biol. Chem.* **107**:225.

Stekol, J. 1934b. Metabolism of l-cystine and dl-cystine in growing dogs maintained on diets of various protein contents. *J. Biol. Chem.* **107**:641.

Stekol, J. A. 1935. Metabolism of L- and DL-methionine in adult and growing dogs maintained on diets of various protein contents. *J. Biol. Chem.* **109**:147.

Sugahara, M., T. Morimoto, T. Kobayashi and S. Ariyoshi. 1967. The nutritional value of D-Amino acid in the chick nutrition. *Agric. Biol. Chem.* **31**:77.

Sullivan, T. W. and H. R. Bird. 1957. Effect of quantity and source of dietary nitrogen on the utilization of the hydroxy analogues of methionine and glycine by chicks. *J. Nutr.* **62**:143.

Summers, J. D., S. Blackman and S. Leeson. 1987. Assay for estimating the potency of various methionine-active sources. *Poult. Sci.* **66**:1779.

Sunde, M. L. 1972. Utilization of D- and DL-amino acids and analogs. *Poult. Sci.* **51**:44.

Thomas, O. P., C. Tamplin, S. D. Crissey, E. Bossard and A. Zuckerman. 1991. An evaluation of methionine hydroxy analog free acid using a nonlinear (exponential) bioassay. *Poult. Sci.* **70**:605.

Tipton, H. C., B. C. Dilworth and E. J. Day. 1965. The relative biological value of DL-methionine and methionine hydroxy analogue in chick diets. *Poult. Sci.* **44**:987.

Tipton, H. C., B. V. Dilworth and E. J. Day. 1966. A comparison of D-, L-, DL-methionine and methionine hydroxy analogue calcium in chick diets. *Poult. Sci.* **45**:381.

Totter, J. R. and C. P. Berg. 1939. The influence of optical isomerism on the utilization of tryptophane, histidine, and lysine for growth in the mouse. *J. Biol. Chem.* **127**:375.

Triebwasser, K. C., P. B. Swan, L. M. Henderson and J. A. Budny. 1976. Metabolism of D- and L-tryptophan in dogs. *J. Nutr.* **106**:642.

van Weerden, E. J., H. L. Bertram and J. B. Schutte. 1982. Comparison of DL-methionine, DL-methionine-Na, DL-methionine hydroxy analogue-Ca and DL-methionine hydroxy analogue free acid in broilers using a crystalline amino acid diet. *Poult. Sci.* **61**:1125.

van Weerden, E. J., J. B. Schutte and H. L. Bertram. 1983. DL-Methionine and DL-methionine hydroxy analogue free acid in broiler diets. *Poult. Sci.* **62**:1269.

Waldroup, P. W., C. J. Mabray, J. R. Blackman, P. J. Slagter, R. J. Short and Z. B. Johnson. 1981. Effectiveness of the free acid of methionine hydroxy analogue as a methionine supplement in broiler diets. *Poult. Sci.* **60**:438.

West, H. D. and H. E. Carter. 1938. Synthesis of α-amino-β-hydroxy-n-butyric acids. VI. Preparation of d- and l-allothreonine and nutritive value of the four isomers. *J. Biol. Chem.* **122**:611.

West, J. W., C. W. Carrick, S. M. Hauge and E. T. Mertz. 1952. The tryptophan requirement of young chickens as influenced by niacin. *Poult. Sci.* **31**:479.

White, J., W. S. Fones and H. A. Sober. 1952. The utilization of D-valine for growth by the rat. *J. Biol. Chem.* **199**:505.

Wilkening, M. C. and B. S. Schweigert. 1947. Utilization of D-tryptophan by the chick. *J. Biol. Chem.* **171**:209.

Winitz, M., J. P. Greenstein and S. M. Birnbaum. 1957. Quantitative nutritional studies with water-soluble chemically defined diets. V. Role of the isomeric arginines in growth. *Arch. Biochem. Biophys.* **72**:448.

Womack, M., B. B. Snyder and W. C. Rose. 1957. The growth effect of D-valine. *J. Biol. Chem.* **224**:793.

Wretlind, K. A. J. 1950. The effect on growth and the toxicity of the two isomers of methionine. *Acta Physiol. Scand.* **20**:1.

Wretlind, K. A. J. 1952. The availability for growth and the toxicity of L- and D-phenylalanine. *Acta Physiol. Scand.* **25**:276.

Wretlind, K. A. J. and W. C. Rose. 1950. Methionine requirement for growth and utilization of its optical isomers. *J. Biol. Chem.* **187**:697.

Zezulka, A. Y. and D. H. Calloway. 1976. Nitrogen retention in men fed isolated soybean protein supplemented with L-methionine, D-methionine, N-acetyl-L-methionine or inorganic sulfate. *J. Nutr.* **106**:1286.

4

METHODS FOR ESTIMATION OF
MINERAL BIOAVAILABILITY

Clarence B. Ammerman

Department of Animal Science
University of Florida
Gainesville, Florida

I. INTRODUCTION

A general discussion of certain methods used in the estimation of mineral element bioavailability is presented in this chapter. More specific and detailed discussion with regard to methodology is presented with individual mineral elements when it is considered appropriate. Age and species of animal, diet and experimental techniques must all be evaluated in selecting a suitable method for estimating bioavailability of a particular mineral element.

II. DIETARY CONSIDERATIONS

It is important that basal diets to be used in bioavailability assays are nutritionally adequate to produce the desired response in the animal. In tests in which the total dietary concentration of the mineral to be tested is less than requirement, it is important that the source of the element of interest represents the major portion of the total dietary concentration of that element. In general, the wider the ratio of test element to basal diet element, the more sensitive the test for measuring bioavailability. For studies in which responses to surfeit dietary concentrations of an element are obtained, concentration of element in the basal diet is relatively less important and the element is generally added at the animal's requirement level rather than below that level.

BIOAVAILABILITY OF NUTRIENTS FOR ANIMALS:
AMINO ACIDS, MINERALS, AND VITAMINS

83

III. ABSORPTION AND CHEMICAL BALANCE

Absorption of a mineral element by an animal may provide an estimate of its bioavailability. The mineral must be absorbed from the gastrointestinal tract, and the assumption is generally made that, once absorbed, the element is available for storage or for use in various physiological processes by the animal. Absorption, however, cannot always be equated to bioavailability. For example, iodine in the form of 3,5-diiodosalicyclic acid was shown to be well utilized by rats but was an ineffective source of the element for cattle (Miller *et al.,* 1964; 1965). The iodine containing compound was absorbed readily by both species, but cattle had a very limited capacity to remove iodine from the organic part of the molecule. Bioavailability of the compound as a source of iodine was high for rats and very low for cattle. As another example, Seal and Heaton (1983) observed that 2-picolinic acid increased zinc absorption in rats by nearly 60%, but at the same time urinary excretion increased so that there was no change in net retention. Although absorption was greater, no greater quantity of zinc was available for potential use at the tissue level. When mineral elements, such as sulfur and selenium, are given to an animal in the form of sulfur or selenium-containing amino acids, absorption and metabolism within the body may differ from that which occurs when other forms of the element are provided. Selenium as sodium selenite and selenomethionine, for example, can be absorbed and metabolized by different pathways, and comparisons in bioavailability of the element based on absorption or tissue deposition may be misleading.

Absorption studies of several days in length have been used most frequently with ruminant animals and generally with macrominerals such as calcium, phosphorus, and magnesium. Similar studies have been done with swine and a few such experiments have been conducted with poultry. Also, absorption studies with the micromineral elements for domestic animals in which intake and fecal excretion of the stable elements are measured are few in number. Reasons for this include the need to feed purified diets, as well as problems resulting from working with such small quantities of the element being absorbed and the serious consequences of even slight contamination.

A. Apparent Absorption

Apparent absorption is used in the evaluation of sources of certain mineral elements and is defined as total intake minus total fecal excretion of the element. Values are usually expressed as a percentage of intake.

$$Apparent\ absorption = \frac{intake\ -\ total\ fecal\ excretion}{intake}\ x\ 100$$

The difference between intake and excretion represents net disappearance of the element from the gastrointestinal tract and does not correct for the portion of the element present in feces that resulted either from abrasion of mucosal cells or from excretion of the element back into the gastrointestinal tract. Apparent absorption is of limited value for elements such as calcium, phosphorus, zinc, manganese, and copper for which the gastrointestinal tract is a major pathway of excretion.

B. True Absorption

True absorption corrects for that portion of the element which has been absorbed into the animal's body and subsequently is excreted back into the gastrointestinal tract. This portion of the total fecal excretion can be designated as "total endogenous fecal excretion" or as sometimes used in the literature, "metabolic fecal excretion." It is composed of the "minimum endogenous excretion" plus the "variable endogenous fraction." Minimum endogenous fecal loss represents the minimal or inevitable loss from the animal's body (ARC, 1980). The remaining endogenous loss can be quite variable in quantity and is influenced in large measure by intake and bioavailability of the mineral element (Fig.1). This portion may not have been involved in essential functions within the animal's body. The two fractions cannot be separated chemically and exist by definition only. The reader needs to be aware that "endogenous" is used frequently in the literature with little clarification whether minimum or total endogenous excretion is involved. True absorption represents total intake minus total fecal excretion (tot. fecal exc.) from which total endogenous has been subtracted.

$$True\ absorption = \frac{intake - (tot.\ fecal\ exc. - tot.\ endogenous\ fecal\ exc.)}{intake} \times 100.$$

The value for true absorption is greater than that for apparent absorption and is a more valid estimate of the amount of a mineral element presented to body tissues for metabolic purposes. Total endogenous fecal excretion can be estimated by use of an appropriate radioisotope (Kleiber et al., 1951; Underwood, 1981). Calculations for determination of total endogenous fecal excretion when using a single isotope are

$$Total\ endogenous\ fecal\ exc. = \frac{specific\ activity\ of\ feces}{specific\ activity\ of\ plasma} \times total\ fecal\ exc.$$

Measurements of true mineral absorption by radioisotope dilution have been limited primarily to the elements calcium and phosphorus for ruminant animals. This method, however, has been applied to zinc absorption in the rat (Weigand and Kirchgessner, 1976; Evans et al., 1979) and manganese absorption in the chick (Wedekind et al., 1991).

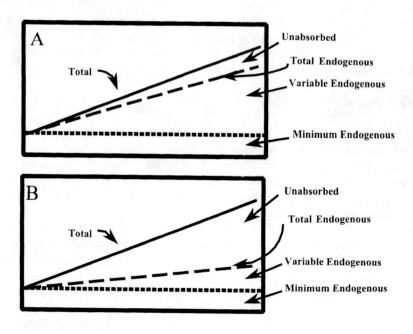

Fig. 1. Illustration of total fecal excretion and its components for mineral elements that have significant excretion by way of the gastrointestinal tract. (A) Readily absorbed mineral source. (B) Relatively unabsorbed mineral source. Total endogenous is also referred to as "metabolic fecal." The variable endogenous fecal excretion fraction can approach zero for those mineral elements excreted primarily by way of the urine.

Estimates of true absorption of certain minerals by ruminants have been obtained without the use of isotopes by using double collections or a comparative technique. The basal diet is fed during the first collection (col.1) and the basal diet plus the mineral compound to be tested is fed during a second collection (col.2). This technique was used by Ammerman *et al.* (1957) to estimate "true" absorption of phosphorus for sheep. The calculation was

$$\frac{(TPI\ col.\ 2 - TPI\ col.\ 1) - (TFP\ col.\ 2 - TFP\ col.\ 1)}{(TPI\ col.\ 2 - TPI\ col.\ 1)} \times 100,$$

where TPI is total phosphorus intake and TFP is total fecal phosphorus. Maintenance of uniform intakes for the same animal between the two collection periods was critical to obtaining meaningful data.   Underwood (1981) discussed a similar technique for estimating bioavailability except that excretion included that in both feces and urine. (See further comment under Section III, D.)

Hintz and Schryver (1973) and Blaney *et al.* (1981) estimated true absorption of magnesium in horses based on a minimum endogenous fecal magnesium excretion of 2.2 mg/kg body wt (BW) daily, and Blaney *et al.* (1982) estimated true absorption in cattle based on a minimum endogenous fecal magnesium excretion of 3.0 mg/kg BW daily (ARC, 1980). Minimum endogenous excretion, as expressed, represents minimal or inevitable loss from the body and estimates of true absorption would approach reality only if dietary intake of magnesium were at requirement or below. As dietary intakes of magnesium increase, especially to levels in excess of the requirement, the variable endogenous excretion represents a greater proportion of total fecal magnesium. Total endogenous fecal excretion (metabolic fecal excretion) is not related to body size and cannot be represented by a constant proportion of body size. It is affected greatly by dietary intake, degree of absorption, and pathway of excretion of the element being tested. In general, true absorption should not be estimated by making use of minimum endogenous fecal excretion levels unless dietary intake of the element is well below requirement.

C. Urinary Excretion

Urine is a major pathway of excretion for some minerals such as magnesium, iodine, and potassium but is a minor pathway for others such as manganese, iron, zinc, and copper.   Urinary excretion is a useful indicator of absorption for magnesium and potassium and other elements with similar excretion characteristics.

D. Net Retention

Net retention, [referred to as "net availability" by Underwood (1981)] is defined as total intake minus total excretion (total fecal plus total urinary) of the element. Collection of urine during absorption studies allows net retention to be calculated. Although this information may be useful in interpreting results, net retention probably has little value in determining bioavailability of a mineral element. In many situations, the mineral element excreted in the urine represents a portion that is potentially nutritionally effective and that has been involved in, or was available for use in, metabolism. It is an error, in such cases, to include the urinary fraction as a part of the unavailable portion of total dietary intake.

IV. GROWTH AND SPECIFIC TISSUE RESPONSE

A. Growth

Growth response in the young chicken has been used as the primary criterion for determining bioavailability of several macro and micromineral elements. A disadvantage of growth rate assays lies in the fact that, for many elements, the method requires use of semipurified diets which increases cost and which also may yield results not entirely applicable when practical diets containing natural ingredients are fed. The young chick with its limited nutrient stores, lack of coprophagy, rapid rate of growth and, thus, high nutrient demand, is an ideal assay animal. Growth response as a criterion for mineral bioavailability has been used with larger domestic animals, but this method becomes less satisfactory because of dietary and labor costs, length of feeding period required, and general insensitivity of growth as a response criterion.

B. Bone Development

Bone development, as usually measured by bone ash response in the very young chicken, has been considered for years as one of the most critical tests for estimating bioavailability of calcium and phosphorus compounds. In general, the bone of choice has been the tibia, and bone ash has been expressed as either total tibia ash or as tibia ash concentration of the dry, fat-free bone. For ease in obtaining tissues from chicks, both beaks and toes have also been used. Although ash values obtained for these tissues are similar to those obtained with the tibia, sensitivity of measurement is greater with the tibia. Bone ash and bone breaking strength (force required to fracture the bone) have also been used widely in swine for phosphorus and also calcium. Bones used most commonly are the metacarpals and metatarsals.

C. Essential Compounds or Enzymes

Functional assays for bioavailability in which the mineral element is necessary for an essential compound (e.g., iron for hemoglobin and cobalt for vitamin B_{12}) have been used. Measurements in tissues of selenium-dependent glutathione peroxidase levels (Combs and Combs, 1986) and cytochrome C oxidase activity as influenced by copper (Price and Chesters, 1985) have been used as indicators for bioavailability of these two elements.

D. Tissue Accumulation

Accumulation of the mineral element in various target organs has been used for many years as a response criterion. Nesbit and Elmslie (1960), for example, indicated that biological availability of iron and copper from various supplemental compounds was related to tissue concentrations of the elements. It was reported by Watson *et al.* (1970) that bone manganese concentrations in chicks fed semipurified diets were more directly related to dietary concentrations of the element than were growth rate or leg development. More recently, the biological availability of several microelements for ruminants and poultry has been estimated by tissue uptake of the elements following high dietary level, short-term supplementation (Henry *et al.*, 1986). As stated by Combs and Combs (1986) in regard to the bioavailability of selenium, this method measures adventitious as well as "critical" (metabolically active) compounds within a tissue. As illustrated in Fig. 2, fewer animals are required to detect statistically significant differences between standard and unknown, or test compound, when greater dietary concentrations are fed.

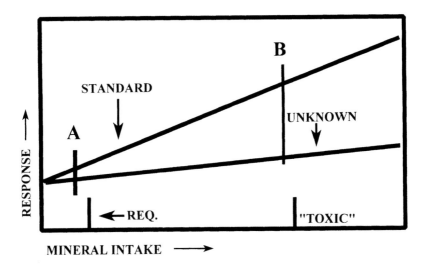

Fig. 2. Illustration of tissue mineral response to dietary addition of a mineral element (Adapted from Henry *et al.*, 1986). (A) Tissue mineral response to dietary intake below requirement. (B) Tissue mineral response to dietary intake near the "toxic" level as defined by decreased feed intake.

The use of elevated dietary mineral levels allows formulation of diets with natural ingredients and, thus, the expression of full genetic growth potential by the animal. Mineral contamination is of less consequence, and the feeding study can be of relatively short duration.

Aoyagi and Baker (1993) with copper and Baker and Oduho (1994) with manganese provided evidence that bioassays using pharmacological dosing (250 to 500 ppm copper; 100 to 1000 ppm manganese) gave the same estimates of relative bioavailability of copper from liver copper accumulation and manganese from tibia manganese accumulation as bioassays involving physiological dosing concentrations (.5 to 1.5 ppm copper; .5 to 10 ppm manganese). In the physiological dosing assays, semipurified diets were fed that resulted in growth and bone manganese responses to supplemental manganese intake and to bile copper increases from supplemental copper intake.

V. USE OF ISOTOPES

Accumulation of radioactive or stable isotopes in appropriate target organs or whole-body retention of an orally administered isotope have been used to estimate absorption of mineral elements from dietary ingredients. Radioisotopes have been used more with food ingredients in tests with laboratory animals than with feed ingredients for domestic animals. Stable isotopes have been used to a limited extent in measuring absorption by humans of mineral elements from foods. Reviews of methods for assessment of mineral utilization in humans and laboratory animals, including the use of stable isotopes and intrinsic and extrinsic labeling with radioisotopes, have been prepared by O'Dell (1984, 1985).

A. Intrinsic and Extrinsic Isotopic Labels

Estimates of absorption of mineral elements from foods and feeds have been obtained using either intrinsic or extrinsic radioactive isotopic labeling (O'Dell, 1984, 1985). Extrinsic labeling is easier to use and is less expensive than intrinsic labeling but may not yield similar information with regard to absorption.

Intrinsic labeling occurs when isotopes are introduced to plants or animals and results in tissues being labeled. When the labeled plant or animal tissue is fed, it is assumed that the isotope and stable element are utilized in the same manner by the animal. Short-term applications of the isotope are sometimes used with growing plants, and this results in the preferential intrinsic labeling of tissues undergoing rapid growth at the time of isotope administration. Under these conditions, distribution of isotope within the total plant tissue may not be representative of that for the stable mineral element (Weaver, 1987).

Extrinsic radioactive labels are usually added directly to the food or feed. Thus, it is necessary to demonstrate that the isotope that has been added is used by the animal identically to the way in which the intrinsic label is utilized. Extrinsic radiolabels have been used to measure absorption for several mineral elements including zinc, iron and selenium. Such labels have generally yielded results considered to be indicative of that for the stable mineral element. Ketelsen *et al.* (1984), however, reported that ^{65}Zn retention was greater in rats from an extrinsically labeled soy flour than from the intrinsically labeled soy product. Also, Gislason *et al.* (1992) labeled sow's milk either intrinsically or extrinsically with ^{59}Fe and observed that different fractions of the milk were being labeled by the two techniques. When measured with pigs, iron retention from the intrinsically labeled milk was considerably greater than that from extrinsically labeled milk.

B. Neutron Activation

Neutron activation of mineral compounds has been used to create radioisotopes that can be used in measuring absorption. Lassiter and Bell (1960), for example, orally administered to sheep ^{64}Cu labeled materials that were obtained by thermal neutron activation of stable copper compounds. However, isotopes other than those desired can also be produced, and these isotopes can interfere with measurement of the appropriate radioactivity. This has been a greater problem with less chemically purified compounds, such as feed grade phosphates, which contain greater quantities of contaminating elements (Ammerman *et al.*, 1963).

C. Compound Synthesis

Chemical compounds containing radioisotopes of the mineral of interest have been synthesized and used in absorption studies following oral administration. Considerable variation occurs frequently with a single oral dose technique used in conjunction with this procedure. One problem with this approach is the difficulty of duplicating compounds in the same form and matrix as they exist in feed grade sources of the mineral element.

VI. OTHER

A. Disappearance from Bags in the Gastrointestinal Tract

Disappearance of mineral elements from feedstuffs suspended in the rumen in nondigestible bags has been used as an indicator of potential utilization by the animal (Emanuele and Staples, 1990). A further refinement of this technique involved removal of dacron bags from the rumen, soaking them in HCl-pepsin for 1 hr to simulate conditions in the abomasum, and reinserting them in a duodenal cannula for collection later from the feces (Emanuele *et al.*, 1989).

VII. *IN VITRO* PROCEDURES

A. Solubility

In vitro solubility of supplemental mineral sources in several solvents has been used to estimate the degree to which the source would be utilized by animals. Solvents have included water, .4% HCl, 2% citric acid, neutral ammonium citrate, ruminal fluid, artificial ruminal fluid, and abomasal fluid. Generally, *in vitro* solubility is a poor indicator of *in vivo* bioavailability.

B. Cellulose Digestibility

In vitro response of ruminal microorganisms to supplementation of phosphorus (Anderson *et al.*, 1956; Chicco *et al.*, 1965) and sulfur (Spears *et al.*, 1976, 1977; Guardiola *et al.*, 1983) from various sources as measured by cellulose digestion has been used as an indicator of their relative bioavailability.

REFERENCES

Agricultural Research Council (ARC). 1980. "The Nutrient Requirements of Ruminant Livestock,"
    p. 183. ARC, Commonwealth Agricultural Bureaux, Slough, UK.
Ammerman, C. B., R. M. Forbes, U. S. Garrigus, A. L. Neumann, H. W. Norton and E. E. Hatfield.
    1957. Ruminant utilization of inorganic phosphates. *J.Anim. Sci.* **16**:796.

Ammerman, C. B., L. R. Arrington, J. T. McCall, J. P. Feaster, G. E. Combs and G. K. Davis. 1963. Inorganic phosphorus utilization by swine as measured by an isotope technique. *J. Anim. Sci.* 22:890.

Anderson, R., E. Cheng and W. Burroughs. 1956. A laboratory technique for measuring phosphorus availability of feed supplements fed to ruminants. *J. Anim. Sci.* 15:489.

Aoyagi, S. and D. H. Baker. 1993. Nutritional evaluation of a copper-methionine complex for chicks. *Poult. Sci.* 72:2309.

Baker, D. H. and G. W. Oduho. 1994. Manganese utilization in the chick: Effects of excess phosphorus on chicks fed manganese-deficient diets. *Poult. Sci.* 73:1162.

Blaney, B. J., R. J. W. Gartner and R. A. McKenzie. 1981. The effects of oxalate in some tropical grasses on the availability to horsess of calcium, phosphorus and magnesium. *J. Agric. Sci. Camb.* 97:507.

Blaney, B. J., R. J. W. Gartner and T. A. Head. 1982. The effects of oxalate in some tropical grasses on calcium, phosphorus and magnesium availability to cattle. *J. Agric. Sci. Camb.* 99:533.

Chicco, C. F., C. B. Ammerman, J. E. Moore, P. A. van Walleghem, L. R. Arrington and R. L. Shirley. 1965. Utilization of inorganic ortho-, meta- and pyrophosphates by lambs and by cellulolytic rumen microorganisms *in vitro*. *J. Anim. Sci.* 24:355.

Combs, G. F., Jr. and S. B. Combs. 1986. "The Role of Selenium in Nutrition." Academic Press, New York.

Emanuele, S. M. and C. R. Staples. 1990. Ruminal release of minerals from six forage species. *J. Anim. Sci.* 68:2052.

Emanuele, S. M., C. R. Staples and C. J. Wilcox. 1991. Extent and site of mineral release from six forage species incubated in mobile dacron bags. *J. Anim. Sci.* 69:801.

Evans, G. W., E. C. Johnson and P. E. Johnson. 1979. Zinc absorption in the rat determined by radioisotope dilution. *J. Nutr.* 109:1258.

Gislason, J., B. Jones, B. Lonnerdal and L. Hambraeus. 1992. Iron absorption differs in piglets fed extrinsically and intrinsically ^{59}Fe-labeled sow's milk. *J. Nutr.* 122:1287.

Guardiola, C. M., G. C. Fahey, Jr., J. W. Spears and U. S. Garrigus. 1983. The effects of sulphur supplementation on cellulose digestion *in vitro* and on nutrient digestion, nitrogen metabolism and rumen characteristics of lambs fed on good quality fescue and tropical star grass hays. *Anim. Feed Sci. Technol.* 8:129.

Henry, P. R., C. B. Ammerman and R. D. Miles. 1986. Bioavailability of manganese sulfate and manganese monoxide in chicks as measured by tissue uptake of manganese from conventional dietary levels. *Poult. Sci.* 65:983.

Hintz, H. F. and H. F. Schryver. 1973. Magnesium, calcium, and phosphorus metabolism in ponies fed varying levels of magnesium. *J. Anim. Sci.* 37:927.

Ketelsen, S. M., M. A. Stuart, C. M. Weaver, R. M. Forbes and J. W. Erdman, Jr. 1984. Bioavailability of zinc to rats from defatted soy flour, acid-precipitated soy concentrate and neutralized soy concentrate as determined by intrinsic and extrinsic labeling techniques. *J. Nutr.* 114:536.

Kleiber, M., A. H. Smith, N. P. Ralston and A. L. Black. 1951. Radiophosphorus (P^{32}) as tracer for measuring endogenous phosphorus in cow's feces. *J. Nutr.* 45:253.

Lassiter, J. W. and M. C. Bell. 1960. Availability of copper to sheep from Cu-labeled inorganic compounds. *J. Anim. Sci.* 19:754.

Meyer, N. R., M. A. Stuart and C. M. Weaver. 1983. Bioavailability of zinc from defatted soy flour, soy hulls and whole eggs as determined by intrinsic and extrinsic labeling techniques. *J. Nutr.* 113:1255.

Miller, J. K., P. W. Aschbacher and E. W. Swanson. 1964. Comparison of the metabolism of sodium iodide and 3,5-diiodosalicyclic acid in dairy cattle. *J. Dairy Sci.* **47**:169.

Miller, J. K., E. W. Swanson and S. M. Hansen. 1965. Effects of feeding potassium iodide, 3,5-diiodosalicyclic acid, or L-thyroxine on iodine metabolism of lactating dairy cows. *J. Dairy Sci.* **48**:888.

Nesbit, A. H. and W. P. Elmslie. 1960. Biological availability to the rat of iron and copper from various compounds. *Trans. Illinois State Acad. Sci.* **53**:101.

O'Dell, B. L. 1984. Bioavailability of trace elements. *Nutr. Rev.* **42**:301.

O'Dell, B. L. 1985. Bioavailability of and interactions among trace elements. *In* "Trace Elements in Nutrition of Children" (R.K. Chandra, Ed.), p. 41. Vevey/Raven Press, New York.

Price, J. and J. K. Chesters. 1985. A new bioassay for assessment of copper availability and its application in a study of the effect of molybdenum on the distribution of available copper in ruminant digesta. *Br. J. Nutr.* **53**:323.

Seal, C. J. and F. W. Heaton. 1983. Chemical factors affecting intestinal absorption of zinc *in vitro* and *in vivo*. *Br. J. Nutr.* **50**:317.

Spears, J. W., L. P. Bush and D. G. Ely. 1977. Influence of nitrate and molybdenum on sulfur utilization by rumen microorganisms. *J. Dairy Sci.* **60**:1889.

Spears, J. W., D. G. Ely, L. P. Bush and R. C. Buckner. 1976. Sulfur supplementation and *in vitro* digestion of forage cellulose by rumen microorganisms. *J. Anim. Sci.* **43**:513.

Underwood, E. J. 1981. "The Mineral Nutrition of Livestock," p. 9. Commonwealth Agricultural Bureaux, Slough, UK.

Watson, L. T., C. B. Ammerman, S. M. Miller and R. H. Harms. 1970. Biological assay of inorganic manganese for chicks. *Poult. Sci.* **49**:1548.

Weaver, C. M. 1987. Biological labeling of foods with isotopes of selenium. *In* "Selenium in Biology and Medicine" (G. F. Combs, Jr., J. E. Spallholz, O. E. Levander and J. E. Oldfield, Eds.), Part A, p. 472. Van Nostrand- Reinhold Company, New York.

Wedekind, K. J., E. C. Titgemeyer, A. R. Twardock and D. H. Baker. 1991. Phosphorus, but not calcium, affects manganese absorption and turnover in chicks. *J. Nutr.* **121**:1776.

Weigand, E. and M. Kirchgessner. 1976. Radioisotope dilution technique for determination of zinc absorption *in vivo*. *Nutr. Metab.* **20**:307.

5

CALCIUM BIOAVAILABILITY

Joseph H. Soares, Jr.

Department of Animal Sciences
Univerity of Maryland
College Park, Maryland

I. INTRODUCTION

Calcium is one of the most abundant elements in the body and is often the major cation in the diet. Ninety-nine percent of the body's calcium is located in the skeleton. The remaining 1% is extremely important in cellular metabolism, blood clotting, enzyme activation, and neuromuscular action. Ionic calcium in blood plasma is maintained precisely by a cascade of regulatory processes centering around the calcium homeostatic hormones. The requirement for calcium varies markedly throughout an animal's life span. The average chick increases its body weight 15-fold from hatching to 3 weeks of age. To achieve this, it must accrete 350 mg calcium/kg body wt daily, and a dairy cow in peak lactation mobilizes 50 mg/kg body wt (Soares, 1987). Except for diets high in legume forages for ruminants, practical diets fed to livestock are almost always deficient in calcium unless supplemented. Typically, an unsupplemented corn-soybean meal diet contains less than .1% calcium. Only that amount of ingested calcium which is actually absorbed and utilized can contribute to an animal's metabolic requirement. Therefore, it is important to know the bioavailability of calcium in dietary ingredients. Calcium in natural feedstuffs from plants quite often exists as complexes with phytate and oxalate, which reduce bioavailability.

BIOAVAILABILITY OF NUTRIENTS FOR ANIMALS:
AMINO ACIDS, MINERALS, AND VITAMINS

95

II. BIOAVAILABILITY STUDIES

A. *In Vivo* Estimates of Bioavailability

Animal weight gain, bone breaking strength, and tibia ash, as well as various parameters of calcium metabolism have been used by many researchers as indicators useful to measure available calcium in the diet. Much more research on relative calcium bioavailability has been conducted with poultry than with other species. Slope ratio assays have been used frequently. The response to added calcium from the feed ingredient is compared to a reference material which is generally assumed to have a bioavailability of 100%. Comparison of slopes of the dose-response curves gives an estimate of relative calcium availability. There are several problems, however, associated with this approach. Combs and Wallace (1962) noted that protein digestibility in pigs was markedly lowered when calcium intake was high. It is generally agreed that diets high in phosphorus or which have extreme calcium to phosphorus ratios reduce calcium availability. It would appear, therefore, that calcium bioavailability assays could be compromised when growth rate was limited by protein or other nutrient needs rather than by calcium intake.

Yoshida and Hoshii (1982a,b,c) fed combinations of calcium and phosphorus to broiler chicks and found that toe ash correlated well with tibia hardness. Their findings indicated, however, that toe ash and tibia hardness were dependent more on phosphorus content of the diet than on calcium concentration. The use of central composite rotatable designs in which dietary concentrations of both calcium and phosphorus have been varied suggests that calcium requirements for optimal bone ash and weight gain are different (Edwards and Lanza, 1981; Roush *et al.*, 1986). In general, the requirement for weight gain is lower than that for maximal bone ash. Bone ash, therefore, was suggested as the response criterion of choice for bioavailability and requirement studies.

In studies with mature fowl, Hurwitz and Bar (1969) used colostomized laying hens to separate fecal and urinary calcium losses and determined that as calcium concentration of the diet increased from .59 to 3.94%, fecal calcium losses increased from 19 to 40% of ingested calcium. This demonstrated that calcium absorption through the intestine is very rapidly modified, and total calcium concentration of the diet could alter physiological factors controlling calcium absorption from a particular source. Similar results were found in poultry and sheep by Damron *et al.* (1974), Braithwaite (1979), and Sibbald (1982).

Myung *et al.* (1983) and Kim *et al.* (1985a,b) used Sibbald's (1982) technique with Japanese quail to determine the availability of calcium in calcium carbonate, calcium sulfate, tricalcium phosphate, dicalcium phosphate, limestone, and oyster shell. They compared the values obtained to those determined using the simpler apparent absorption technique. The Sibbald method is based on forced feeding of specific quantities of feed and collection of feces. The two methods were close in their respective estimations of calcium availability from each of the sources. The availability of calcium from limestone and oyster shell, two commonly used calcium supplements, was only 72 and 68%, respectively (Kim *et al.*, 1985a). Calcium availability was found to be influenced by particle size of the supplement (optimal at 40 to 80 mesh) and age of birds (availability decreased with age). The metabolic fecal and endogenous urinary calcium losses were estimated to account for less than .2% of the total requirement (Myung *et al.*, 1983).

Radioisotopes have been quite useful to determine the availability of calcium from several sources (Hurwitz, 1964; Hurwitz and Bar, 1965; Hertoghe *et al.*, 1967). Yttrium[91] has been used as a nonabsorbed dietary marker to estimate relative absorption of calcium and phosphorus throughout the gastrointestinal tract (Hurwitz, 1964; Hurwitz and Bar, 1965). Calcium[45] and [47]Ca have been used for direct estimation of calcium uptake (Hertoghe *et al.*, 1967). When only one isotope, such as [45]Ca, is used, availability values ignore the endogenous losses which are not adequately accounted for during absorption studies. Extrinsically labeled calcium is assumed to be freely exchangeable with feed calcium. Most studies support this concept (Schwartz, 1988; Buchouski *et al.*, 1989), but some food sources, such as spinach, have been shown to be nonexchangeable (Weaver *et al.*, 1987; Schwartz, 1988). Using whole-body radioactivity methods, Hertoghe *et al.* (1967) compared the accuracy of balance trials to direct measurement or uptake of radioactive calcium in rats. Their results showed that balance trials gave lower estimates of the availability of calcium from calcium chloride compared to their estimation from whole-body radioactivity after a gavage of labeled calcium.

In ruminant studies of calcium bioavailabilty, calcium absorption or retention is frequently determined (Tables I and II). Since absorption of calcium is quite low, a balance study combined with intravenous administration of radioactive calcium can be an effective way to estimate endogenous losses as well as to improve the accuracy of the balance trial (Chrisp and Sykes, 1989a,b).

III. FACTORS INFLUENCING BIOAVAILABILITY

A. Dietary Factors

Several factors, in addition to those mentioned already, have been shown to influence absorption of calcium from the gut. For example, the estimation of calcium availability from a feedstuff is affected greatly by the calcium to phosphorus ratio of the diet (Kim et al., 1985b; Albanese et al., 1986; Lopes and Perry, 1986; Roush et al., 1986). Interestingly, ruminants can tolerate relatively high calcium to phosphorus ratios if magnesium is not high in the diet (Chester-Jones et al., 1990).

Calcium is absorbed in the ionic form, and factors which reduce the concentration of ionic calcium (oxalate, phytate, phosphate, and excessive sulfate) reduce its uptake in animals (Harrison, 1959; Nelson, 1967; Nelson et al., 1968; Ward et al., 1972; Nelson and Kirby, 1987; Poneros-Schneirer and Erdman, 1989). Ward et al. (1984) demonstrated an excellent correlation between the nonoxalate calcium concentration in the diet and tibia ash expressed on a dry, fat-free basis. Oxalate-bound calcium was found to be as high as 20 to 33% of total calcium in samples of alfalfa meal (Ward et al., 1979; Hintz et al., 1984; Cromwell, 1989). When oxalate concentrations are high in horse diets, calcium absorption appeared to be reduced (Swartzman et al., 1978; McKenzie et al., 1981; Blaney et al., 1981). It was suggested by Weaver et al. (1987) that the oxalate content of spinach is the factor reducing calcium bioavailability.

Phytic acid reduces calcium bioavailability provided at least five phosphate groups are present on the molecule (Lonnerdal et al., 1989). Consequently, many studies have shown that cereal grain-based diets, alfalfa and various grasses and hays have low calcium bioavailability (Mudd, 1970; Negi, 1971; Ward et al., 1979; Sykes and Geenty, 1986; Chrisp et al., 1989a; Cromwell, 1989; Martz et al., 1990).

Additions of lactose (Baker et al., 1967; Moser et al., 1977; Rayssiquier and Poncet, 1980; Greger et al., 1989; Buchowski and Miller, 1991), casein (Chrisp et al., 1989a), anion:cation ratio (Lomba et al., 1978), or source of protein (Boila and Phillips, 1988) have been reported to increase calcium absorption and retention in both ruminants and nonruminants. However, Allen et al. (1990) reported that calcium absorption is reduced in sheep when aluminum citrate was added to the diet. Citrate alone did not alter calcium absorption, suggesting that aluminum was the primary factor. Aluminum has been reported by others to reduce calcium balance in the rat and sheep (Alder and Berlyne, 1985; Allen et al., 1990). Adding ascorbic acid to diets fed to rats, on the other hand, did not change calcium availability in several foods and feeds (Poneros and Erdman, 1988; Poneros-Schneirer and Erdman, 1989). Similarly the calcium ionophore, monensin, was reported by Greene et al. (1988) to not alter absorption of calcium by steers, but it did increase urinary calcium excretion (Kirk et al., 1985). However, Sticker et al. (1991) reported that lysocellin and tetronasin reduced blood calcium in steers.

Absorption of calcium in the anterior small intestine is both an active (mediated by vitamin D) and a passive process (DeLuca, 1974; Norman, 1987). While both vitamin D_2 and D_3 can be used by most species, vitamin D_3 is the only form that has activity in avians. Furthermore, it is known that there are limited stores of this nutrient in the body (Tsang *et al.*, 1988). The form and the quantity of vitamin D available to an animal can significantly influence calcium absorption in poultry (Kaetzel and Soares, 1979; Lofton and Soares, 1986) and dairy cattle (Hibbs and Conrad, 1983). This in turn would influence the availability of calcium in a feedstuff. Finally, there are a number of reports showing young animals retain more calcium than mature animals (Hansard *et al.*, 1954, 1957; Harrison, 1959; Horst *et al.*, 1978). This emphasizes the importance of using animals of similar age when comparing the relative availability of calcium in feedstuffs.

Several workers have demonstrated that availability of calcium from commonly used calcium supplements varies according to particle size. McNaughton *et al.* (1974) reported maximal calcium availability for growth and tibia ash in chicks when medium ground (16 mesh) particles were fed. Roland (1986) reviewed 44 papers that compared the availability of calcium from fine granular limestone with that of oyster shell: over one-third of these studies showed oyster shell to be a more available source of calcium, one report presented data showing limestone to be more available than oyster shell and the remaining papers reported no differences. Several reports were reviewed showing that when limestone and oyster shell of similar particle size were fed, there were no detectable differences between the two sources. This would indicate that comparable particle size is of importance when comparing oyster shell calcium with calcium from limestone.

Several reports have indicated that particle size is a major determinant of calcium and phosphorus availability in defluorinated phosphates (Scott *et al.*, 1971; Roland and Harms, 1973; Roland *et al.*, 1974; Miur *et al.*, 1975.; Kuhle *et al.*, 1977; Watkins *et al.*, 1977; Brister *et al.*, 1981; Roland, 1986). Recently, however, Burnell *et al.* (1990) conducted studies with day-old broiler chicks fed a defluorinated phosphate which had been ground to produce samples of various particle sizes ranging from .05 to 2.0 mm. Using the slope ratio method to determine calcium and phosphorus availability, the authors estimated that the availabilities ranged from 90 to 101% relative to monosodium phosphate monohydrate and calcium carbonate standards. There were no significant differences among the samples tested and, therefore, the authors suggested that particle size is not an important factor within the range of particle size used. These results are supported by data from Pond *et al.* (1982) and Ross *et al.* (1984) who determined calcium availability in limestone samples having fine to coarse particles. Weanling pigs fed practical diets were observed to utilize similar amounts of calcium from the three sources based on growth, bone ash, feed efficiency, and serum alkaline phosphatase.

Greger *et al.* (1987) determined apparent calcium absorption for several common calcium sources using the weanling rat. When dried skim milk was considered to be 100% available, there was similar availability of calcium in dicalcium phosphate (93%), amino acid chelated calcium (110%), oyster shell (102%), calcium lactate

(104%) and calcium carbonate (102%). Dolomite (81%) or any of the limestone sources with high magnesium had significantly lower calcium availability.

In other studies with lactating cows or sheep, the true absorption of calcium from common grasses, such as timothy, fescue, and ryegrass averaged about 30% (Mudd, 1970, Sykes and Geenty, 1986; Chrisp et al., 1989a,b). In general, adding casein (Chrisp et al., 1989a), increasing anion:cation ratio (Lomba et al., 1978) or previous use of nitrogen fertilizers to stimulate grass growth (Mudd, 1970) increased dietary calcium availability. Calves fed bermudagrass forage with or without dicalcium phosphate had an apparent calcium absorption of 42 vs 48%, respectively (Gutierrez et al., 1984). Although calcium oxalate depresses calcium availability in nonruminant diets, Negi (1971) showed that steers averaged 60% absorption of calcium in the oxalate form.

B. Animal Factors

Calcium availability, as determined by radiocalcium recoveries from pair-fed 25-kg barrows, was 42% in a cereal grain-based diet (Whittemore et al., 1972). Using total balance or radioisotopic balance techniques, Hansard et al. (1957) showed that the greatest differences in calcium availability were due to age (growing heifers vs mature cattle). Nevertheless, the calcium in bone meal, calcium chloride, and dicalcium phosphate was most available. Defluorinated phosphate, ground limestone, and hay had significantly less bioavailable calcium. Mature cattle averaged 47% true calcium absorption for the inorganic sources vs 56% for growing cattle. Interestingly, three sources of hay, alfalfa, lespedeza, and orchardgrass, averaged 35% true calcium absorption for mature cattle vs 47% for growing calves. Langemann et al. (1957) used similar methods to show that calves absorbed 89% of milk calcium and 28% of the calcium in an orchardgrass-grain diet. In contrast, a mature nonlactating cow absorbed 23 and 8%, respectively, of the calcium from milk and orchardgrass-grain sources. Cymbaluk et al. (1989) estimated the true absorption of calcium in growing horses decreased from 70% at 8 months to 42% at 24 months of age.

IV. SUMMARY

Feedstuffs that are considered to have relative calcium bioavailability values for both nonruminant and ruminants of 95% or more in comparison to calcium carbonate include aragonite, bone meal, calcium gluconate, dicalcium phosphate, ground egg shell, ground limestone, ground oyster shell, calcium sulfate, nonfat dry milk, and tricalcium phosphate. In addition, when compared to dried skim milk, calcium lactate, calcium carbonate, chelated calcium, and oyster shell had relative bioavailabilities of 100%. Slightly less available (85 to 95%) but still considered excellent calcium sources are alfalfa hay, defluorinated phosphate, low fluorine rock phosphate, anhydrous calcium chloride, calcium citrate, and soybean meal. However, high oxalate alfalfa can have significantly lower calcium availability for horses. Those feedstuffs generally having less than 80% calcium bioavailability include calcium oxalate, dolomitic limestone, soft rock phosphate, and grass hays such as rye, timothy, and orchardgrass.

Table I. Bioavailability of calcium sources for animals[a]

Source	RV	Standard	Response criterion	Meth cal	Type diet	Added level, %	Reference
Chickens							
Alfalfa hay	88	Calcium carbonate	Bone ash	SC	N	.16-.68	Ward et al. (1984)
Bone meal	100	Calcium carbonate	Bone ash	TP	SP	NG	Blair et al. (1965)
Calcium gluconate	>100	Calcium carbonate	Shell ash	MR	N	NG	Hunter et al. (1933)
Calcium gluconate	100	Calcium carbonate	Growth & Bone ash	SC	N	.3-.7	Waldroup et al. (1964)
Calcium gluconate	>100	Calcium carbonate	Bone ash	MR	N	NG	Hunter et al. (1933)
Calcium sulfate	90	Calcium carbonate	Carcass & Bone Ca	SR	N	1.90-3.56	Hurwitz and Rand (1965)
Calcium sulfate	100	Calcium carbonate	Growth & Bone ash	SC	N	.3-.7	Waldroup et al. (1964)
Defluorinated phosphate	93	Calcium carbonate	Growth & Bone ash	SC	N	.45-1.13	Dilworth and Day (1964)
Defluorinated phosphate (.05-2.0 mm)	94	Calcium carbonate	Bone ash & BBS	SR	N	.47-.74	Burnell et al. (1990)
Egg shell, crushed	100	Limestone	Shell quality	MR	N	NG	Meyer et al. (1973)
Limestone, ground	100	Calcium carbonate	Growth & Bone ash	SC	N	.3-.7	Waldroup et al. (1964)
Limestone, ground	87	Calcium carbonate	Shell thickness	SR	N	.4-1	Reid and Weber (1976)
Limestone, ground	89	Calcium carbonate	Growth & Bone ash	SR	N	.4-1	Reid and Weber (1976)

102

Limestone, dolomitic	64-68	Calcium carbonate	Growth & Bone ash	MR	N	.5-1.1	Stillmak and Sunde (1971)
Low F rock phosphate	90	Calcium carbonate	Growth & Bone ash	SC	N	.45-1.13	Dilworth and Day (1964)
Oyster shell	>100	Calcium carbonate	Shell quality	MR	N	3.00-3.75	Roland (1986)
Oyster shell, ground	100	Calcium carbonate	Growth & Bone ash	SC	N	.3-.7	Waldroup et al. (1964)
Oyster shell, ground	108	Calcium carbonate	Growth & Bone ash	SR	N	.4-1	Reid and Weber (1976)
Oyster shell, ground	100	Calcium carbonate	Shell thickness	SR	N	.4-1	Reid and Weber (1976)
Soft rock phosphate	68	Calcium carbonate	Growth & Bone ash	SC	N	.45-1.13	Dilworth and Day (1964)
Steel slag	50	Limestone	Egg prod	MR	N	3.3-3.88	Leach (1985)
Tricalcium phosphate	100	Calcium carbonate	Balance	-	SP	NG	Blair et al. (1965)

Swine

Alfalfa meal	16-25	Calcium carbonate	BBS	SR	N	.1, .2	Cromwell et al. (1983)
Aragonite	93-102	Calcium carbonate	BBS	SR	N	.35-.70	Ross et al. (1984)
Calcium carbonate FG	80	Calcium carbonate RG	Ca ret	MR	SP	.4	Kuznetsov et al. (1987)
Calcium chloride	94	Calcium carbonate	Ca ret	MR	SP	.4	Kuznetsov et al. (1987)
Calcium chloride, anhydrous	86	Calcium carbonate	Ca ret	MR	SP	.4	Kuznetsov et al. (1987)
Calcium citrate	90	Calcium carbonate	Ca ret	MR	SP	.4	Kuznetsov et al. (1987)

Table I. (continued)

Source	RV	Standard	Response criterion	Meth cal	Type diet	Added level, %	Reference
Calcium oxalate	65	Calcium carbonate	Ca ret	MR	SP	.4	Kuznetsov et al. (1987)
Calcium succinate	96	Calcium carbonate	Ca ret	MR	SP	.4	Kuznetsov et al. (1987)
Calcium sulfate	100	Calcium carbonate	Growth	MR	N	NG	McCampbell and Aubel (1934)
Calcium sulfate	83	Calcium carbonate	Ca ret	MR	SP	.4	Kuznetsov et al. (1987)
Gypsum	98	Calcium carbonate	BBS	SR	N	.35-.70	Ross et al. (1984)
Limestone	99	Calcium carbonate	BBS	SR	N	.35-.70	Ross et al. (1984)
Limestone (fine to coarse)	42[b]	-	True abs	-	N	.9-3.1	Whittemore et al. (1972)
Limestone, dolomitic	78	Calcium carbonate	BBS	SR	N	.35-.70	Ross et al. (1984)
Marble dust	98	Calcium carbonate	BBS	SR	N	.35-.70	Ross et al. (1984)
Oyster shell, ground	98	Calcium carbonate	BBS	SR	N	.35-.70	Ross et al. (1984)
Cattle							
Albacar	49[b]		True abs	-	N	1.0-1.6%	Wholt et al. (1986)
Alfalfa hay	41[b]		True abs	-	N	.33	Hansard et al. (1957)
Alfalfa hay	31[b]		True abs	-	N	.33	Hansard et al. (1957)
Alfalfa hay	25[b]		True abs	-	N	.51	Martz et al. (1990)
Alfalfa hay/corn	42[b]		True abs	-	N	.51	Martz et al. (1990)
Aragonite	49[b]		True abs	-	N	1.0-1.6	Wholt et al. (1986)
Bermudagrass	52[b]		App abs	-	N	NG	Gutierrez et al. (1984)

Bone meal	63	Calcium carbonate	App abs	MR	N	NG	Agrawal and Talapatra (1971)
Bone meal	133	Calcium carbonate	True abs	MR	N	.33	Hansard et al. (1957)
Bone meal	138	Calcium carbonate	True abs	MR	N	.33	Hansard et al. (1957)
Calcium chloride RG	132	Calcium carbonate	True abs	MR	N	.33	Hansard et al. (1957)
Calcium chloride FG	120	Calcium carbonate	True abs	MR	N	.33	Hansard et al. (1957)
Calcium chloride, dihyd FG	71[b]	-	True abs	-	N	.25-1.11	Goetsch and Owens (1985)
Calcium carbonate RG	40[b]	-	True abs	-	N	.33	Hansard et al. (1957)
Calcium carbonate RG	51[b]	-	True abs	-	N	.33	Hansard et al. (1957)
Calcium carbonate RG	100	Calcium carbonate	True abs	MR	N	.33	Hansard et al. (1957)
Calcium carbonate RG	100	Calcium carbonate	True abs	MR	N	.33	Hansard et al. (1957)
Calcium carbonate RG	85[b]	-	True abs	-	N	.25-1.11	Goetsch and Owens (1985)
Calcite flow	49[b]	-	True abs	-	N	1.0-1.6	Wohlt et al. (1986)
Dicalcium phosphate RG	126	Calcium carbonate	True abs	MR	N	.33	Hansard et al. (1957)
Dicalcium phosphate	125	Calcium carbonate	True abs	MR	N	.33	Hansard et al. (1957)
Dicalcium phosphate	56[b]	-	App abs	-	N	NG	Agrawal and Talapatra (1971)
Dicalcium phosphate FG	116	Calcium carbonate	True abs	MR	N	.33	Hansard et al. (1957)
Dicalcium phosphate FG	124	Calcium carbonate	True abs	MR	N	.33	Hansard et al. (1957)
Defluorinated phosphate	108	Calcium carbonate	True abs	MR	N	.33	Hansard et al. (1957)
Defluorinated phosphate	100	Calcium carbonate	True abs	MR	N	.33	Hansard et al. (1957)
Lespedeza, hay	98	Calcium carbonate	True abs	MR	N	.33	Hansard et al. (1957)

Table I. (continued)

Source	RV	Standard	Response criterion	Meth cal	Type diet	Added level, %	Reference
Lespedeza, hay	90	Calcium carbonate	True abs	MR	N	.33	Hansard et al. (1957)
Limestone	88	Calcium carbonate	True abs	MR	N	.33	Hansard et al. (1957)
Limestone	93	Calcium carbonate	True abs	MR	N	.33	Hansard et al. (1957)
Milk, dried skim	89[b]	-	True abs	-	SP	NG	Lengemann et al. (1957)
Milk, dried skim	23[b]	-	True abs	-	SP	NG	Lengemann et al. (1957)
Monocalcium phosphate RG	120	**Calcium carbonate**	**True abs**	**MR**	N	.33	**Hansard et al. (1957)**
Monocalcium phosphate RG	140	Calcium carbonate	True abs	MR	N	.33	Hansard et al. (1957)
Orchardgrass, hay	100	Calcium carbonate	True abs	MR	N	NG	Hansard et al. (1957)
Orchardgrass, hay	98	Calcium carbonate	True abs	MR	N	NG	Hansard et al. (1957)
Timothy and fescue, prefertilization	31[b]	-	App abs	-	N	.34-.95	Mudd (1970)
Timothy and fescue, post-fertilization (N)	39[b]	-	App abs	-	N	.34-.95	Mudd (1970)
Sheep							
Bromegrass, smooth	37[b]	-	App abs	-	N	.33	Powell et al. (1978)
Bromegrass	18[b]	-	App abs	-	N	1.1	Harmon and Britton (1983)
Calcium phytate	52[b]	-	True abs	-	SP	.24	Tillman and Brethour (1958)
Clover, white	24[b]	-	App abs	-	N	.87-1.54	Grace et al. (1974)

Fescue, tall	21[b]	-	App abs	-	N	.41	Powell et al. (1978)
Milk, sheep	96[b]	-	App abs	-	N	NG	Dillion and Scott (1979)
Monocalcium phosphate	49[b]	-	True abs	-	SP	.24	Tillman and Brethour (1958)
Orchardgrass	38[b]	-	App abs	-	N	.35	Powell et al. (1978)
Orchardgrass, hay	10[b]	-	App abs	-	N	.45	Giduck and Fontenot (1987)
Poultry manure	**2[h]**	**-**	**App abs**	**-**	**N**	**15.5 g/day**	**Ben-Ghedalia et al. (1982)**
Ryegrass, perennial	42[b]	-	App abs	-	N	.39	Powell et al. (1978)
Ryegrass, perennial	22[b]	-	App abs	-	N	.87-1.54	Grace et al. (1974)
Ryegrass, short rotation	32[b]	-	App abs	-	N	.87-1.54	Grace et al. (1974)
Soybean meal	15[h]	-	App abs	-	N	6.27 g/day	Ben-Ghedalia et al. (1982)
Goats							
Alfalfa, full-bloom	47[b]	-	True abs	-	N	.9-1.10	Fredeen (1989)
Alfalfa, vegetative stage	**56[b]**	**-**	**True abs**	**-**	**N**	**.9-1.10**	**Fredeen (1989)**
Horses							
Alfalfa, high oxalate	76[h]	-	True abs	-	N	.15	Hintz et al. (1984)
Alfalfa, low oxalate	80[h]	-	True abs	-	N	.15	Hintz et al. (1984)
Bone meal, steamed	71[b]	-	True abs	-	N	.30-.44	Hintz and Schryver (1972)
Calcium oxalate	6[b]	-	Ret	-	N	.17-.27	Blaney et al. (1981)
Dicalcium phosphate	73[h]	-	True abs	-	N	.30-.44	Hintz and Schryver (1972)
Limestone, ground	67[b]	-	True abs	-	N	.15	Hintz and Schryver (1972)

Table I. (continued)

Rats

Source	RV	Standard	Response criterion	Meth cal	Type diet	Added level, %	Reference
Alfalfa	85[b]	-	Ret	-	SP	1.43-1.73	Armstrong and Thomas (1952)
Alfalfa	85[b]	-	Ret	-	N	NG	Armstrong et al. (1957)
Alfalfa, dry, ground	76[b]	-	Ret	-	SP	NG	Sur and Subrahmanyan (1952)
Bread, white	99	Calcium sulfate	Bone Ca	SR	SP	2.01-2.72	Ranhotra et al. (1981)
Calcium lactate	104	Milk, dried skim	App abs	MR	N	1.7-4.4	Greger et al. (1987)
Calcium carbonate	102	Milk, dried skim	App abs	MR	N	1.7-4.4	Greger et al. (1987)
Calcium carbonate	27[b]	-	True abs	-	SP	NG	Weaver et al. (1987)
Calcium carbonate and magnesium	81	Milk, dried skim	App abs	MR	N	1.7-4.4	Greger et al. (1987)
Casein	91[b]	-	App abs	-	SP	.05	Greger et al. (1989)
Casein	85[b]	-	App abs	-	SP	.05	Greger et al. (1989)
Casein-lactose hydrolized milk	70[b]	-	App abs	-	SP	.05	Greger et al. (1989)
Chelated calcium	98	Milk, dried skim	App abs	MR	N	1.7-4.4	Greger et al. (1987)
Chelated calcium and magnesium	90	Milk, dried skim	App abs	MR	N	1.7-4.4	Greger et al. (1987)
Calcium carbonate	100	CaCO₃	Bone Ca	MR	SP	.15-.18	Poneros and Erdman (1988)
Calcium carbonate	100	CaCO₃	Bone Ca	MR	SP	.15-.18	Poneros-Schneier and Erdman (1989)

108

Calcium chloride	30[b]	-	True abs	-	SP	NG	Weaver et al. (1987)
Calcium oxalate	3[b]	-	True abs	-	SP	NG	Weaver et al. (1987)
Clover, red	83[b]	-	Ret	-	SP	1.43-1.73	Armstrong and Thomas (1952)
Clover, red	80[b]	-	Ret	-	N	NG	Armstrong et al. (1957)
Clover, white	79[b]	-	Ret	-	SP	1.45-1.73	Armstrong and Thomas (1952)
Dicalcium phosphate	82[b]	-	App abs	-	SP	.05	Greger et al. (1989)
Dicalcium phosphate	93	Milk, dried skim	App abs	MR	N	1.7-4.4	Greger et al. (1987)
Kale	29[b]	-	True abs	-	SP	NG	Weaver et al. (1987)
Limestone, dolomitic	66[b]	-	App abs	-	SP	.05	Greger et al. (1989)
Limestone, dolomitic	81	Milk, dried skim	App abs	MR	N	1.7-4.4	Greger et al. (1987)
Milk	74[b]	-	App abs	-	SP	.05	Greger et al. (1989)
Milk, dry or milk, dried/skim	81[b]	-	Ret	-	SP	NG	Sur and Subrahmanyan (1952)
Milk, dry, non-fat or milk, dried/skim	54[b]	-	App abs	-	N	1.7-4.4	Greger et al. (1987)
Milk, dry, non-fat or milk, dried/skim	77[b]	-	App abs	-	N	1.7-4.4	Greger et al. (1987)
Milk, dry, non-fat or milk, dried/skim	95	Calcium carbonate	B ash & Bone Ca	MR	SP	.15-.18	Poneros-Schneier and Erdman (1989)
Milk, dry, non-fat or milk, dried/skim	95	Calcium carbonate	Bone Ca	MR	SP	.15-.18	Poneros and Erdman (1988)

Table I. (continued)

Source	RV	Standard	Response criterion	Meth cal	Type diet	Added level, %	Reference
Milk, dry, non-fat or milk dried/skim	100	Calcium carbonate	Bone Ca	MR	SP	.15-.18	Poneros-Schneier and Erdman (1989)
Milk, dry, non-fat or milk, dried/skim	113	Calcium sulfate	Bone Ca	SR	SP	2.01-2.72	Ranhotra et al. (1981)
Milk, dry, non-fat or milk, dried/skim	100	Calcium carbonate	Bone ash & bone Ca	MR	SP	.15-.18	Poneros-Schneier and Erdman (1989)
Milk, lactose - hydrolized	60[b]	-	App abs	-	SP	.05	Greger et al. (1989)
Orchardgrass	69[b]	-	Ret	-	N	NG	Armstrong et al. (1957)
Oyster shell	102	Milk, dried skim	App abs	MR	N	1.7-4.4	Greger et al. (1987)
Oyster shell and magnesium	92	Milk, dried skim	App abs	MR	N	1.7-4.4	Greger et al. (1987)
Ryegrass, perennial	77[b]	-	Ret	-	N	NG	Armstrong et al. (1957)
Sesame seeds	65	Calcium carbonate	Bone ash & bone Ca	MR	SP	.15-.18	Poneros and Erdman (1989)
Sesame seeds	65	Calcium carbonate	Bone Ca	MR	SP	.15-.18	Poneros-Schneier and Erdman (1989)
Spinach	47	Calcium carbonate	Bone Ca	MR	SP	.15-.18	Poneros-Schneier and Erdman (1989)
Spinach	3[b]	-	True abs	-	SP	NG	Weaver et al. (1987)
Timothy	79[b]	-	Ret	-	N	NG	Armstrong et al. (1957)
Wheat bread, whole	104	Calcium sulfate	Bone Ca	SR	SP	2.01-2.72	Ranhotra et al. (1981)

110

| Wheat bread, whole | 95 | Calcium carbonate | Bone ash & bone Ca | MR | SP | .15-.18 | Poneros-Schneier and Erdman (1989) |

[a]Abbreviations can be found in Appendix I. Chemical formula for a compound given only if provided by the author; RG indicates reagent grade, FG indicates feed grade.

[b]Percentage absorption or retention, not relative value.

Table II. Relative bioavailability of supplemental calcium sources[a]

Source	Poultry	Swine	Cattle	Horses
Calcium carbonate	100	100	100	100
Aragonite	-	95 (1)	-	-
Bone meal	100 (1)	-	110 (3)	70 (1)
Calcium chloride	-	90 (2)	125 (2)	-
Calcium citrate	-	90 (1)	-	-
Calcium gluconate	100 (3)	-	-	-
Calcium oxalate	-	65 (1)	-	5 (1)
Calcium succinate	-	95 (1)	-	-
Calcium sulfate	95 (2)	95 (3)	-	-
Defluorinated phosphate	95 (2)	-	-	-
Dicalcium phosphate	-	-	110 (5)	75 (1)
Limestone	95 (3)	-	90 (2)	70 (1)
Limestone, dolomitic	65 (1)	80 (1)	-	-
Low fluorine rock phosphate	90 (1)	-	-	-
Marble dust	-	100 (1)	-	-
Monocalcium phosphate	-	-	130 (2)	-
Oystershell	100 (4)	100 (1)	-	-
Soft rock phosphate	70 (1)	-	-	-
Tricalcium phosphate	100 (1)	-	-	-

[a]Average values rounded to nearest "5" and expressed relative to response with calcium carbonate. Number of studies or samples involved indicated within parentheses. Sources are identified according to AAFCO (1994).

REFERENCES

Agrawal, B. L. and S. K. Talapatra. 1971. Biological availability of calcium in feedstuffs. V. Availability of calcium from mineral salts. *Indian J. Anim. Sci.* **41**:11.

Albanese, A. A., E. J. Lorenze, A. H. Edelson, A. Tarlow, E. H. Wein and L. Carroll. 1986. Effects of dietary calcium: phosphorus ratios on utilization of dietary calcium for bone synthesis in women 20-75 years. *Nutr. Rep. Int.* **33**:879.

Alder, A. J. and G. M. Berlyne. 1985. Duodenal aluminum absorption in the rat. Effect of vitamin D. *Am. J. Physiol.* **249**:G209.

Allen, V. G., J. P. Fontenot and S. H. Rahnema. 1990. Influence of aluminum citrate and citric acid on mineral metabolism in wether sheep. *J. Anim. Sci.* **68**:2496.

Armstrong, R. H. and B. Thomas. 1952. The availability of calcium in three legumes of grassland. *J. Agric. Sci.* **42**:454.

Armstrong, R. H., B. Thomas and D. G. Armstrong. 1957. The availability of calcium in three grasses. *J. Agric. Sci. Camb.* **49**:446.

Association of American Feed Control Officials (AAFCO). 1994. Official publication. AAFCO, Atlanta, GA.

Baker, D. H., D. E. Becker, A. H. Jensen and B. G. Harmon. 1967. Response of the weanling rat to alpha- or beta-lactose with or without an excess of dietary phopshorus. *J. Dairy Sci.* **50**:1314.

Ben-Ghedalia, D., H. Tagari, A. Geva and S. Zamwel. 1982. Availability of macroelements from a concentrate diet supplemented with soybean meal or poultry manure fed to sheep. *J. Dairy Sci.* **65**:1760.

Blair, R., P. R. English and W. Michie. 1965. Effect of calcium source on calcium retention in the young chick. *Br. Poult. Sci.* **6**:355.

Blaney, B. J., R. J. W. Gartner and R. A. McKenzie. 1981. The inability of horses to absorb calcium from calcium oxalate. *J. Agric. Sci. Camb.* **97**:639.

Boila, R. J. and G. D. Phillips. 1988. Effects of faunation, protein source and surgical modification of the intestinal tract upon flows of calcium, phosphorus, and magnesium in the digestive tract of sheep. *Can. J. Anim. Sci.* **68**:853.

Braithwaite, G. D. 1979. The effect of dietary intake of calcium and phosphorus on their absorption and retention by mature Ca-replete sheep. *J. Agric. Sci. Camb.* **92**:337.

Braithwaite, G. D. and Sh. Riazuddin. 1971. The effect of age and level of dietary calcium intake on calcium metabolism in sheep. *Br. J. Nutr.* **26**:215.

Brister R. D., S. S. Linton and C. R. Greger. 1981. Effects of dietary calcium sources and particle size on laying hen performance. *Poult. Sci.* **60**:2648.

Buchowski, M. J. and D. D. Miller. 1991. Lactose, calcium source and age affect calcium bioavailability in rats. *J. Nutr.* **121**:1746.

Buchowski, M. J., K. C. Sowizral, F. W. Lengemann, D. van Campen and D. D. Miller. 1989. A comparison of intrinsic and extrinsic tracer methods for estimating calcium bioavailability to rats from dairy foods. *J. Nutr.* **119**:228.

Burnell, T. W., G. L. Cromwell and T. S. Stahly. 1990. Effects of particle size on the biological availability of calcium and phosphorus in defluorinated phosphate for chicks. *Poult. Sci.* **69**:1110.

Chester-Jones, H., J. P. Fontenot and H. P. Veit. 1990. Physiological and pathological effects of feeding high levels of magnesium to steers. *J. Anim. Sci.* **68**:4400.

Chrisp, J. S., A. R. Sykes and N. D. Grace. 1989a. Kinetic aspects of calcium metabolism in lactating sheep offered herbages with different Ca concentrations and the effect of protein supplementation. *Br. J. Nutr.* **61**:45.

Chrisp, J. S., A. R. Sykes and N. D. Grace. 1989b. Faecal endogenous loss of calcium in young sheep. *Br. J. Nutr.* **61**:59.

Combs, G. E. and H. D. Wallace. 1962. Growth and digestibility studies with young pigs fed various levels and sources of calcium. *J. Anim. Sci.* **21**:734.

Cromwell, G. L. 1989. An evaluation of the requirements and biological availability of calcium and phosphorus for swine. *In* "Proceedings of the TexasGulf Nutrition Symposium." Raleigh, NC.

Cromwell, G. L., T. S. Stahly and H. J. Monegue. 1983. Bioavailability of the calcium and phosphorus in dehydrated alfalfa meal for growing pigs. *J. Anim. Sci.* **57**(Suppl. 1):242 [Abstract].

Cymbaluk, N. F., G. I. Christison and D. H. Leach. 1989. Nutrient utilization by limit-and ad libitum-fed growing horses. *J. Anim. Sci.* **67**:414.

Damron, B. L., T. L. Andrews and R. H. Harms. 1974. Effect of diet composition upon the performance of laying hens receiving Curacao Island phosphate. *Poult. Sci.* **53**:99.

DeLuca, H. F. 1974. Vitamin D: The vitamin and the hormone. *Fed. Proc.* **33**:2211.

Dillon, J. and D. Scott. 1979. Digesta flow and mineral absorption in lambs before and after weaning. *J. Agric. Sci. Camb.* **92**:289.

Dilworth, B. C. and E. J. Day. 1964. Phosphorus availability studies with feed grade phosphates. *Poult. Sci.* **43**:1039.

Edwards, H. M. and G. M. Lanza. 1981. Calcium and phosphorus requirement studies with broiler and leghorn type chickens. *Poult. Sci.* **60**:1650 [Abstract].

Fredeen, A. H. 1989. Effect of maturity of alfalfa (*Medicago sativa*) at harvest on calcium absorption in goats. *Can. J. Anim. Sci.* **69**:365.

Giduck, S. A. and J. P. Fontenot. 1987. Utilization of magnesium and other macrominerals in sheep supplemented with different readily-fermentable carbohydrates. *J. Anim. Sci.* **65**:1667.

Goetsch A. L. and F. N. Owens. 1985. Effects of calcium sources and level on site of digestion and calcium levels in the digestive tract of cattle fed high-concentrate diets. *J. Anim. Sci.* **61**:995.

Grace, N. D., M. J. Ulyatt and J. C. MaCrae. 1974. Quantitative digestion of fresh herbage by sheep. III. The movement of Mg, Ca, P, K, and Na in the digestive tract. *J. Agric. Sci. Camb.* **82**:321.

Greene, L. W., B. J. May, G. T. Scheling and F. M. Byers. 1988. Site and extent of apparent magnesium and calcium absorption in steers fed monensin. *J. Anim. Sci.* **66**:2987.

Greger, J. L., C. M. Gutkowski and R. R. Khazen. 1989. Interactions of lactose with calcium, magnesium, and zinc in rats. *J. Nutr.* **119**:1691.

Greger, J. L., C. E. Krzykowski, R. R. Khazen and C. L. Krashoc. 1987. Mineral utilization by rats fed various commercially available calcium supplements or milk. *J. Nutr.* **117**:717.

Gutierrez, O., C. M. Geerken and A. Diaz. 1984. Apparent digestibility and retention of Ca and P in calves fed forage diets alone or supplemented with dicalcium phosphate. *Cuban J. Agric. Sci.* **18**:157.

Hansard, S. L., C. L. Comar and M. P. Plumlee. 1954. The effects of age upon calcium utilization and maintenance requirements in the bovine. *J. Anim. Sci.* **13**:25.

Hansard, S. L., H. M. Crowder and W. A. Lyke. 1957. The biological availability of calcium in feeds for cattle. *J. Anim. Sci.* **16**:437.

Harmon, D. L. and R. A. Britton. 1983. Balance and urinary excretion of calcium, magnesium and phosphorus in response to high concentrate feeding and lactate infusion in lambs. *J. Anim, Sci.* **57**:1306.

Harrison, H. E. 1959. Factors influencing calcium absorption. *Fed. Proc.* **18**:1085.

Hertoghe, J .J., S. B. Phinney and M. E. Rubini. 1967. Intestinal absorption and body retention of ^{47}Ca in rats: Evaluation of the method. *J. Nutr.* **93**:454.

Hibbs, J. W. and H. R. Conrad. 1983. The relation of calcium and phosphorus intake and digestion and the effects of vitamin D feeding on the utilization of calcium and phosphorus by lactating dairy cows. *Ohio Agric. Res. Dev. Center Res. Bull.* **1150**.

Hintz, H. F. and H. F. Schryver. 1972. Availability to ponies of calcium and phosphorus from various supplements. *J. Anim. Sci.* **34**:979.

Hintz, H. F., H. F. Schryver, J. Doty, C. Lakin and R. A. Zimmerman. 1984. Oxalic acid content of alfalfa hays and its influence on the availability of calcium, phosphorus and magnesium to ponies. J. Anim. Sci. **58**:939.

Horst, R. L., H. F. DeLuca and N. A. Jorgensen. 1978. The effect of age on calcium absorption and accumulation of 1,25-dihydroxyvitamin D_3 in intestinal mucosa of rats. *Metab. Bone Dis. Relat. Res.* **1**:29.

Hunter, J. E., R. A. Dutcher and H. C. Knandel. 1933. Relative utilization of calcium from calcium carbonate and calcium gluconate by chickens. *Proc. Soc. Exp. Biol.* **31**:70.

Hurwitz, S. 1964. Bone composition and Ca^{45} retention in fowl as influenced by egg formation. *Am. J. Physiol.* **206**:198.

Hurwitz, S. and A. Bar. 1969. Intestinal calcium absorption in the laying hen, and its importance in calcium homeostasis. *Am. J. Clin. Nutr.* **22**:391.

Hurwitz, S. and A. Bar. 1965. Absorption of calcium and phosphorus along the gastrointestinal tract of the laying fowl as influenced by dietary calcium and egg shell formation. *J. Nutr.* **86**:433.

Hurwitz, S. and N. T. Rand. 1965. Utilization of calcium from calcium sulfate by chicks and laying hens. *Poult. Sci.* **44**:177.

Kaetzel, D. M., Jr. and J. H. Soares, Jr. 1979. Effects of cholecalciferol steroids on bone and eggshell calcification in Japanese quail. *J. Nutr.* **109**:1601.

Kim, Y. S., S. S. Sun and K. H. Myung. 1985a. A comparison of true available calcium with apparent available calcium values using 6 calcium supplements for breeding Japanese quail. *Korean J. Anim. Sci.* **27**:297.

Kim, Y. S., S. S. Sun and K. H. Myung. 1985b. The effects of level and method of calcium input, age, and particle size on true available calcium value in breeding Japanese quail. *Korean J. Anim. Sci.* **27**:286.

Kirk, D. J., L. W. Greene, G. T. Schelling and F. M. Byers. 1985. Effects of monensin on Mg, Ca, P, and Zn metabolism and tissue concentrations in lambs. *J. Anim. Sci.* **60**:1485.

Kuhle, H. J., Jr., D. P. Holder and T. W. Sullivan. 1977. Influence of dietary calcium level, source and particle size on performance of laying chickens. *Poult. Sci.* **56**:605.

Kuznetsov, S. G., B. D. Kal'nitskii and A. P. Bataeva. 1987. Biological availability of calcium from chemical compounds for young pigs. *Soviet Agric. Sci.* **3**:48.

Leach, R. M., Jr. 1985. Steel making slag as a source of dietary calcium for the laying hen. *Nutr. Rep. Int.* **32**:475.

Lengemann, F.W ., C. L. Comar and R. H. Wasserman. 1957. Absorption of calcium and strontium from milk and nonmilk diets. *J. Nutr.* **61**:571.

Lofton, J. T. and J. H. Soares, Jr. 1986. The effects of vitamin D_3 on leg abnormalities in broilers. *Poult. Sci.* **65**:749.

Lomba, F., G. Chauvaux, E. Teller, L. Lengele and V. Bienfet. 1978. Calcium digestibility in cows as influenced by the excess of alkaline ions over stable acid ions in their diets. *Br. J. Nutr.* **39**:425.

Lonnerdal, B., A. Sandberg, B. Sanstrom and C. Kunz. 1989. Inhibitory effects of phytic acid and other inositol phosphates on zinc and calcium absorption in suckling rats. *J. Nutr.* **119**:211.

Lopes, H. O. S. and T. W. Perry. 1986. Effect of dietary phosphorus and roughage levels on calcium, magnesium and potassium utilization by sheep. *J. Anim. Sci.* **63**:1983.

Martz, F. A., A. T. Belo, M. F. Weiss and R. L. Belyea. 1990. True absorption of calcium and phosphorus from alfalfa and corn silage when fed to lactating cows. *J. Dairy Sci.* **73**:1288.

McCampbell, C. W. and C. E. Aubel. 1934. Calcium carbonate vs. calcium sulphate in swine rations. *Am. Soc. Anim. Prod.* **34**:189.

McKenzie, R. A., B. J. Blaney and R. J. W. Gartner. 1981. The effect of dietary oxalate on calcium, phosphorus and magnesium balances in horses. *J. Agric. Sci. Camb.* **97**:69.

McNaughton, J. L., B. C. Dilworth and E. J. Day. 1974. Effect of particle size on the utilization of calcium supplements by the chick. *Poult. Sci.* **53**:1024.

Meyer, R., R. C. Baker and M. L. Scott. 1973. Effects of hen egg shell and other calcium sources upon egg shell strength and ultrastructure. *Poult. Sci.* **52**:949.

Miur, F. V., R. W. Gerry and P. C. Harris. 1975. Effect of various sources and sizes of calcium carbonate on egg quality and laying house performance of Red x rock sex-linked females. *Poult. Sci.* **54**:1898.

Mudd, A. J. 1970. The influence of heavily fertilized grass on mineral metabolism of dairy cows. *J. Agric. Sci. Camb.* **74**:11.

Moser, R. L., E. R. Peo, Jr., T. D. Crenshaw and P. J. Cunningham. 1977. Effect of dietary lactose on gain, feed conversion, blood, bone and intestinal parameters in postweaning rats and swine. *J. Anim. Sci.* **51**:89.

Myung, K. H., S. Sunn, and Y. S. Kim. 1983. Studies on the calcium bioavailability by the true available mineral methodology. 1. Measurement of calcium requirements in breeding Japanese quail. *Korean J. Anim. Sci.* **25**:680.

Negi, S. S. 1971. Calcium assimilation in relation to metabolism of soluble and insoluble oxalates in the ruminant system: A reappraisal. *Indian J. Anim. Sci.* **41**:913.

Nelson, T. S. 1967. The utilization of phytate phosphorus by poultry - A review. *Poult. Sci.* **46**:862.

Nelson, T. S. and L. K. Kirby. 1987. The calcium binding properties of natural phytate in chick diets. *Nutr. Rep. Int.* **35**:949.

Nelson, T. S., T. R. Shieh, R. J. Wodzinski and J. H. Ware. 1968. The availability of phytate phosphorus in soybean meal before and after treatment with a mold phytase. *Poult. Sci.* **47**:1842.

Norman, A. W. 1987. Studies on the vitamin D endocrine system in the avian . *J. Nutr.* **117**:797.

Pond, W. G., J. T. Yen, W. E. Wheeler and D. A. Hill. 1982. Calcium bioavailability from limestones of differing particle size and rate of reactivity for growing nonruminants. *Nutr. Rep. Int.* **26**:1027.

Poneros, A. G. and J. W. Erdman, Jr. 1988. Bioavailability of calcium for tofu, tortillas, nonfat dry milk and mozzarella cheese in rats: Effect of supplemental ascorbic acid. *J. Food Sci.* **53**:208.

Poneros-Schneier, A. G. and J. W. Erdman, Jr. 1989. Bioavailability of calcium from sesame seeds, almond powder, whole wheat bread, spinach and nonfat dry milk in rats. *J. Food Sci.* **54**:150.

Powell, K., R. L. Reid and J. A. Balasko. 1978. Performance of lambs on perennial ryegrass, smooth bromegrass, orchardgrass and tall fescue pastures. II. Mineral utilization, *in vitro* digestibility and chemical composition of herbage. *J. Anim. Sci.* **46**:1503.

Ranhotra G. S., J. A. Celroth, F. A. Torrence, M. A. Bocks and G. L. Winterringer. 1981. Bread (white and whole wheat) and nonfat dry milk sources of bioavailable calcium for rats. *J. Nutr.* **111**:2081.

Rayssiquier, Y. and C. Poncet. 1980. Effect of lactose supplement on digestion of lucerne hay by sheep. II. Absorption of magnesium and calcium in the stomach. *J. Anim. Sci.* **51**:186.

Reid, B. L. and C. W. Weber. 1976. Calcium availability and trace mineral composition of feed grade calcium supplements. *Poult. Sci.* **55**:600.

Roland, D. A., Sr. 1986. Eggshell quality: Oystershell versus limestone and the importance of particle size or solubility of calcium source. *World Poult. Sci.* **42**:166.

Roland, D. A., Sr. and R. H. Harms. 1973. Calcium metabolism in the laying hen. 5. Effect of various sources and sizes of calcium carbonate on shell quality. *Poult. Sci.* **52**:369.

Roland, D. A.,Sr., D. R. Sloan and R. H. Harms. 1974. Effects of various levels of calcium with and without pullet-sized limestone on shell quality. *Poult Sci.* **53**:662.

Ross, R. D., G. L. Cromwell and T. S. Stahly. 1984. Effects of source and particle size on the biological availability of calcium in calcium supplements for growing pigs. *J. Anim. Sci.* **59**:125.

Roush, W. B., M. Mylet, J. L. Rosenberger and J. Derr. 1986. Investigation of calcium and available phosphorus requirements for laying hens by response surface methodology. *Poult. Sci.* **65**:964.

Schwartz, R., M. Topley and J. B. Russell. 1988. Effect of tricarballylic acid, a nonmetabolizable rumen fermentation product of trans-aconitic acid, on Mg, Ca and Zn utilization of rats. *J. Nutr.* **118**:183

Scott, M. L., S. J. Hull and P. A. Mullenhoff. 1971. The calcium requirements of laying hens and effects of dietary oyster shell upon egg shell quality. *Poult. Sci.* **50**:1055.

Sibbald, I. R. 1982. Measurement of mineral bioavailability: Extension of true metabolizable energy methodology. *Poult. Sci.* **61**:485.

Soares, J. H. 1987. Metabolic aspects of calcification in avians. *J. Nutr.* **117**:783.

Sticker, L. S., L. D. Bunting, W. E. Wyatt and G. W. Wolfrom. 1991. Effect of supplemental lysocellin and tetronasin on growth, ruminal and blood metabolites and ruminal proteolytic activity in steers grazing ryegrass. *J. Anim. Sci.* **69**:4273.

Stillmak, S. J. and M. L. Sunde. 1971. The use of high magnesium limestone in the diet of the laying hen. *Poult. Sci.* **50**:564.

Sur, B. K. and V. Subrahmanyan. 1952. Availability of calcium in lucerne and its value in nutrition. *Indian J. Med. Res.* **40**:481.

Swartzman, J. A., H. F. Hintz and H. F. Schryver. 1978. Inhibition of calcium absorption in ponies fed diets containing oxalic acid. *Am. J. Vet. Res.* **39**:1621.

Sykes, A. R. and K. G. Geenty. 1986. Calcium and phosphorus balances of lactating ewes at pasture. *J. Agric. Sci. Camb.* **106**:369.

Tillman, A. D. and J. R. Brethour. 1958. Utilization of phytin phosphorus by sheep. *J. Anim. Sci.* **17**:104.

Tsang, C. P. W., A. A. Grunder, J. H. Soares, Jr. and R. Narbaitz. 1988. Effects of cholecalciferol or calcium deficiency on oestrogen metabolism in the laying hen. *Br. Poult. Sci.* **29**:753.

Waldroup, P. W., C. B. Ammerman and R. H. Harms. 1964. The utilization by the chick of calcium from different sources. *Poult. Sci.* **43**:212.

Ward, G., R. C. Dobson and J. R. Dunham. 1972. Influences of calcium and phosphorus intakes, vitamin D supplement, and lactation on calcium and phosphorus balances. *J. Dairy Sci.* **55**:768.

Ward, G., L. H. Harbers and J. J. Blaha. 1979. Calcium-containing crystals in alfalfa: Their fate in cattle. *J. Dairy Sci.* **62**:715.

Ward, G., L. H. Harbers, A. Kahrs and A. Dayton. 1984. Availability of calcium from alfalfa for chicks. *Poult. Sci.* **63**:82.

Watkins, R. M., B. C. Dilworth and E. J. Day. 1977. Effect of calcium supplement particle size and source on the performance of laying chickens. *Poult. Sci.* **56**:1641.

Weaver, C. M., B. R. Martin, J. S. Ebner and C. A. Krueger. 1987. Oxalic acid decreases calcium absorption in rats. *J. Nutr.* **117**:1903.

Whittemore, C. T., W. C. Smith and A. Thompson. 1972. The availability and absorption of calcium and phosphorus in the young growing pig. *Anim. Prod.* **15**:265.

Wohlt, J. E., D. E. Ritter and J. L. Evans. 1986. Calcium sources for milk production in holstein cows via changes in dry matter intake, mineral utilization, and mineral source buffering potential. *J. Dairy Sci.* **69**:2815.

Yoshida, M. and H. Hoshii. 1982a. Re-evaluation of requirement of calcium and available phosphorus for starting meat-type chicks. *Jpn. Poult. Sci.* **19**:101.

Yoshida, M. and H. Hoshii. 1982b. Re-evaluation of requirement of calcium and available phosphorus for starting egg-type chicks. *Jpn. Poult. Sci.* **19**:93.

Yoshida, M. and H. Hoshii. 1982c. Relationship between ash content of the toe and hardness of the tibia bone of meat-type chicks. *Jpn. Poult. Sci.* **19**:126.

6

COBALT BIOAVAILABILITY

Pamela R. Henry

Department of Animal Science
University of Florida
Gainesville, Florida

I. INTRODUCTION

Gastrointestinal microflora of livestock synthesize vitamin B_{12} and its analogs from dietary cobalt, and for ruminants and certain other animals the quantities synthesized can be great enough to meet the host animal's vitamin B_{12} requirement. Nonruminants, in general, require dietary vitamin B_{12}. Vitamin B_{12} contains approximately 4% cobalt, and Smith (1987) recently reviewed the synthesis and metabolism of the vitamin and its analogs. Signs of cobalt deficiency in ruminants include loss of appetite, weight loss, weakness, emaciation, and anemia. A deficiency of the element is recognized worldwide among grazing ruminants (Underwood, 1977); thus, there is a widespread need for the use of supplemental cobalt in livestock production.

II. BIOAVAILABILITY STUDIES

A. *In Vitro* Measures of Bioavailability

Cobalt may be the one mineral element for which an *in vitro* assay may be more indicative of true availability than *in vivo* methods because vitamin B_{12} production by the microflora is the actual physiological response to cobalt. Assays that use vitamin B_{12} activity as a response criterion should be considered carefully. The determination of vitamin B_{12} exclusive of its various analogs, which include B_{12}-Factor (III), pseudovitamin B_{12}, Factor A, Factor B, and Factor C (Smith, 1987), is difficult. Of the microbiological assays, only that using *Ochromonas malhamensis* is specific for vitamin B_{12}, whereas those using *Lactobacillus leichmannii*, *Euglena*

BIOAVAILABILITY OF NUTRIENTS FOR ANIMALS:
AMINO ACIDS, MINERALS, AND VITAMINS
Copyright © 1995 by Academic Press, Inc.

gracilis, and *Escherichia coli* also indicate activity for some of the analogs as well (Ford, 1953; Guttman, 1963). The early assays using isotope dilution required rigorous isolation and purification of vitamin B_{12} (Guttman, 1963). More recently, liver and serum vitamin B_{12} concentrations in lambs have been determined with a competitive protein-binding assay that utilized $^{57}Co\text{-}B_{12}$ as the tracer (Daugherty *et al.*, 1986). In the assay, purified porcine intrinsic factor was used as the vitamin B_{12}-binding protein and analogs were separated during preparation (Kolhouse *et al.*, 1978). However, only one report that attempted to use this technique was found.

Allen (1986) measured vitamin B_{12} production during continuous ruminal cultures that had been supplemented with cobalt. Vitamin B_{12} flows were similar (73, 72, 71, and 65 mg/day), from fermentors treated as control (no added cobalt) or 1 mg cobalt/kg DM as cobalt glucoheptonate, cobalt dextrolactate, and cobalt sulfate. Thus, no measurable response due to added cobalt was demonstrated.

B. *In Vivo* Measures of Bioavailability

Few studies exist in which comparisons in bioavailability among cobalt sources were made. In general, studies with cobalt sources have consisted of supplementing deficient animals with a single source, possibly at a few added levels, often under field conditions. Several authors have suggested that various cobalt compounds would be suitable as supplemental sources without providing research data. Smith and Loosli (1957) and Ammerman and Miller (1972) suggested that cobalt sulfate, chloride, nitrate, or carbonate were appropriate supplemental sources of the element. Latteur (1962) suggested that cobalt sulfate, chloride, and nitrate were suitable, but that phosphate was not.

Toxicity of a mineral element is related to its bioavailability and Ely *et al.* (1948) fed calves 500 mg of cobalt daily as cobalt chloride, sulfate, and carbonate for 30 days. They concluded that the three forms were equally toxic and therefore equally available based on their ability to induce anorexia. Loss of appetite is also a sign of cobalt deficiency. When cobalt sulfate or cobalt carbonate was administered to cobalt-deficient sheep, either by oral administration in a water solution or by capsule twice weekly, the length of time required for appetite recovery was similar (Keener *et al.*, 1950).

Andrews *et al.* (1966) supplemented cobalt-deficient sheep with 300 mg of cobalt in capsules monthly as anhydrous cobalt sulfate or cobalt oxide predominantly as Co_3O_4. Growth and serum and liver vitamin B_{12} concentrations were similar for the two sources.

No studies were found in which radiolabeled [^{60}Co]-cobalt sources were compared, but absorption of several labeled cobalt compounds has been reported. Radiolabeled cobalt administered orally as carbonate (Keener *et al.*, 1951), chloride

(Monroe *et al.*, 1952), and oxide as Co_2O_3 (Mittler, 1954) were all absorbed and found in tissues. Mittler (1954) postulated that cobalt oxide reacted with HCl in the digestive tract to form chloride, which was readily absorbed.

Ammerman *et al.* (1982) suggested liver accumulation of cobalt as an indicator of its solubility in the rumen and thus its availability to ruminal microorganisms for vitamin B_{12} synthesis. Tissue cobalt concentrations are not necessarily correlated with vitamin B_{12} activity but the more soluble sources, however, may be more readily available to ruminal microflora and also may be absorbed more rapidly and accumulated by various tissues. In sheep fed for 20 days, liver cobalt concentrations were lower in animals fed 40 ppm cobalt as cobaltous oxide (CoO) or cobaltic-cobaltous oxide (Co_3O_4) than in those fed cobaltous carbonate ($CoCO_3$) and cobaltous sulfate ($CoSO_4 \cdot 7H_2O$; Ammerman *et al.*, 1982). Cobalt glucoheptonate averaged 86% as available as $CoSO_4 \cdot 7H_2O$ based on liver and kidney cobalt concentrations in sheep fed 20, 40, or 60 ppm cobalt from either source for 16 days (Kawashima *et al.*, 1989) (Tables I and II).

Mills (1987) discussed the use of physiological responses to vitamin B_{12} that may be used to assess cobalt status and may also be applicable to cobalt bioavailability studies. Adenosyl-cobalamin serves as a cofactor for the enzyme methylmalonyl CoA mutase, which is necessary for the conversion of propionate to succinate. A rise in plasma methylmalonate seems to be a useful indicator of physiologically - marginal cobalt intake; however, it can be influenced by variations in normal ruminal propionate supply (McMurray *et al.*, 1985). Cobalamin is also a cofactor for tetrahydrofolate methyltransferase, which is involved in methyl group transfer reactions in which methyltetrahydrofolate and homocysteine are substrates (Mills, 1987). A secondary consequence of the failure of this enzyme is a depletion of tissue tetrahydrofolate which, in turn, inhibits the breakdown of formiminoglutamic acid, a normal metabolite of histidine. Increased urinary formiminoglutamic acid may also be a useful indicator of early cobalt deficiency (Gawthorne, 1968). Urinary collections under pasture conditions to determine early deficiency problems are difficult at best, but this method may have application for determining availability of supplemental sources when animals can be held in metabolism cages.

Cobalt has also been supplied to ruminant animals in the form of cobalt oxide pellets as described by Dewey *et al.* (1958). These pellets can supply cobalt for extended periods; however, they can be regurgitated from the reticulorumen and lost, and sometimes become coated with calcium phosphate which reduces their effectiveness. A more recent method for providing slow release of cobalt in the rumen is a soluble glass pellet which can also provide other trace elements (Allen *et al.*, 1978; Judson *et al.*, 1988). Also, boluses containing multiple trace elements including cobalt sulfate and prepared under pressure have been an effective source of cobalt for cattle (Ritchie *et al.*, 1991).

III. FACTORS INFLUENCING BIOAVAILABILITY

A. Dietary Factors

Dietary factors that seem to have the greatest effect on ruminal production of vitamin B_{12} are cobalt concentration, roughage content of the diet, and total feed intake (Sutton and Elliot, 1972; Hedrich *et al.*, 1973; Allen, 1986). Increasing cobalt and roughage:concentrate ratio or decreasing digestible DM intake increased production of vitamin B_{12} by sheep ruminal microflora. There was no difference in the total cobalt excretion by sheep given [^{60}Co]Cl$_2$ via capsule or ^{60}Co as an intrinsic label on alfalfa or timothy hay (Looney *et al.*, 1976). Sheep fed alfalfa hay excreted radioactive cobalt more rapidly but retained more in the body 11 days after administration than sheep fed timothy hay regardless of whether the cobalt dose was given orally by capsule or as intrinsic label on the forage.

Dietary addition of inorganic sulfate or cyanide in sheep decreased liver cobalt stores, but added dietary molybdenum increased liver cobalt (Spais *et al.*, 1966). It has been suggested that iron and cobalt share a common intestinal transport pathway governed by the same mechanism (Smith, 1987).

Additional dietary cysteine and methionine alleviated the growth depression in chicks brought about by high dietary cobalt (250 ppm) and decreased the accumulation of cobalt in liver and kidney (Southern and Baker, 1981).

IV. SUMMARY

Very few critical tests of bioavailability of cobalt sources for ruminants have been made. The carbonate, chloride, sulfate, nitrate, and glucoheptonate forms of cobalt have been indicated to be effective supplemental sources of cobalt for ruminants but not always with support of comparative data. When compared with the sulfate form, the oxides as either Co_3O_4 or CoO were not well absorbed by sheep when tissue accumulation of cobalt was used as an indicator of utilization. Orally administered heavy pellets made of cobalt oxide and clay, which remain in the reticulorumen for several months have been effective in supplying cobalt to sheep and cattle. Problems have been observed with loss through regurgitation and with coating of the pellets.

Table I. Bioavailability of cobalt sources for animals[a]

Source	RV	Standard	Response criterion	Meth cal	Type diet	Added level, ppm	Reference
Sheep							
Cobaltous carbonate RG ($CoCO_3$)	98	Cobaltous sulfate RG ($CoSO_4 \cdot 7H_2O$)	Liv Co	SC	N-.18 ppm	40	Ammerman et al. (1982)
$CoCO_3$ FG	122	$CoSO_4 \cdot 7H_2O$ RG	Liv Co	SC	N-.18 ppm	40	Ammerman et al. (1982)
Cobaltic-cobaltous oxide RG (Co_3O_4)	13	$CoSO_4 \cdot 7H_2O$ RG	Liv Co	SC	N-.18 ppm	40	Ammerman et al. (1982)
Co_3O_4 FG	31	$CoSO_4 \cdot 7H_2O$ RG	Liv Co	SC	N-.18 ppm	40	Ammerman et al. (1982)
Cobaltous oxide by-product, FG (CoO)	53	$CoSO_4 \cdot 7H_2O$ RG	Liv Co	SC	N-.18 ppm	40	Ammerman et al. (1982)
Cobalt glucoheptonate	80	$CoSO_4 \cdot 7H_2O$ RG	Liv Co	SR	N-.17 ppm	20, 40, 60	Kawashima et al. 1989
Cobalt glucoheptonate	92	$CoSO_4 \cdot 7H_2O$ RG	Kid Co	SR	N-.17 ppm	20, 40, 60	Kawashima et al. 1989

[a]Abbreviations can be found in Appendix I. Chemical formula for a compound given only if provided by the author; RG indicates reagent grade, FG indicates feed grade.

Table II. Relative bioavailability of supplemental cobalt sources[a]

Source	Sheep
Cobaltous sulfate	100
Cobalt chloride[b]	-
Cobalt glucoheptonate	85 (1)
Cobalt nitrate[b]	-
Cobaltic-cobaltous oxide (Co_3O_4)	20 (2)
Cobaltous carbonate	110 (2)
Cobaltous oxide (CoO)	55 (1)

[a]Average values rounded to nearest "5" and expressed relative to response obtained with cobaltous sulfate. Number of studies or samples involved indicated within parentheses.

[b]Indicated as effective source of cobalt. No comparative data available.

REFERENCES

Allen, M. J. 1986. Effects of cobalt supplementation on carbohydrate and nitrogen utilization by ruminal bacteria in continuous culture. M.S. Thesis. Univ. of Minnesota, St. Paul.

Allen W. M., B. F. Sansom, C. F. Drake and D. C. Davies. 1978. A new method for the prevention of trace element deficiencies. *Vet. Sci. Commun.* **2**:73.

Ammerman, C. B., P. R. Henry and P. R. Loggins. 1982. Cobalt bioavailability in sheep. *J. Anim. Sci.* **55**(Suppl. 1):403 [Abstract].

Ammerman, C. B. and S. M. Miller. 1972. Biological availability of minor mineral ions: A review. *J. Anim. Sci.* **35**:681.

Andrews, E. D., B. J. Stephenson, C. E. Isaacs and R. H. Register. 1966. The effects of large doses of soluble and insoluble forms of cobalt given at monthly intervals on cobalt deficiency disease in lambs. *N.Z. Vet. J.* **14**:191.

Daugherty, M. S., M. L. Galyean, D. M. Hallford and J. H. Hageman. 1986. Vitamin B_{12} and monensin effects on performance, liver and serum vitamin B_{12} concentrations and activity of propionate metabolizing hepatic enzymes in feedlot lambs. *J. Anim. Sci.* **62**:452.

Dewey, D. W., H. J. Lee and H. R. Marston. 1958. The provision of cobalt to ruminants by means of heavy pellets. *Nature* **181**:1367.

Ely, R. E., K. M. Dunn and C. F. Huffman. 1948. Cobalt toxicity in calves resulting from high oral administration. *J. Anim. Sci.* **7**:239.

Ford, J. E. 1953. The microbiological assay of "vitamin B_{12}." The specificity of the requirement of *Ochromonas malhamensis* for cyanocobalamin. *Br. J. Nutr.* **7**:299.

Gawthorne, J. M. 1968. Excretion of methylmalonic acid and formiminoglutamic acid during the induction and remission of vitamin B_{12} deficiency in sheep. *Aust. J. Biol. Sci.* **21**:789.

Guttman, H. N. 1963. Vitamin B_{12} and congeners. *In* " Analytical Microbiology" (F. Kavanagh, Ed.), Academic Press, New York.

Hedrich, M. F., J. M. Elliot and J. E. Lowe. 1973. Response in vitamin B_{12} production and absorption to increasing cobalt intake in the sheep. *J. Nutr.* **103**:1646.

Judson, G. J., T. H. Brown, B. R. Kempe and R. K. Turnbull. 1988. Trace element and vitamin B_{12} status of sheep given an oral dose of one, two or four soluble glass pellets containing copper, selenium and cobalt. *Aust. J. Exp. Agric.* **28**:299.

Kawashima, T., C. B. Ammerman and P. R. Henry. 1989. Tissue uptake of cobalt from glucoheptonate in sheep. *J. Anim. Sci.* **67**(Suppl. 1):503 [Abstract].

Keener, H. A., R. R. Baldwin and G. P. Percival. 1951. Cobalt metabolism studies with sheep. *J. Anim. Sci.* **10**:428.

Keener, H. A., G. P. Percival, G. H. Ellis and K. C. Beeson. 1950. A study of the function of cobalt in the nutrition of sheep. *J. Anim. Sci.* **9**:404.

Kolhouse, J. F., H. Kondo, N. C. Allen, E. Podell and R. H. Allen. 1978. Cobalamin analogues are present in human plasma and can mask cobalamin deficiency because current radioisotope dilution assays are not specific for true cobalamin. *N. Engl. J. Med.* **299**:785.

Latteur, J. P. 1962. " Cobalt Deficiencies and Sub-Deficiencies in Ruminants". Centre d'Information du Cobalt, Brussels, Belgium.

Looney, J. W., G. Gille, R. L. Preston, E. R. Graham and W. H. Pfander. 1976. Effects of plant species and cobalt intake upon cobalt utilization and ration digestibility by sheep. *J. Anim. Sci.* **42**:693.

McMurray, C. H., D. A. Rice, M. McLoughlin and W. J. Blanchflower. 1985. Cobalt deficiency and the potential of methylmalonic acid as a diagnostic and prognostic indicator. *In* "Trace Elements in Man and Animals - 5" (C. F. Mills, I. Bremner and J. K. Chesters, Eds.), p. 603. Commonwealth Agricultural Bureaux, Slough, U.K.

Mills, C. F. 1987. Biochemical and physiological indicators of mineral status in animals: Copper, cobalt and zinc. *J. Anim. Sci.* **65**:1702.

Mittler, S. 1954. Nutritional availability of cobaltic oxide, Co_2O_3. *Nature* **174**:88.

Monroe, R. A., H. E. Sauberlich, C. L. Comar and S. L. Hood. 1952. Vitamin B_{12} biosynthesis after oral and intravenous administration of inorganic Co^{60} to sheep. *Proc. Soc. Exp. Biol. Med.* **80**:250.

Ritchie, N. S., D. C. Lawson and J. J. Parkins. 1991. A multiple trace element and vitamin sustained release bolus for cattle. *In* "Trace Elements in Man and Animals-7" (B. Momcilovic, Ed.). Institute for Medical Research and Occupational Health, University of Zagreb, Zagreb, Croatia.

Smith, R. M. 1987. Cobalt. *In* "Trace Elements in Human and Animal Nutrition" (W. Mertz, Ed.), 5th ed. Academic Press, New York.

Smith, S. E. and J. K. Loosli. 1957. Cobalt and vitamin B_{12} in ruminant nutrition. A review. *J. Dairy Sci.* **40**:1215.

Southern, L. L. and D. H. Baker. 1981. The effect of methionine or cysteine on cobalt toxicity in the chick. *Poult. Sci.* **60**:1303.

Spais, A., A. Papasteriadis, A. Agiannidis and T. Lazaridis. 1966. Action of inorganic sulphate, sulphide, cyanide and molybdenum on liver cobalt in lambs. *Ann. Rep. Vet. Fac. Aristotelian Univ. Thessaloniki* **7**:167.

Sutton, A. L. and J. M. Elliot. 1972. Effect of ratio of roughage to concentrate and level of feed intake on ovine ruminal vitamin B_{12} production. *J. Nutr.* **102**:1341.

Underwood, E. J. 1977. "Trace Elements in Human and Animal Nutrition," 4th ed. Academic Press, New York.

7

COPPER BIOAVAILABILITY

David H. Baker

Department of Animal Sciences and
Division of Nutritional Sciences
University of Illinois
Urbana, Illinois

Clarence B. Ammerman

Department of Animal Science
University of Florida
Gainesville, Florida

I. INTRODUCTION

The first conclusive evidence of biological essentially for copper was provided by Hart *et al.* (1928) when it was demonstrated that the element was required for recovery from anemia in rats. Copper deficiency has detrimental effects on numerous organs and tissues, including the hematopoietic system, cardiovascular system, central nervous system, and the integumentum. Copper is an essential component of several metalloenzymes whose functional deficits give rise to the pathology associated with copper deficiency. Some of these enzymes can be directly associated with specific pathology, e.g., tyrosinase and lack of pigmentation, lysyl oxidase, and cardiovascular defects. Other copper metalloenzymes, such as cytochrome c oxidase, Cu,Zn-superoxide dismutase and dopamine-β-monoxygenase, play key roles in metabolism, but it is difficult to assign specific pathology to decreases in their activities. The anemia of copper deficiency results from impairment of iron metabolism and is particularly manifested when dietary iron is borderline, but the specific copper-dependent enzyme or protein involved in iron metabolism is unclear. The metabolic functions of copper, which have been

BIOAVAILABILITY OF NUTRIENTS FOR ANIMALS:
AMINO ACIDS, MINERALS, AND VITAMINS
Copyright © 1995 by Academic Press, Inc.

127

described (O'Dell, 1976), serve as indices of copper status and of copper bioavailability.

Copper deficiency is a serious problem for grazing ruminants in many countries of the world. This is due both to low concentrations of the element in forage as well as to elevated amounts of molybdenum and sulfur, which interfere with copper utilization. Despite the fact that most practical diets contain adequate copper for swine and poultry, the element is still generally supplemented to complete diets for these species. Copper may be limiting in certain human diets and particularly at risk are the premature infant and the exclusively breast-fed infant (NRC, 1989).

II. BIOAVAILABILITY STUDIES

A. *In Vitro* Estimates of Bioavailability

Fischer *et al.* (1981) prepared everted duodenal sacs from immature rats to investigate the effect of zinc on copper absorption. The washed sacs were filled with copper-free, Krebs-Ringer buffer (KRB) and incubated in Waymouth's medium containing copper; absorption was expressed as ng of copper transported to the KRB medium. In a slight variation of this method (Fischer *et al.*, 1983), duodenal segments were filled with Waymouth's medium to which [67]Cu was added. The sac was incubated in KRB and the radioactivity released used as a measure of copper transfer.

Aoyagi (1992) evaluated solubility of several copper salts in various solvents. It was concluded that *in vitro* solubility is not a good index of *in vivo* copper bioavailability. For example, cuprous oxide (Cu_2O) was only 9% soluble in dilute HCl, whereas cupric oxide (CuO) was 50% soluble, but cuprous oxide was as bioavailable as cupric sulfate ($CuSO_4 \cdot 5H_2O$; 100% soluble in dilute HCl), whereas cupric oxide was unavailable. Also, cuprous chloride (CuCl) was about 50% soluble in dilute acid solutions (HCl at pH 1.3 or citric acid at pH 2.3) compared with 100% for cupric sulfate, but cuprous chloride was 143% bioavailable relative to cupric sulfate.

B. *In Vivo* Estimates of Bioavailability

Since the early studies of Schultze *et al.* (1934), the soluble salts, primarily cupric sulfate or chloride, have been used as reference standards for comparative evaluation of the absorption and bioavailability of copper. Recently, cupric sulfate pentahydrate, $CuSO_4 \cdot 5H_2O$, has been the most commonly used reference standard (Suttle, 1974a; Lonnerdal et al., 1985; Johnson et al., 1988) although $CuCO_3$ has also served this role (Lo et al.,1984). Quantitative data related to the relative copper bioavailability in feedstuffs and supplements are presented in Table I.

1. Copper Radioisotopes

Whole-body retention of ^{67}Cu has been used to evaluate copper absorption by rats (Stuart and Johnson, 1986; Johnson et al., 1988). In this method, which is analogous to the one used by Heth and Hoekstra (1965) to measure zinc absorption, whole-body radioactivity is determined repeatedly for a period of time after absorption of the isotope is complete. The period must be sufficiently long to allow measurement of copper turnover or endogenous loss; the plot of whole-body radioactivity expressed as logarithm of the percentage of original activity vs time must be linear. By extrapolation of the linear portion of the curve to zero time, initial retention is evaluated. True absorption can be calculated by correcting for the loss of a comparable parenteral dose of radioactive copper. Foodstuffs are labeled either extrinsically or intrinsically with ^{67}Cu and the absorption compared to that of ^{67}Cu-labeled cupric sulfate.

In a variation of this method, nursing rats were administered by gastric intubation ^{64}Cu-labeled milk and compared to controls given aqueous solutions of labeled cupric sulfate. The uptake of radioactivity into various organs of 14-day-old rat pups was measured after 6 hr (Lonnerdal et al., 1985). A similar technique has been used in nearly mature rats to compare the effect of different carbohydrates on copper absorption (Fields et al., 1986). Using ligated segments of rat intestine maintained in situ and ^{64}Cu as a tracer, van Campen and Mitchell (1965) developed a method to estimate copper absorption. The percentage of a radioactive dose found in blood and various organs 3 hr after introduction of the isotope was used as an index of absorption. The highest rate of absorption occurred in the stomach segment, followed by duodenum and ileum. A similar technique has been used in the chick (Starcher, 1969). Oestreicher and Cousins (1985) used the vascularly perfused rat intestine to measure copper as well as zinc absorption.

Two studies with ruminants have been conducted with single doses of ^{64}Cu-labeled products obtained by thermal neutron activation of stable compounds. The data from these studies do not readily lend themselves to calculation of relative biological availability values. Lassiter and Bell (1960) reported similar plasma and whole blood uptake of radioactive copper in sheep when radioactive cupric chloride ($CuCl_2$), cupric sulfate, or cupric nitrate [$Cu(NO_3)_2$] were administered. Copper from cupric oxide needles was considerably less well absorbed. In another phase of the same study, radioactive copper from cupric carbonate was better absorbed than that from cupric oxide, either as needles or powder, or cuprous oxide. Copper as metal wire was almost completely unavailable. In similar research in which radioactive copper compounds were administered as single doses to steers (Chapman and Bell, 1963), radioactive copper from cupric nitrate and cupric carbonate gave similar responses in radioactive copper levels in plasma; cupric sulfate and cupric chloride gave similar, but somewhat lower, absorption values. Significantly less copper absorption occurred from cuprous oxide, with very limited absorption of radioactive copper from cupric oxide either as powder or needles or from metalic copper wire.

2. Plethoric Dietary Supplementation

A less direct evaluation of copper absorption is the use of high dietary concentrations of copper and measurement of copper accumulation in tissues. The practical use of plethoric amounts of dietary copper first arose when high levels of copper were observed to improve swine performance (Bowland et al., 1961). Under these conditions, high concentrations of copper accumulate in the liver and other tissues. Liver copper concentration has been used to compare the relative bioavailability of copper from various supplements (Table I) for chickens (Norvell et al., 1974; Ledoux et al., 1991; Baker et al., 1991), pigs (Bunch et al., 1961; Bowland et al., 1961; Cromwell et al., 1978), cattle (Ivan et al., 1990), sheep (Dalgarno and Mills, 1975; Charmley and Ivan, 1989), and rats (Kirchgessner and Grassman, 1970; Lo et al., 1984).

To compare the relative bioavailability of copper at plethoric vs deficient dietary concentrations, Aoyagi and Baker (1993a,b,c,d) and Aoyagi et al. (1993; 1995) examined a number of criteria indicative of copper status in chicks. Copper-depleted chicks were fed casein-soy concentrate diets containing graded concentrations of copper (.5 to 16 ppm) from 1 to 3 weeks posthatching. Between .5 and 2.5 ppm copper, liver copper concentration increased by 30%, but total gall bladder or bile copper concentration increased sevenfold. A comparison was made between use of bile copper accumulation after dosing a deficient diet with 0 or 1 ppm of the element and liver copper accumulation after plethoric dietary additions at 300 to 500 ppm. In direct comparisons of the low vs high-dose bioassays, relative availablity values were not significantly different. The standard, cupric sulfate, cupric basic carbonate, cuprous oxide, copper-methionine, and copper-lysine were all utilized similarly, whereas cuprous chloride was more available, and cupric oxide was unavailable. The unavailability of copper in cupric oxide has also been shown in pigs (Cromwell et al., 1989), and Kegley and Spears (1993) have suggested that cupric oxide administered orally was poorly available to growing cattle.

A gall bladder uptake bioassay was used to evaluate copper bioavailability in several feedstuffs (Aoyagi et al., 1993; 1995). Feed ingredients were found to have widely varying bioavailability relative to cupric sulfate. In general, the copper in fresh beef, sheep, or poultry liver was highly available, but that in pork liver was totally unavailable.   Autoclaving raw pork liver increased relative copper bioavailability to 32% (Aoyagi *et al.*, 1995). Copper in meat and bone meal was found to have lower availablity than that in poultry by-product meal, whereas that in soybean meal and cottonseed meal was 40 to 50% that of cupric sulfate.

3. Physiological Dietary Supplementation

   a. Tissue Concentrations of Copper.   Suttle (1974a) applied the principle of depletion-repletion to determine copper bioavailability in sheep. Ewes were made hypocupremic, less than .35 ppm copper in plasma, then given graded levels of copper for 33 days; the increase in plasma copper was the criterion of bioavailability. This technique was used to compare cupric sulfate, cupric sulfide (CuS), and cupric sulfate fed with variable levels of dietary sulfur (Suttle, 1974b).   Liver copper concentration has also been used to assess copper bioavailability in rats (Lo *et al.*, 1984) and chicks (Izquierdo and Baker, 1986; Zanetti *et al.*, 1991).   Total liver copper in rats responded linearly to graded levels of copper from cupric carbonate and soybean protein.   Liver copper accumulation in response to dietary copper concentration varies with species. The differences for sheep, cattle, swine, poultry, and rats are illustrated in Fig.1.   The diet to which copper is supplemented can also have a marked effect on liver uptake of copper (Waibel *et al.*, 1964; Funk and Baker, 1991).   Funk and Baker (1991) fed chicks graded doses of copper (0, 100, 200, 400, and 800 ppm) from cupric sulfate in a corn-soybean meal diet or a semipurified dextrose diet. Liver copper concentration began increasing at 100 ppm added copper in chicks fed the casein diet but it required 400 ppm for the same effect in those fed the corn-soybean meal diet.   At doses of 400 or 800 ppm copper, liver copper concentration was five times greater in chicks fed the casein diet than in those fed the corn-soybean meal diet.

   b.   Metalloprotein Biosynthesis and Enzymatic Activity.   Copper has a direct effect on iron metabolism and, thus, indirectly affects hemoglobin biosynthesis. The first sign of copper deficiency experimentally observed was anemia in rats fed cow's milk supplemented with iron. In those early studies hemoglobin regeneration was used to estimate the bioavailability of various copper compounds (Schultze *et al.*, 1934; 1936) and more recently to evaluate copper-amino acid and copper-peptide complexes (Kirchgessner and Grassman, 1970).
   The activities of ceruloplasmin, Cu,Zn-superoxide dismutase (SOD), and cytochrome c oxidase have been used as indices of copper status (L'Abbe and Fischer, 1984) and are useful measures of relative absorption and utilization in

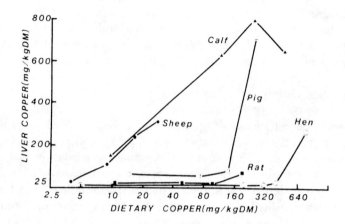

Fig. 1. Species differences in responses in liver copper stores to increases in dietary copper supply as summarized by Suttle (1987). Reprinted with permission from "Copper in Animals and Man" (J. McC. Howell and J. M. Gawthorne, Eds.), Vol. 1. p.27. CRC Press, Boca Raton, FL. Copyright CRC Press, Boca Raton, FL.

depleted animals. Lee *et al.* (1988) measured and compared liver copper concentration, liver SOD, serum ceruloplasmin, and serum copper concentrations as indicators of copper bioavailability. The most linear response and the best statistical fit of the data were provided by liver copper, followed by liver SOD. The enzyme methodology has been refined to compare the ratio of a cupro-metalloenzyme to that of another enzyme whose activity was not affected by copper status (Price and Chesters, 1985). In this method the activities of cytochrome c oxidase and NADH dehydrogenase in duodenal mucosa were measured and the ratios plotted against copper dose. The linear response curves allowed comparison of natural product copper to that of cupric sulfate.

c. Other Criteria. Conventional balance techniques are generally inadequate for measurement of copper bioavailability, particularly in ruminants (Suttle, 1974a). Growth rate has also been found to be relatively insensitive to dietary copper additions.

C. Slow Release Supplements for Ruminants

Supplemental copper for ruminants grazing copper-deficient areas has frequently been provided as a copper salt mixed with other mineral compounds and offered to grazing animals on a free-choice basis. In general, this has been a satisfactory means of copper supplementation but variable and sometimes insufficient intake of the mineral mixture can result in inadequate intakes of the element. Other forms of supplemental copper have been developed to alleviate this problem and to provide for situations in which copper is very much limiting production compared to the other elements.

Injectable forms of copper-containing compounds have been shown to be effective in preventing copper deficiency in ruminants. Sutherland et al. (1955) in Australia and Allcroft and Uvarov (1959) in Great Britain reported that copper glycinate injected subcutaneously was an effective source of copper for sheep and cattle. Their studies indicated a fairly wide margin of safety with this method of copper administration and suggested that multiple injections yearly would be effective in maintaining normal copper nutrition for animals grazing copper- deficient forages. Injectable copper as copper glycinate, copper-calcium-EDTA or copper methionate was effective in maintaining normal blood and liver copper in pregnant ewes (Hemingway et al., 1970). Suttle (1981) found copper as diethylamino oxyquinoline sulfonate was more effective than that as calcium-copper-EDTA in sheep, whereas the reverse was true in cattle. In the same studies, copper methionate resulted in marked reactions at, and slow translocation from, the injection site. Judson et al. (1984) reported that subcutaneous injections of copper as copper diethylamino oxyquinoline sulfonate gave transient increases in liver copper in grazing sheep.

Copper glycinate and, in particular, copper methionate, caused severe localized reactions at the site of injection, a condition observed to a much lesser degree with copper-EDTA (Ishmael et al., 1970; Boila et al., 1984a; Bohman et al., 1984). The positive but short-term effects on copper nutrition of injectable copper forms, in general, have been reported by numerous investigators (Boila et al., 1984b; Richards et al., 1985; Trengove and Judson, 1985; Givens et al., 1988; Rogers and Poole, 1988). The need for frequently repeated treatments with the injectable copper forms due to the transitory positive response and the adverse reactions at the site of injection results in added stress on the animal and has discouraged use of this procedure.

A single dose of copper oxide needles (oxidized copper wire particles) to cattle and sheep was suggested by Judson et al. (1981) and others to be effective in maintaining normal copper nutrition in animals for several months. Judson et al. (1984) reported that liver copper concentrations in sheep given an oral dose of 3 g of copper oxide needles were significantly greater than those of untreated sheep for a period of 80 weeks. Richards *et al.* (1985) tested supplemental copper sources under field conditions with more than 500 head of cattle. Animals were treated either orally with 24 g copper oxide needles, subcutaneously with 100 mg copper as calcium-copper-EDTA, or left unsupplemented as controls. Following the grazing season of 133 to 194 days, average liver copper concentration was 178, 45, and 42 ppm on a dry tissue basis for the copper oxide needles, calcium-copper-EDTA, and the control group, respectively. Similar findings were obtained by Deland *et al.* (1986) when oral copper oxide needles were compared with injected copper glycinate for grazing cattle. Rogers and Poole (1988) summarized the results from 12 studies in which oral copper oxide needles were administered to cattle and concluded that single treatments could be effective in increasing bovine copper status for 6 to 8 months.

Telfer and Zervas (1982) and Knott *et al.* (1985) described a soluble glass that could serve as a carrier for microminerals and could be formed into a heavy bolus suitable for administration to ruminant animals. Once the bolus was located in the reticulorumen, glass was solubilized slowly and release of microminerals occurred. The soluble glass bolus developed for commercial use contained cobalt, selenium, and copper and, in early studies, positive responses to copper and cobalt were observed in sheep and cattle (Allen *et al.*, 1985; Judson *et al.*, 1985a) or positive responses to all three elements were observed (Care *et al.*,1985; Carlos *et al.*, 1985; Judson *et al.*, 1985b). In general, the slow release, soluble glass boluses seem to be effective in promoting normal copper nutrition in ruminant animals. Variations in their length of effectiveness may be influenced by factors such as differences in solubility rate of the glass and decrease in release rate of copper from the glass due to a reduction in surface area as dissolution occurs.

Trengove and Judson (1985) found glass boluses, oxidized copper particles, or copper-calcium-EDTA subcutaneous injections to give similar positive responses in liver copper concentrations of sheep. Koh and Judson (1987) found soluble glass boluses and oxidized copper particles were equally effective in maintaining adequate liver copper levels in young cattle for an extended period of time. In other studies, however, Langlands *et al.* (1986) observed that the glass boluses were less effective with sheep and cattle than either copper particles or injected copper-calcium-EDTA.

Givens *et al.* (1988) observed with calves grazing pasture containing less than 2 ppm copper on a DM basis that two soluble glass boluses containing a total of 28 g copper given orally yielded a positive response equal to that of monthly subcutaneous injections of copper diethylamino oxyquinoline sulfonate providing 12 mg copper per 50 kg live weight at each injection time. According to McFarlane *et al.* (1991), 28 g copper as cupric oxide in glass pellets administered orally maintained adequate copper status in growing heifers for at least 44 weeks whereas 16 g copper as cupric oxide particles given orally or 120 mg copper as copper glycinate in a subcutaneous injection were effective for much shorter periods of time. It was suggested that the considerable individual variability in response to copper as glass pellets or particles observed in this study was due to regurgitation of portions of the orally adminstered dose.

Lawson *et al.* (1989, 1990) described a sustained release bolus for cattle composed of compressed cupric oxide powder, other trace elements, and certain vitamins with an expected life in the reticulorumen of about 300 days. The minerals and vitamins are released from one end of a polymer-coated cylinder. Additional studies (Lawson *et al.*, 1991; Ritchie *et al.*, 1991) demonstrated positive effects on copper status of cattle with continuous release rates over an 8-month period. Pellets from cement produced by reacting finely powdered cupric oxide with phosphoric acid and administered orally were found to remain in the reticulorumen and to supply adequate copper to cattle and sheep to meet their needs for at least 3 months (Manston *et al.*, 1985). The indicated composition of the compound was $CuHPO_4$, and rates of copper release were decreased with higher curing temperatures.

III. FACTORS INFLUENCING BIOAVAILABILITY

A. Dietary Factors

1. Chelating Agents.

Davis *et al.* (1962) observed that supplemental copper or EDTA stimulated hematopoiesis in chicks fed a diet, based on soybean protein, that contained 14 ppm copper. The results suggested that soybean protein contained a copper-binding component that was counteracted by EDTA. This effect of EDTA would be analogous to its effect in counteracting the zinc-phytate interaction. The concept was supported by the observed effect of phytate in decreasing copper retention in rats (Davies and Nightingale, 1975). However, others have not observed an effect of soybean protein, which is rich in phytate, on copper absorption and utilization (Lo *et al.*, 1984). In fact, Lee *et al.* (1988) observed that phytate increased copper bioavailability, presumably by eliminating the copper antagonistic effect of zinc.

2. Metal-Ion Interactions.

Smith and Larson (1946) first showed that excess dietary zinc is antagonistic to copper and leads to an anemia that is alleviated by copper supplementation. The observation has been confirmed and extended to rats (van Reen, 1953; Magee and

Matrone, 1962; Murthy *et al.*, 1974) and other species, including chicks (Hill and Matrone, 1962; Southern and Baker, 1983), swine (Ritchie *et al.*, 1963; Hill *et al.*, 1983), and sheep (Saylor and Leach, 1980). The interaction of zinc and copper has also been observed in rats fed diets extremely low in zinc. In rats that were severely zinc-deficient, plasma, muscle, and testis copper concentrations were elevated above normal (O'Dell *et al.*, 1976). Copper status is highly sensitive to zinc intake, much more so than the reverse interaction.

The zinc-copper antagonism is mediated primarily through the absorption process as shown by ligated intestinal segments (van Campen and Scaife, 1967) and the vascularly perfused intestine (Oestreicher and Cousins, 1985). Apparently, zinc induces high concentrations of metallothionein in the intestinal mucosa and this protein binds copper more strongly than zinc. In rats fed high levels of zinc, most of the absorbed copper replaced zinc bound to metallothionein because of its higher affinity. The copper bound to metallothionein was not absorbed but sloughed off with the mucosal cells (Hall *et al.*, 1979; Fischer *et al.*, 1983). Whether there is impairment of copper utilization beyond the point of absorption in animals fed excess zinc is unknown, but it is clear that the activities of copper metalloenzymes are depressed. Heart and liver SOD as well as cytochrome c oxidase activities were depressed by excess dietary zinc (L'Abbe and Fischer, 1984).

Another essential element, molybdenum, also interacts strongly with copper to decrease its bioavailability. This interaction involves sulfur and anionic molybdenum. Sulfur exacerbates the detrimental effect of molybdenum in ruminants (Dick, 1952) while alleviating the effect in rats (Gray and Daniels, 1964; Bremner and Young, 1978). See Suttle (1974c) for review of earlier literature. Absorption of copper by sheep was decreased when they were given increasing dietary levels of both molybdenum and sulfur, separately and additively. In 1975, Dick *et al.* proposed a mechanism for the copper-molybdenum-sulfur interaction that involved the formation of insoluble copper thiomolybdates, $Cu(MoO_nS_{4-n})^2$, in the rumen. More recently, Allen and Gawthorne (1987) found that the solid phase of ruminal digesta was involved in the interaction. They observed that thiomolybdate was bound to proteins in the digestive tract and postulated that this complex sequestered copper more tenaciously than thiomolybdate alone.

Several nonessential elements interact with copper, notably cadmium, silver, and lead. Cadmium was toxic to chicks in the dietary range of 25 to 400 ppm and copper supplementation decreased cadmium-induced mortality (Hill *et al.*, 1963). This suggests that copper, as well as zinc antagonism, is a component of cadmium toxicosis. Silver also accentuated copper deficiency in chicks and the effect was prevented by copper supplementation (Hill *et al.*, 1964). Lead-induced anemia in rats was alleviated by copper, suggesting that lead interferes with copper in regard to iron metabolism and, thus, hemoglobin biosynthesis (Klauder and Petering, 1977).

3. Other Dietary Components

Substances of high chelating and reducing potential tend to decrease copper bioavailability, perhaps by converting cupric to cuprous ion. Two such compounds, ascorbic acid and fructose, have been studied in several species. Ascorbic acid decreased copper absorption and utilization in chicks (Carlton and Henderson, 1965; Hill and Starcher, 1965; Aoyagi and Baker, 1993), rats (van Campen and Gross, 1968), miniature pigs (Voelker and Carlton, 1969), and guinea pigs (Smith and Bidlack, 1980).

Compared to starch, sucrose reduced copper bioavailability in rats (Fields *et al.*, 1983; Johnson and Hove, 1986). At least one monosaccharide component of sucrose, fructose, also accentuated low copper status (Fields *et al.*, 1984; reviewed by O'Dell, 1990). The mechanism by which fructose acts is unclear, but higher retention of ^{67}Cu in the intestinal tract of rats fed fructose, compared to those fed starch, suggested impairment of absorption (Fields *et al.*, 1986). This is consistent with the observation that the metabolism of intraperitoneally administered copper was not affected by dietary carbohydrate source (Holbrook *et al.*, 1986).

The effect of fructose on copper status of pigs fed low copper diets is much less, if any. Sholfield *et al.* (1990) fed pigs for 10 weeks low copper diets containing 20% of the metabolizable energy in the form of glucose or fructose. There was no carbohydrate-copper interaction on body weight gain or serum copper concentration, but fructose increased relative heart weight and aortic lysyl oxidase activity. Severe copper deficiency was not observed in this experiment. Schoenemann *et al.* (1990) fed weanling pigs for 10 weeks diets containing 59% sucrose or cornstarch and low or adequate copper. Copper deficiency occurred in both groups fed low copper as shown by decreased body weight, erythrocyte SOD activity, and tissue copper concentrations and increased heart weight. However, source of carbohydrate did not influence the indices of copper status, showing no evidence of carbohydrate-copper interaction.

Cysteine added to diets at 4000 ppm markedly reduced copper absorption in chicks (Robbins and Baker, 1980a,b; Aoyagi and Baker, 1994). Oral cysteine was more antagonistic to copper utilization than oral cystine or methionine (Baker and Czarnecki-Mauldin, 1987). Cysteine may be acting as a reducing agent in the gut, but it is also likely that cysteine binds copper (*via* SH and NH_3 moieties) and forms a complex that is absorbed poorly. Methylated cysteine compounds, such as D-penicillamine and dimercaptopropanol, are used as prescription drugs to ameliorate copper toxicoses, such as those found with copper poisoning and in Wilson's disease and Indian childhood cirrhosis (Baker and Czarnecki-Mauldin, 1987).

Some organic arsenicals, used as feed additives, decrease absorption of copper. When added to a practical-type broiler diet containing 1000 ppm copper, 3-nitro-4-hydroxyphenylarsonic acid at 50 to100 ppm markedly reduced liver copper concentration in chicks 1 to 3 weeks of age (Czarnecki and Baker, 1985). Similar observations have been made in pigs and rats (Czarnecki *et al.*, 1984).

IV. SUMMARY

The bioavailability of copper has been evaluated by slope ratio analysis of data obtained by use of indicators, such as liver or bile copper concentration, cytochrome c oxidase, or SOD activities, in animals fed low copper diets that induce suboptimal copper status. Most of the bioavailability data for copper supplements presented, however, were obtained by feeding dietary copper levels well beyond the requirement (Table II). Cupric sulfate has served most frequently as the standard source of copper. In general, the copper of plant source feedstuffs is only about 50% as available as that in animal source feed ingredients. Of the copper compounds used as supplements, most are well absorbed. Cupric oxide and cupric sulfide are exceptions, both being extremely poorly absorbed by all species. Cupric oxide needles administered orally to ruminants, however, are effective sources of copper for an extended period of time. Cupric carbonate is intermediate in absorption, but basic cupric carbonate [$CuCO_3 \cdot Cu(OH)_2$] is well absorbed. Limited research with copper amino acids and copper proteinate suggests somewhat greater absorption of copper than that obtained with cupric sulfate.

Table I. Bioavailability of copper sources for domestic animals[a]

Source	RV	Standard	Response criterion	Method cal	Type diet	Added level, ppm	Reference
Chickens							
Copper-lysine	99	Cupric sulfate RG ($CuSO_4 \cdot 5H_2O$)	Liv Cu	SR	N-11 ppm	150, 300, 450	Pott et al. (1994)
Copper-lysine	116	Cupric sulfate	Liv Cu	SR	N-290 ppm	75, 150	Baker et al. (1991)
Copper-lysine	120	Cupric sulfate	Bile Cu	SR	SP- 5 ppm	.5, 1	Aoyagi and Baker (1993b)
Copper-methionine	96	Cupric sulfate	Bile Cu	SR	SP-.5 ppm	.5, 1	Aoyagi and Baker (1993d)
Copper-methionine	88	Cupric sulfate	Liv Cu	SR	N-308	100, 200	Aoyagi and Baker (1993d)
Corn gluten meal	48	Cupric sulfate	Bile Cu	SR	SP-.5 ppm	1	Aoyagi et al. (1993)
Cottonseed meal	41	Cupric sulfate	Bile Cu	SR	SP-.5 ppm	1	Aoyagi et al. (1993)
Cupric acetate	188	Cupric sulfate	Liv Cu	TP	N-16 ppm	720	Norvell et al. (1974)
Cupric acetate	99	Cupric sulfate FG	Liv Cu	SR	N-11 ppm	150–450	Ledoux et al. (1991)
Cupric basic carbonate ($CuCO_3 \cdot Cu(OH)_2$)	113	Cupric sulfate	Bile Cu	SR	SP-.5 ppm	.5, 1	Aoyagi and Baker (1993a)
Cupric carbonate FG	66	Cupric acetate RG	Liv Cu	SR	N-5 ppm	5, 10, 20	Zanetti et al. (1991)
Cupric carbonate FG	68	Cupric acetate RG	Liv Cu	SR	N-11 ppm	150, 300, 450	Ledoux et al. (1991)
Cupric chloride	110	Cupric sulfate	Liv Cu	TP	N-16 ppm	720	Norvell et al. (1974)
Cupric chloride	106	Cupric sulfate	Liv Cu	TP	N-15 ppm	720	Norvell et al. (1975)
Cupric chloride, tribasic FG [$Cu_2(OH)_3Cl$]	100	Cupric sulfate RG	Liv Cu	SR	N	200, 400, 600	Miles et al. (1994)
$Cu_2(OH)_3Cl$ FG	106	Cupric sulfate RG	Liv Cu	SR	N-26	150, 300, 450	Ammerman et al. (1995)

Table 1. (continued)

Source	RV	Standard	Response criterion	Meth cal	Type diet	Added level, ppm	Reference
Cupric oxide FG	<1	Cupric acetate RG	Liv Cu	SR	N-11 ppm	150, 300, 450	Ledoux et al. (1991)
Cupric oxide	<1	Cupric sulfate	Liv Cu	SR	N-290 ppm	75, 150	Baker et al. (1991)
Cupric oxide	0	Cupric sulfate	Bile Cu	SR	SP-.5 ppm	1, 2	Aoyagi and Baker (1993a)
Cupric oxide	0	Cupric sulfate	Liv Cu	TP	N-15 ppm	720	Norvell et al. (1975)
Cupric oxide RG	1	Cupric sulfate RG	Liv Cu	TP	N-14 ppm	750	Jackson and Stevenson (1981)
Cupric sulfate FG	98	Cupric acetate RG	Liv Cu	SR	N-11 ppm	150, 300, 450	Ledoux et al. (1991)
Cuprous chloride	143	Cupric sulfate	Bile Cu	SR	SP-.5 ppm	.5, 1	Aoyagi and Baker (1993a)
Cuprous chloride	145	Cupric sulfate	Liv Cu	SR	N-308 ppm	50, 100	Aoyagi and Baker (1993d)
Cuprous iodide	46	Cupric sulfate	Liv Cu	TP	N	1, 2	McNaughton et al. (1974)
Cuprous oxide	92	Cupric sulfate	Liv Cu	SR	N-290 ppm	75-150	Baker et al. (1991)
Cuprous oxide	98	Cupric sulfate	Bile Cu	SR	SP-.5 ppm	.5, 1	Aoyagi and Baker (1993a)
Feather meal	<1	Cupric sulfate	Bile Cu	SR	SP-.5 ppm	.5	Aoyagi et al. (1995)
Hair meal, swine	9	Cupric sulfate	Bile Cu	SR	SP-.5 ppm	1	Aoyagi et al. (1995)
Liver, beef	82	Cupric sulfate	Bile Cu	SR	SP-.5 ppm	1	Aoyagi et al. (1993)
Liver, pork	<1	Cupric sulfate	Bile Cu	SR	SP-.5 ppm	1	Aoyagi et al. (1993)
Liver, poultry	105	Cupric sulfate	Bile Cu	SR	SP-.5 ppm	1	Aoyagi et al. (1993)
Liver, sheep	113	Cupric sulfate	Bile Cu	SR	SP-.5 ppm	1	Aoyagi et al. (1993)
Meat and bone meal, beef	4	Cupric sulfate	Bile Cu	SR	SP-.5 ppm	1	Aoyagi et al. (1995)
Meat and bone meal, mixed	28	Cupric sulfate	Bile Cu	SR	SP-.5 ppm	1	Aoyagi et al. (1995)

Meat and bone meal, pork	53	Cupric sulfate	Bile Cu	SR	SP-.5 ppm	1	Aoyagi et al. (1995)
Peanut hulls	44	Cupric sulfate	Bile Cu	SR	SP-.5 ppm	1	Aoyagi et al. (1993)
Poultry by-product meal	67	Cupric sulfate	Bile Cu	SR	SP-.5 ppm	1	Aoyagi et al. (1993)
Soybean meal	38	Cupric sulfate	Bile Cu	SR	SP-.5 ppm	1	Aoyagi et al. (1993)
Soybean mill run	47	Cupric sulfate	Bile Cu	SR	SP-.5 ppm	1	Aoyagi et al. (1993)
Swine feces	36	Cupric sulfate	Liv Cu	SR	SP 20 ppm	250-748	Izquierdo and Baker (1986)

Swine

Copper citrate + sodium molybdate	93	Cupric sulfate	Liv Cu	MR	N	20	Dowdy and Matrone (1968)
Copper citrate + sodium molybdate	74	Cupric sulfate	Cer	MR	N	20	Dowdy and Matrone (1968)
Copper methionine	107	Cupric sulfate	Liv Cu	TP	N-10+ ppm	250	Bunch et al. (1965)
Copper-molybdenum complex	68	Cupric sulfate	Liv Cu	MR	N	20	Dowdy and Matrone (1968)
Copper-molybdenum complex	0	Cupric sulfate	Cer	MR	N	20	Dowdy and Matrone (1968)
Cupric carbonate	62	Cupric sulfate	Liv Cu	TP	N	250	Allen et al. (1961)
Cupric carbonate	111	Cupric sulfate	^{64}Cu WB	MR	N-15 ppm	SOD-10 mg	Buescher et al. (1961)
Cupric oxide	89	Cupric sulfate	^{64}Cu WB	MR	N-15 ppm	SOD	Buescher et al. (1961)
Cupric oxide	15	Cupric sulfate	Liv Cu	MR	N-3 ppm	250	Bunch et al. (1961)
Cupric oxide	27	Cupric sulfate	Liv Cu	TP	N-10 ppm	250	Bunch et al. (1963)
Cupric oxide	0	Cupric sulfate	Liv Cu	MR	N-30 ppm	250	Cromwell et al. (1989)
Cupric sulfide	0	Cupric sulfate	Liv Cu	TP	N	250	Barber et al. (1960)

Table 1. (continued)

Source	RV	Standard	Response criterion	Meth cal	Type diet	Added level, ppm	Reference
Cupric sulfide	33	Cupric sulfate	Cu^{64} upt	MR	N	250	Bowland et al. (1961)
Cupric sulfide	23	Cupric sulfate	Cu^{64} upt	MR	N	250	Bowland et al. (1961)
Cupric sulfide	0	Cupric sulfate	Liv Cu	MR	N	250	Barber et al. (1961)
Cupric sulfide	**<1**	**Cupric sulfate**	**Liv Cu**	**MR**	**N**	**250**	**Cromwell et al. (1978)**
Cattle							
Copper-lysine	100	Cupric sulfate	Pla Cu	TP	N	30 mg/day	Kegley and Spears (1993)
Copper proteinate	112	Cupric sulfate	Pla Cu[b]	MR	N	14	Kincaid et al. (1986)
Copper proteinate	147	Cupric sulfate	Liv Cu[b]	MR	N	14	Kincaid et al. (1986)
Copper proteinate	102	Cupric sulfate	Liv Cu	MR	N	10	Wittenberg et al. (1990)
Na$_2$CuEDTA·3H$_2$O	91	Cupric sulfate	Liv Cu	MR	N-7 ppm	105 mg/day	Miltimore et al. (1978)
Na$_2$CuEDTA·3H$_2$O	104	Cupric sulfate	Liv Cu	MR	N-7 ppm	105 mg/day	Miltimore et al. (1978)
Cupric chloride	121	Cupric sulfate	Liv Cu	TP	N-6 ppm	14-16	Ivan et al. (1990)
Cupric chloride	114	Cupric sulfate	Liv Cu	TP	N-6 ppm	14-16	Ivan et al. (1990)
Cupric oxide	25	Cupric sulfate	Liv Cu	TP	N-7 ppm	18	Xin et al. (1991)
Cupric oxide	0	Cupric sulfate	Pla Cu	TP	N	30 mg/day	Kegley and Spears (1993)
Sheep							
Copper EDTA	96	Cupric sulfate	Liv Cu	TP	N	70 mg Cu 1x/wk	MacPherson and Hemingway (1968)
Copper glycine	96	Cupric sulfate	Liv Cu	TP	N	70 mg Cu 1x/wk	MacPherson and Hemingway (1968)

Cupric chloride	123	Cupric sulfate	Liv Cu	TP	N-6.7 ppm	29	Charmley and Ivan (1989)
Cupric chloride	105	Cupric sulfate	Liv Cu	TP	N-8.6 ppm	5, 10	Ivan et al. (1990)
Cupric sulfide	35	Cupric sulfate	Liv Cu	MR	N	30 mg/day	Dick (1954)
Cupric sulfide	11	Cupric sulfate	Pla Cu reg	MR	SP-1.5 ppm	5	Suttle (1974b)
Cuprous acetate	98	Cupric sulfate	Liv Cu	TP	N-6.7 ppm	29	Charmley and Ivan (1989)
Swine feces	35	Cupric sulfate	Liv Cu	MR	NG	30, 60	Prince et al. (1975)
Swine feces	70	Cupric sulfate	Liv Cu	MR	N	4	Dalgarno and Mills (1975)
Swine feces	60	Cupric sulfate	Pla Cu	MR	N	4	Dalgarno and Mills (1975)
Swine feces	80	Cupric sulfate	Pla Cu	TP	SP	8	Suttle and Price (1976)
Swine feces	75	Cupric sulfate	Pla Cu	TP	SP	4	Suttle and Price (1976)
Swine feces	25	Cupric sulfate	Liv Cu	TP	N-7.9 ppm	13 - 16	Poole et al. (1990)

Rats

Beef, cooked	100	Cupric sulfate	Ext lab	MR	P-2.6 ppm	8-11 g	Johnson et al. (1988)
Copper-amino acids							
Copper-(D-alanine)	112	Cupric sulfate	Liv Cu	TP	P	3.18	Kirchgessner and Grassman (1970)
Copper-(L-alanine)$_2$	103	Cupric sulfate	Liv Cu	TP	P	3.18	Kirchgessner and Grassman (1970)
Copper-(L-alanine)$_2$	146	Cupric sulfate	Liv Cu	TP	P	3.18	Kirchgessner and Grassman (1970)
Copper-(L-alanyl-L-alanine)	126	Cupric sulfate	Liv Cu	TP	P	3.18	Kirchgessner and Grassman (1970)
Copper-(L-arginine)$_2$	105	Cupric sulfate	Liv Cu	TP	P	3.18	Kirchgessner and Grassman (1970)

Table I. (continued)

Source	RV	Standard	Response criterion	Meth cal	Type diet	Added level, ppm	Reference
Copper-(L-aspartate)	86	Cupric sulfate	Liv Cu	TP	P	3.18	Kirchgessner and Grassman (1970)
Copper aspartate	110	Cupric sulfate	Hb reg	MR	N	.01 mg/day	Shultze et al. (1936)
Copper-(L-cystine)	111	Cupric sulfate	Liv Cu	TP	P	3.18	Kirchgessner and Grassman (1970)
Copper-(L-glutamate)	94	Cupric sulfate	Liv Cu	TP	P	3.18	Kirchgessner and Grassman (1970)
Copper-(L-isoleucine)₂	126	Cupric sulfate	Liv Cu	TP	P	3.18	Kirchgessner and Grassman (1970)
Copper-(DL-leucine)₂	162	Cupric sulfate	Liv Cu	TP	P	3.18	Kirchgessner and Grassman (1970)
Copper-(DL-leucyl-DL-leucine)	146	Cupric sulfate	Liv Cu	TP	P	3.18	Kirchgessner and Grassman (1970)
Copper-(L-leucine)₂	247	Cupric sulfate	Liv Cu	TP	P	3.18	Kirchgessner and Grassman (1970)
Copper-(L-leucyl-L-leucine)	183	Cupric sulfate	Liv Cu	TP	P	3.18	Kirchgessner and Grassman (1970)
Copper-(L-leucyl-L-leucyl-L- leucine)	157	Cupric sulfate	Liv Cu	TP	P	3.18	Kirchgessner and Grassman (1970)
Copper-(L-lysine)₂	118	Cupric sulfate	Liv Cu	TP	P	3.18	Kirchgessner and Grassman (1970)
Copper-(L-methionine)₂	114	Cupric sulfate	Liv Cu	TP	P	3.18	Kirchgessner and Grassman (1970)
Copper-(L-phenylalanine)₂	129	Cupric sulfate	Liv Cu	TP	P	3.18	Kirchgessner and Grassman (1970)

Compound		Standard	Criterion			Value	Reference
Copper-(poly-D-alanine)	141	Cupric sulfate	Liv Cu	TP	P	3.18	Kirchgessner and Grassman (1970)
Copper-(poly-L-alanine)	123	Cupric sulfate	Liv Cu	TP	P	3.18	Kirchgessner and Grassman (1970)
Copper-(L-serine)$_2$	112	Cupric sulfate	Liv Cu	TP	P	3.18	Kirchgessner and Grassman (1970)
Copper-(L-threonine)$_2$	95	Cupric sulfate	Liv Cu	TP	P	3.18	Kirchgessner and Grassman (1970)
Copper-(L-tryptophane)$_2$	114	Cupric sulfate	Liv Cu	TP	P	3.18	Kirchgessner and Grassman (1970)
Copper-(L-tyrosine)$_2$	122	Cupric sulfate	Liv Cu	TP	P	3.18	Kirchgessner and Grassman (1970)
Copper-(L-valine)$_2$	127	Cupric sulfate	Liv Cu	TP	P	3.18	Kirchgessner and Grassman (1970)
Copper carbonate ore	100	Cupric sulfate	Hb reg	MR	N	.03 mg/day	Elmslie et al. (1942)
Copper citrate	106	Cupric sulfate	Hb reg	MR	N	.01 mg/day	Shultze et al. (1936)
Copper citrate	99	Cupric sulfate	Liv Cu	TP	P	3.18	Kirchgessner and Grassman (1970)
Copper EDTA	121	Cupric sulfate	Liv Cu	TP	P	3.18	Kirchgessner and Grassman (1970)
Copper fumarate	108	Cupric sulfate	Liv Cu	TP	P	3.18	Kirchgessner and Grassman (1970)
Copper nucleinate	95	Cupric sulfate	Hb reg	MR	N	.01 mg/day	Schultze et al. (1936)
Copper oxalate	112	Cupric sulfate	Liv Cu	TP	P	3.18	Kirchgessner and Grassman (1970)
Copper pyrophosphate	75	Cupric sulfate	Hb reg	MR	N	.01 mg/day	Schultze et al. (1936)

Table I. (continued)

Source	RV	Standard	Response criterion	Meth cal	Type diet	Added level, ppm	Reference
Copper pyrophosphate	49	Cupric sulfate	Liv Cu	MR	N	500	Nesbit and Elmslie (1960)
Copper sulfide ore	0	Cupric sulfate	Hb reg	MR	N	.03 mg/day	Elmslie et al. (1960)
Cupric oxide	27	Cupric sulfate	Liv Cu	MR	N	250, 500	Nesbit and Elmslie (1960)
Cuprous cysteine mercaptide	95	Cupric sulfate	Hb reg	MR	N	.01 mg/day	Schultze et al. (1936)
Garbanzo beans, cooked	65	Cupric sulfate	Ext lab	MR	P-2.6 ppm	8-11 μg	Johnson et al. (1988)
Grass dried (6-7 ppm Cu)	75	Cupric sulfate	Cyt c oxidase	MR	SP-.4-.8 ppm	10 μg/day	Price and Chesters (1985)
Heart, pork, dried	80	Cupric sulfate	Hb reg	MR	N	.01 mg/day	Schultze et al. (1936)
Liver, chicken, cooked	72	Cupric sulfate	Ext lab	MR	P-2.6 ppm	8-11 g	Johnson et al. (1988)
Liver, pork, dried	80	Cupric sulfate	Hb reg	MR	N	.01 mg/day	Schultze et al. (1936)
Milk, human	25[c]	-	^{64}Cu liv	-	NG	-	Lonnerdal et al. (1985)
Milk, cow's	18[c]	-	^{64}Cu liv	-	NG	-	Lonnerdal et al. (1985)
Milk, cow's formula	23[c]	-	^{64}Cu liv	-	NG	-	Lonnerdal et al. (1985)
Peanuts, roasted	89	Cupric sulfate	Ext lab	MR	P-2.6 ppm	8-11 μg	Johnson et al. (1988)
Shrimp, cooked	109	Cupric sulfate	Ext lab	MR	P-2.6 ppm	8-11 μg	Johnson et al. (1988)
Soybean protein - A	112	Copper carbonate	Liv Cu	SR	P-.53 ppm	.5, 1.0, 1.5, 2.0	Lo et al. (1984)
Soybean protein - B	101	Copper carbonate	Liv Cu	SR	P-.53 ppm	.5, 1.0, 1.5, 2.0	Lo et al. (1984)
Soybean protein - C	107	Copper carbonate	Liv Cu	SR	P-.53 ppm	.5, 1.0, 1.5, 2.0	Lo et al. (1984)
Sunflower seeds, roasted	100	Cupric sulfate	Ext lab	MR	P-2.6 ppm	8-11 μg	Johnson et al. (1988)

Wheat	21[c]	-	Int & ext lab	-	N-5 ppm	-	Johnson and Lykken (1983)
Wheat	13[c]	-	Ext lab	-	N-5 ppm	-	Johnson and Lykken (1983)
Wheat germ	100	Cupric sulfate	Hb reg	MR	N	.01 mg/day	Schultze et al. (1936)
Yeast, brewer's	90	Cupric sulfate	Hb reg	MR	N	.01 mg/day	Schultze et al. (1936)

[a]Abbreviations can be found in Appendix I. Chemical formula for a compound given only if provided by the author; RG indicates reagent grade, FG indicates feed grade.

[b]Value for standard source was ≤ that for unsupplemented control group.

[c]Percentage absorption, not relative value.

Table II. Relative bioavailability of supplemental copper sources[a]

	Species			
Source	Poultry	Swine	Cattle	Sheep
Cupric sulfate	100	100	100	100
Copper EDTA	-	-	95 (1)	120 (1)
Copper-lysine	105 (2)	-	100 (1)	-
Copper-methionine	90 (2)	110 (1)	-	-
Copper proteinate	-	-	-	130 (1)
Cupric acetate	100 (3)	-	-	-
Cupric basic carbonate	115 (1)	-	-	-
Cupric carbonate	65 (2)	85 (2)	-	-
Cupric chloride	110 (2)	-	115 (2)	115 (1)
Cupric chloride, tribasic	105 (2)	-	-	-
Cupric oxide[b]	0 (4)	30 (4)	15 (2)	-
Cupric sulfide	-	10 (4)	25 (2)	-
Cuprous acetate	-	-	100 (1)	-
Cuprous chloride	145 (2)	-	-	-
Cuprous oxide	100 (1)	-	-	-

[a]Average values rounded to nearest "5" and expressed relative to response obtained with cupric sulfate. Number of studies or samples involved indicated within parentheses.

[b]Cupric oxide needles which are retained for extended periods within the intestinal tract of ruminants have been shown to be an effective source of copper.

REFERENCES

Allcroft, R. and O. Uvarov. 1959. Parental administration of copper compounds to cattle with special reference to copper glycine (copper amino-acetate). *Vet. Res.* **71**:797.

Allen, J. D. and J. M. Gawthorne. 1987. Involvement of the solid phase of rumen digesta in the interaction between copper, molybdenum and sulfur in sheep. *Br. J. Nutr.* **58**:265.

Allen, M. M., R. S. Barber, R. Braude and K. C. Mitchell. 1961. Further studies on various aspects of the use of high-copper supplements for growing pigs. *Br. J. Nutr.* **15**:507.

Allen, W. M., C. F. Drake and M. Tripp. 1985. Use of controlled release systems for supplementation during trace element deficiency - The administration of boluses of controlled release glass (CRG) to cattle and sheep. *In* "Trace Elements in Man and Animals-5" (C. F. Mills, I. Bremner and J. K. Chesters, Eds.), p. 19. Commonwealth Agricultural Bureaux, Slough, UK.

Ammerman, C. B., P. R. Henry, X. G. Luo and R. D. Miles. 1995. Bioavailability of copper from tribasic cupric chloride for nonruminants. *In* "Proc. Am. Soc. Anim. Sci., Southern Section," p. 18 [Abstract].

Aoyagi, S. 1992. Bioavailability of copper in inorganic and organic copper supplements for young chicks. MS Thesis. University of Illinois, Urbana.

Aoyagi, S. and D. H. Baker. 1993a. Bioavailability of copper in analytical-grade and feed-grade inorganic copper sources when fed to provide copper at levels below the chicks requirement. *Poult. Sci.* **72**:1075.

Aoyagi, S. and D. H. Baker. 1993b. Nutritional evaluation of copper-lysine and zinc-lysine complexes for chicks. *Poult. Sci.* **72**:165.

Aoyagi, S. and D. H. Baker. 1993c. Bioavailability of copper in chicken bile. *J. Nutr.* **123**:870.

Aoyagi, S. and D. H. Baker. 1993d. Nutritional evaluation of a copper-methionine complex for chicks. *Poult. Sci.* **72**:2309.

Aoyagi, S. and D. H. Baker. 1994. Copper-amino acid complexes are partially protected against inhibitory effects of L-cysteine and L-ascorbate. *J. Nutr.* **124**:388.

Aoyagi, S., K. M. Hiney and D. H. Baker. 1995. Copper bioavailability in pork liver and in various animal by-products as determined by chick bioassay. *J. Anim. Sci.* **73**:799.

Aoyagi, S., K. J. Wedekind and D. H. Baker. 1993. Estimates of copper bioavailability from liver of different animal species and from feed ingredients derived from plants and animals. *Poult. Sci.* **72**:1746.

Baker, D. H. and G. L. Czarnecki-Mauldin. 1987. Pharmacologic role of cysteine in ameliorating or exacerbating mineral toxicities. *J. Nutr.* **117**:1003.

Baker, D. H., J. Odle, M. A. Funk and T. M. Wieland. 1991. Research note: Bioavailability of copper in cupric oxide, cuprous oxide, and in a copper-lysine complex. *Poult. Sci.* **70**:177.

Barber, R. S., J. P. Bowland, R. Braude, K. G. Mitchell and J. W. G. Porter. 1961. Copper sulphate and copper sulphide (CuS) as supplements for growing pigs. *Br. J. Nutr.* **15**:189.

Barber, R. S., R. Braude, K. C. Mitchell and J. W. C. Porter. 1960. Copper sulphate and copper sulphide (CuS) as supplements for growing pigs. *Proc. Nutr. Soc.* **9**:xxvi [Abstract].

Bohman, V. R., E. L. Drake and W. C. Behrens. 1984. Injectable copper and tissue composition of cattle. *J. Dairy Sci.* **67**:1468.

Boila, R. J., T. J. Devlin, R. A. Drysdale and L. E. Lillie. 1984a. Injectable Cu complexes as supplementary Cu for grazing cattle. *Can. J. Anim. Sci.* **64**:365.

Boila, R. J., T. J. Devlin, R. A. Drysdale and L. E. Lillie. 1984b. Supplementary copper for grazing beef cattle - injectable copper glycinate, and copper sulfate in free-choice mineral supplements. *Can. J. Anim. Sci.* **64**:675.

Bowland, J. P., R. Braude, A. G. Chamberlain, R. F. Glascock and K. G. Mitchell. 1961. The absorption, distribution and excretion of labelled copper in young pigs given different quantities, as sulphate or sulphide, orally or intravenously. *Br. J. Nutr.* **15**:59.

Bremner, I. and B. W. Young. 1978. Effects of dietary molybdenum and sulfur on the distribution of copper in plasma and kidneys of sheep. *Br. J. Nutr.* **39**:325.

Buescher, R. G., S. A. Griffin and M. C. Bell. 1961. Copper availability to swine from Cu^{64} labelled inorganic compounds. *J. Anim. Sci.* **20**:529.

Bunch, R. J., J. T. McCall, V. C. Speer and V. W. Hays. 1965. Copper supplementation for weanling pigs. *J. Anim. Sci.* **24**:995.

Bunch, R. J., V. C. Speer, V. W. Hays, J. H. Hawbaker and D. V. Catron. 1961. Effects of copper sulfate, copper oxide and chlortetracycline on baby pig performance. *J. Anim. Sci.* **20**:723.

Bunch, R. J., V. C. Speer, V. W. Hays and J. T. McCall. 1963. Effects of high levels of copper and chlortetracyline on performance of pigs. *J. Anim. Sci.* **22**:56.

Care, A. D., P. J. B. Anderson, D. V. Illingworth, G. Zervas and S. B. Telfer. 1985. The effect of soluble-glass on the copper, cobalt and selenium status of Suffolk cross lambs. *In* "Trace Elements in Man and Animals-5" (C. F. Mills, I. Bremner, and J. K. Chesters, Eds.), p. 717. Commonwealth Agricultural Bureaux, Slough, UK.

Carlos, C., G. Zervas, P. M. Driver, P. J. B. Anderson, D. V. Illingworth, S. A. Al-Tekrity and S. B. Telfer. 1985. The effect of soluble-glass boluses on the copper, cobalt and selenium status of Scottish blackface ewes. *In* "Trace Elements in Man and Animals-5" (C. F. Mills, I. Bremner, and J. K. Chesters, Eds.), p. 714. Commonwealth Agricultural Bureaux, Slough, UK.

Carlton, W. W. and W. Henderson. 1965. Studies in chickens fed a copper-deficient diet supplemented with ascorbic acid, reserpine and diethylstilbestrol. *J. Nutr.* **85**: 67.

Chapman, H. L. and M. C. Bell. 1963. Relative absorption and excretion by beef cattle of copper from various sources. *J. Anim. Sci.* **22**: 82.

Charmley, L. L. and M. Ivan. 1989. The relative accumulation of copper in the liver and kidneys of sheep fed corn silage supplemented with copper chloride, copper acetate or copper sulfate. *Can. J. Anim. Sci.* **69**:205.

Cromwell, G. L., T. S. Stahly and H. J. Monegue. 1989. Effects of source and level of copper on performance and liver copper stores in weanling pigs. *J. Anim. Sci.* **67**:2996.

Cromwell, G. L., V. W. Hays and T. L. Clark. 1978. Effects of copper sulfate, copper sulfide and sodium sulfide on performance and copper stores of pigs. *J. Anim. Sci.* **46**:692.

Czarnecki, G. L. and D. H. Baker. 1985. Reduction of liver copper concentration by the organic arsenical 3-nitro-4-hydroxyphenyl-arsonic acid. *J. Anim. Sci.* **60**:40.

Czarnecki, G. L., M. S. Edmonds, O. A. Izquierido and D. H. Baker. 1984. Effect of 3-nitro-4-hydroxyphenylarsonic acid on copper utilization by the pig, rat and chick. *J. Anim. Sci.* **59**:997.

Dalgarno, A. C. and C. F. Mills. 1975. Retention by sheep of copper from aerobic digests of pig faecal slurry. *J. Agric. Sci. Camb.* **85**:11.

Davies, N. T., and R. Nightingale. 1975. The effects of phytate on intestinal absorption and secretion of zinc, and whole-body retention of Zn, copper, iron and manganese in rats. *Br. J. Nutr.* **34**:243.

Davis, P. N., L. C. Norris and F. H. Kratzer. 1962. Interference of soybean proteins with the utilization of trace minerals. *J. Nutr.* **77**:217.

Deland, M. P. B., D. Lewis, P. R. Cunningham and D. W. Dewey. 1986. Use of orally administered oxidized copper wire particles for copper therapy in cattle. *Aust. Vet. J.* **63**:1.

Dick, A. T. 1952. The effect of diet and of molybdenum on copper metabolism in sheep. *Aust. Vet. J.* **28**:30.

Dick, A. T. 1954. Studies on the assimilation and storage of copper in crossbred sheep. *Aust. J. Agric. Res.* **5**:511.

Dick, A. T., D. W. Dewey and J. M. Gawthorne. 1975. Thiomolybdates and the copper-molybdenum-sulfur interaction in ruminant nutrition. *J. Agric. Sci. Camb.* **85**: 567.

Dowdy, R. P. and G. Matrone. 1968. A copper-molybdenum complex: Its effects and movement in the piglet and sheep. *J. Nutr.* **95**:197.

Elmslie, W. P., W. R. Bunting, R. A. Sturdy and P. R. Cutter. 1942. New sources of mineral elements in animal nutrition. *Trans. Illinois State Acad. Sci.* **35**:95.

Fields, M., R. J. Ferretti, J. C. Smith and S. Reiser. 1983. Effect of copper deficiency on metabolism and mortality in rats fed sucrose or starch diets. *J. Nutr.* **113**:1335.

Fields, M., R. J. Ferretti, J. C. Smith and S. Reiser. 1984. The interactions of type of dietary carbohydrates with copper deficiency. *Am. J. Clin. Nutr.* **39**:289.

Fields, M., J. Holbrook, D. Scholfield, J. C. Smith and S. Reiser. 1986. Effect of fructose or starch on copper-67 absorption and excretion by the rat. *J. Nutr.* **16**:625.

Fischer, P. W. F., A. Giroux, and M. R. L'Abbe. 1981. The effect of dietary zinc on intestinal copper absorption. *Am. J. Clin. Nutr.* **34**:1670.

Fischer, P. W. F., A. Giroux and M. R. L'Abbe. 1983. Effects of zinc on mucosal copper binding and on the kinetics of copper absorption. *J. Nutr.* **113**:462.

Funk, M. A. and D. H. Baker. 1991. Toxicity and tissue accumulation of copper in chicks fed casein and soy-based diets. *J. Anim. Sci.* **69**:4505.

Givens, D. I., G. Zervas, V. R. Simpson and S. B. Telfer. 1988. Use of soluble glass rumen boluses to provide a supplement of copper for suckled calves. *J. Agric. Sci. Camb.* **110**:199.

Gray, L. F. and L. J. Daniels. 1964. Effect of the copper status of the rat on the copper-molybdenum-sulfate interaction. *J. Nutr.* **84**:31.

Hall, A. C., B. W. Young and I. Bremner. 1979. Intestinal metallothionein and the mutual antagonism between copper and zinc in the rat. *J. Inorg. Biochem.* **11**:57.

Hart, E. B., H. Steenbock, J. Waddell and C. A. Elvehjem. 1928. Iron in nutrition. VI. Copper as a supplement to iron for hemoglobin building in the rat. *J. Biol. Chem.* **77**:797.

Hemingway, R. G., A. MacPherson and N. S. Ritchie. 1970. Improvement in the copper status of ewes and their lambs resulting from the use of injectable copper compounds. *In* " Trace Element Metabolism in Animals" (C. F. Mills, Ed.), p. 264. Livingstone, Edinburgh, Scotland.

Heth, D. A. and W. G. Hoekstra. 1965. Zinc-65 absorption and turnover in rats I. A procedure to determine zinc-65 absorption and the antagonistic effect of calcium in a practical area. *J. Nutr.* **85**:367.

Hill, C. H. and G. Matrone. 1962. A study of copper and zinc interrelationships. *In* "Proceedings of the 12th World's Poultry Congress," p. 219. Bloxam and Chambers, Sydney, Australia..

Hill, C. H., G. Matrone, W. L. Payne and C. W. Barber. 1963. *In vivo* interactions of cadmium and copper, zinc and iron. *J. Nutr.* **80**:227.

Hill, C. H. and B. Starcher. 1965. Effect of reducing agents on copper deficiency in the chick. *J. Nutr.* **85**:271.

Hill, C. H., B. Starcher and G. Matrone. 1964 . Mercury and silver interrelationships with copper. *J. Nutr.* **83**:107.

Hill, G. M., P. K. Ku, E. R. Miller, D. E. Ullrey, T. A. Losty and B. L. O'Dell. 1983. A copper deficiency in neonatal pigs induced by a high zinc maternal diet. *J. Nutr.* **113**:867.

Holbrook, J., M. Fields, J. C. Smith and S. Reiser. 1986. Tissue distribution and excretion of copper-67 intraperitoneally administered to rats fed fructose or starch. *J. Nutr.* **116**: 831.

Ishmael, J., P. J. Treeby and J. McC. Howell. 1970. Lesions found in ewes which have died following the administration of copper calcium edetate for prevention of swayback. *In* "Trace Element Metabolism in Animals" (C.F. Mills, Ed.), p. 68. Livingstone, Edinburgh, Scotland.

Ivan, M., J. G. Proulx, R. Morales, H. C. V. Codagnone and M. de S. Dayrell. 1990. Copper accumulation in the liver of sheep and cattle fed diets supplemented with copper sulfate or copper chloride. *Can. J. Anim. Sci.* **70**:727.

Izquierdo, O. A. and D. H. Baker. 1986. Bioavailability of copper in pig feces. *Can. J. Anim. Sci.* **66**:1145.

Jackson, N. and M. H. Stevenson. 1981. A study of the effects of dietary added cupric oxide on the laying, domestic fowl and a comparison with the effects of hydrated copper sulphate. *Br. J. Nutr.* **45**:99.

Johnson, M. A. and S. S. Hove. 1986. Development of anemia in copper-deficient rats fed high levels of dietary iron and sucrose. *J. Nutr.* **116**:1225.

Johnson, P. E. and G. I. Lykken. 1983. Absorption by rats of intrinsic and extrinsic copper labels from wheat. *Fed. Proc.* **42**:528. [Abstract].

Johnson, P. E., M. A. Stuart, and T. D. Bowman. 1988. Bioavailability of copper to rats from various foodstuffs and in the presence of different carbohydrates. *Proc. Soc. Exp. Biol. Med.* **187**: 44.

Judson, G. J., T. H. Brown and D. W. Dewey. 1985a. Trace element supplements for sheep: Evaluation of copper oxide and a soluble glass bullet, impregnated with copper and cobalt. *In* "Trace Elements in Man and Animals-5" (C. F. Mills, I. Bremner, and J. K. Chesters, Eds.), p. 729. Commonwealth Agricultural Bureaux, Slough, UK.

Judson, G. J., D. W. Dewey, J. D. McFarlane and M. J. Riley. 1981. Oxidised copper wire for oral copper therapy in cattle. *In* "Trace Element Metabolism in Man and Animals-4" (J. McC. Howell, J. M. Gawthorne, and C. L. White, Eds.), p. 187. Australian Academy of Science, Canberra, Australia.

Judson, G. J., T.-S. Koh, J. D. McFarlane, R. K. Turnbull and B. R. Kempe. 1985b. Copper and selenium supplements for cattle: Evaluation of the selenium bullet, copper oxide and the soluble glass bullet. *In* "Trace Elements in Man and Animals-5" (C. F. Mills, I. Bremner, and J. K. Chesters, Eds.), p. 725. Commonwealth Agricultural Bureaux, Slough, UK.

Judson, G. J., C. L. Trengove, M. W. Langman and R. Vandergraaff. 1984. Copper supplementation of sheep. *Aust. Vet. J.* **61**:40.

Kegley, E. B. and J. W. Spears. 1993. Bioavailability of feed grade copper sources (oxide, sulfate or lysine) in growing cattle. *J. Anim. Sci.* **71** (Suppl. 1):27 [Abstract].

Kincaid, R. L., R. M. Blauwiekel and J. D. Cronrath. 1986. Supplementation of copper as copper sulfate or copper proteinate for growing calves fed forages containing molybdenum. *J. Dairy Sci.* **69**:160.

Kirchgessner, M. and E. Grassman. 1970. Dynamics of copper absorption. *In* "Trace Element Metabolism in Animals" (C. F. Mills, Ed.), p. 227. Livingston, Edinburgh, Scotland.

Klauder, D. S. and H. G. Petering. 1977. Anemia of lead intoxication: a role for copper. *J. Nutr.* **107**: 1779.

Knott, P., B. Algar, G. Zervas and S. B. Telfer. 1985. Glass-A medium for providing animals with supplementary trace elements. In: "Trace Elements in Man and Animals-5" (C.F. Mills, I. Bremner, and J.K. Chesters, Eds.), p. 708. Commonwealth Agricultural Bureaux, Slough, UK.

Koh, T.-S. and G. J. Judson. 1987. Copper and selenium deficiency in cattle: An evaluation of methods of oral therapy and an observation of a copper-selenium interaction. *Vet. Res. Commun.* **11**:133.

L'Abbe, M. R. and P. W. F. Fischer. 1984. The effect of high dietary zinc and copper deficiency on the activity of copper requiring metalloenzymes in the growing rat. *J. Nutr.* **114**: 813.

Langlands, J. P., J. E. Bowles, C. E. Donald and A .J. Smith. 1986. Trace element nutrition of grazing ruminants. II. Hepatic copper storage in young and adult sheep and cattle given varying quantities of oxidized copper particles and other copper supplements. *Aust. J. Agric. Res.* **37**:189.

Lassiter, J. W. and M. C. Bell. 1960. Availability of copper to sheep from Cu-labeled inorganic compounds. *J. Anim. Sci.* **19**:754.

Lawson, D. C., R. G. Hemingway, J. J. Parkins and N. S. Ritchie. 1990. Field trials with multi-trace element/vitamin boluses for grazing cattle. *J. Sci. Food Agric.* **50**:282.

Lawson, D. C., N. S. Ritchie, R. G. Hemingway and J. J. Parkins. 1989. A novel, sustained-release rumen bolus for cattle, containing trace elements and vitamins. *Proc. Nutr. Soc.* **48**:89A.

Lawson, D. C., N. S. Ritchie and J. J. Parkins. 1991. The use of a multiple trace element and vitamin bolus in cattle under conditions of low selenium or low copper status. In: "Trace Elements in Man and Animals-7" (B. Momcilovic, Ed.), p. 15-8. Institute for Medical Research and Occupational Health, University of Zagreb, Zagreb, Yugoslavia.

Ledoux, D. R., P. R. Henry, C. B. Ammerman, P. V. Rao and R. D. Miles. 1991. Estimation of the relative bioavailability of inorganic copper sources for chicks using tissue uptake of copper. *J. Anim. Sci.* **69**:215.

Lee, D-Y., J. Schroeder and P. T. Gordon. 1988. Enhancement of Cu bioavailability in the rat by phytic acid. *J. Nutr.* **118**:712.

Lo, G. S., S. L. Settle and F. H. Steinke. 1984. Bioavailability of copper in isolated soybean protein using the rat as an experimental model. *J. Nutr.* **114**: 320.

Lonnerdal, B., J. G. Bell and C. L. Keen. 1985. Copper absorption from human milk, cow's milk, and infant formulas using a suckling rat model. *Am. J. Clin. Nutr.* **42**:836.

McFarlane, J. D., G. J. Judson, R. K. Turnbull and B. R. Kempe. 1991. An evaluation of copper-containing soluble glass pellets, copper oxide particles and injectable copper as supplements for cattle and sheep. *Aust. J. Exp. Agr.* **31**:165.

McNaughton, J. L., E. J. Day, B. C. Dilworth and B. D. Lott. 1974. Iron and copper availability from various sources. *Poult. Sci.* **53**:1325.

MacPherson, A. and R. G. Hemingway. 1968. Effects of liming and various forms of oral copper supplementation on the copper status of grazing sheep. *J. Sci. Food Agric.* **19**:53.

Magee, A. C. and G. Matrone. 1962. Studies on growth, copper metabolism and iron metabolism of rats fed high levels of zinc. *J. Nutr.* **72**:233.

Manston, R., B. F. Sansom, W. M. Allen, H. J. Prosser, D. M. Groffman, P. J. Brant and A. D. Wilson. 1985. Reaction cements as materials for the sustained release of trace elements into the digestive tract of cattle and sheep. 1. Copper release. *J. Vet. Pharmacol. Therap.* **8**:368.

Miles, R. D. , C. B. Ammerman, P. R. Henry, and S. F. O'Keefe. 1994. The influence of high dietary copper supplementation from two feed-grade inorganic sources on broiler performance, tissue copper accumulation and dietary prooxidant activity. *Poult. Sci.* **73**(Suppl. 1): 114 [Abstract].

Miltimore, J. E., C. M. Kalnin and J. B. Clapp. 1978. Copper storage in the livers of cattle supplemented with injected copper and with copper sulfate and chelated copper. *Can. J. Anim. Sci.* **58**:525.

Murthy L., L. M. Klevay and H. G. Petering. 1974. Interrelationships of zinc and copper nutriture in the rat. *J. Nutr.* **104**:1458.

Nesbit, A. H. and W. P. Elmslie. 1960. Biological availability to the rat of iron and copper from various compounds. *Trans. Illinois State Acad. Sci.* **53**:101.

Norvell, M. J., M. C. Thomas, W. D. Coatcher, D. A. Gable and C. C. Calvert. 1974. Some effects of high dietary levels of various salts of copper in broiler chickens. *In* " Trace Substances in Environmental Health-8" (D. D. Hemphill, Ed.). Univesity of Missouri, Columbia, MO.

Norvell, M. J., D. A. Cable and M. C. Thomas. 1975. Effects of feeding high levels of various copper salts to broiler chickens. *In* "Trace Substances in Environmental Health - 9" (D. D. Hemphill, Ed.). University of Missouri, Columbia, MO.

National Research Council (NRC). 1989. " Recommended Dietary Allowances". 10th ed. National Academy Press, Washington, DC.

O'Dell, B. L. 1976. Biochemistry and physiology of copper in vertebrates. *In* "Trace Elements in Human Health and Disease" (A. S. Prasad and D. Oberleas, Ed.), Vol 1, p. 15. Academic Press, New York.

O'Dell, B. L. 1990. Dietary carbohydrate source and copper bioavailability. *Nutr. Rev.* **48**:425.

O'Dell, B. L., P. G. Reeves and R. F. Morgan. 1976. Interrelationships of tissue copper and zinc concentrations in rats nutritionally deficient in one or the other of these elements. *In* "Trace Sustances in Envirorunental Health" (D. D. Hemphill, Ed.), p. 411. University of Missouri, Columbia, MO.

Oestreicher, P. and R. J. Cousins. 1985. Copper and zinc absorption in the rat: Mechanism of mutual antagonism. *J. Nutr.* **115**:159.

Poole, D. B. R., D. McGrath, G. A. Fleming and W. Moore. 1990. Effects of applying copper-rich pig slurry to grassland. 4. Sheep feeding experiments. *Irish J. Agric. Res.* **29**:35.

Price, J. and J. K. Chesters. 1985. A new bioassay for assessment of copper availability and its application in a study of the effect of molybdenum on the distribution of available copper in ruminant digesta. *Br. J. Nutr.* **53**:323.

Prince, T. J., V. W. Hays and G. L. Cromwell. 1975. Environmental effects of high copper pig manure on pastures for sheep. *J. Anim. Sci.* **41**:326 [Abstract].

Pott, E. B., P. R. Henry, C. B. Ammerman, A. M. Merritt, J. B. Madison and R. D. Miles. 1994. Relative bioavailability of copper in a copper-lysine complex for chicks and lambs. *Anim. Feed Sci. Technol.* **45**:193.

Richards, D. H., G. R. Hewett, J. M. Parry and C. H. Yeoman. 1985. Bovine copper deficiency: Use of copper oxide needles. *Vet. Rec.* **116**:618.

Ritchie, H. D., R. W . Luecke, B. W. Baltzer, E. R. Miller, D. E. Ullrey and J. A. Hoefer. 1963. Copper and zinc interrelationships in the pig. *J. Nutr.* **79**:117.

Ritchie, N. S., D. C. Lawson and J. J. Parkins. 1991. A multiple trace element and vitamin sustained release bolus for cattle. *In* "Trace Elements in Man and Animals-7" (B. Momcilovic, Ed.), p. 15-12. Institute for Medical Research and Occupational Health, University of Zagreb, Zagreb, Yugoslavia.

Robbins, K. R. and D. H. Baker. 1980a. Effect of high-level copper feeding on sulfur amino acid need of chicks fed corn-soybean meal and purified crystalline amino acid diets. *Poul. Sci.* **59**:1099.

Robbins, K. R. and D. H. Baker. 1980b. Effect of sulfur amino acid level and source on the performance of chicks fed high levels of copper. *Poult. Sci.* **59**:1246.

Rogers, P. A. M. and D. B. R. Poole. 1988. Copper oxide needles for cattle: A comparison with parental treatment. *Vet. Rec.* **123**:147.

Saylor, W. W. and R. M. Leach. 1980. Intracellular distribution of copper and zinc in sheep: Effect of age and dietary levels of the metals. *J. Nutr.* **110**: 448.

Schoenemann, H. M., M. L. Failla and N. C. Steele. 1990. Consequences of severe copper deficiency are independent of dietary carbohydrate in young pigs. *Am. J. Clin. Nutr.* **52**:147.

Schultze, M. O., C. A. Elvehjem and E. B. Hart. 1934. The availability of copper in various compounds as a supplement to iron in bemoglobin formation. *J. Biol. Chem.* **106**:735.

Schultze, M. O., C. A. Elvehjem and E. B. Hart. 1936. Further studies on the availability of copper from various sources as a supplement to iron in hemoglobin formation. *J. Biol. Chem.* **115**: 453.

Sholfield, D. J., S. Reiser, M. Fields, N. C. Steele, J. C. Smith, S. Darcey and K. Ono. 1990. Dietary copper, simple sugars, and metabolic changes in pigs. *J. Nutr. Biochem.* **1**:362.

Smith, C. B. and W. R. Bidlack. 1980. Interrelationship of dietary ascorbic acid and iron on the tissue distribution of ascorbic acid, iron and copper in female guinea pigs. *J. Nutr.* **110**:1398.

Smith, S. E. and E. J. Larson. 1946. Zinc toxicity in rats. Antagonistic effects of copper and liver. *J. Biol. Chem.* **163**:29.

Southern, L. L. and D. H. Baker. 1983. Zinc toxicity, zinc deficiency and zinc- copper interrelationship in *Eimera acervulina*-infected chicks. *J. Nutr.* **113**:688.

Starcher, B. C. 1969. Studies on the mechanism of copper absorption in the chick. *J. Nutr.* **97**:321.

Stuart, M. A. and P. E. Johnson. 1986. Copper absorption and copper balance during consecutive periods for rats fed varying levels of dietary copper. *J. Nutr.* **116**:1028.

Sutherland, A. K. , G. R. Moule and J. M. Harvey. 1955. On the toxicity of copper aminoacetate injection and copper sulphate drench for sheep. *Aust. Vet. J.* **1**:141.

Suttle, N. F. 1974a. A technique for measuring the biological availability of copper to sheep, using hypocupremic ewes. *Br. J. Nutr.* **32**:395.

Suttle, N. F. 1974b. Effects of organic and inorganic sulphur on the availability of dietary copper to sheep. *Br. J. Nutr.* **32**: 559.

Suttle, N. F. 1974c. Recent studies of the copper-molybdenum antagonism. *Proc. Nutr. Soc.* **33**: 299.

Suttle, N. F. 1981. Comparison between parenterally administered copper complexes of their ability to alleviate hypocupraemia in sheep and cattle. *Vet. Rec.* **109**:304.

Suttle, N. F. 1987. The nutritional requirement for copper in animals and man. *In* "Copper in Animals and Man" (J. McC. Howell and J. M. Gawthorne, Eds.), Vol. I, p. 21. CRC Press, Boca Raton, FL.

Suttle, N. F. and J. Price. 1976. The potential toxicity of copper-rich animal excreta to sheep. *Anim. Prod.* **23**:233.

Telfer, S. B. and G. Zervas. 1982. The release of copper from soluble glass bullets in the reticulorumen of sheep. *Anim. Prod* . **34**:379.

Trengove, C. L. and G. J. Judson. 1985. Trace element supplementation of sheep: Evaluation of various copper supplements and a soluble glass bullet containing copper, cobalt and selenium. *Aust. Vet. J.* **62**:321.

van Campen, D. and E. Gross. 1968. Influence of ascorbic acid on the absorption of copper by rats. *J. Nutr.* **95**:617.

van Campen, D. R. and E. A. Mitchell. 1965. Absorption of Cu , Zn , Mo99 and Fe from ligated segments of the rat gastrointentinal tract. *J. Nutr.* **86**:120.

van Campen, D. R. and P. U. Scaife. 1967. Zinc interference with copper absorption in rats. *J. Nutr.* **91**:473.

van Reen, R. 1953. Effects of excessive dietary zinc in the rat and the interrelationship with copper. *Arch. Biochem. Biophys.* **46**:337.

Voelker, R. W. and W. W. Carlton. 1969. Effect of ascorbic acid on copper deficiency in miniature swine. *Am. J. Vet. Res.* **30**:1825.

Waibel, P. E., D. C. Snetsinger, R. A. Ball and J. H. Sautter. 1964. Variation in tolerance of turkeys to dietary copper. *Poult. Sci.* **43**:504.

Wittenberg, K. M., R. J. Boila and M. A. Shariff. 1990. Comparison of copper sulfate and copper proteinate as copper sources for copper-depleted steers fed high molybdenum diets. *Can. J. Anim. Sci.* **70**:895.

Xin, Z., D. F. Waterman, R. W. Hemken, R. J. Harmon and J. A. Jackson. 1991. Effects of copper sources and dietary cation-anion balance on copper availability and acid-base status in dairy calves. *J. Dairy Sci.* **74**:3167.
Zanetti, M. A., P. R. Henry, C. B. Ammerman and R. D. Miles. 1991. Estimation of the relative bioavailability of copper sources in chicks fed conventional dietary levels. *Br. Poult. Sci.* **32**:583.

8

IODINE BIOAVAILABILITY

Elwyn R. Miller

Department of Animal Science
Michigan State University
East Lansing,Michigan

Clarence B. Ammerman

Department of Animal Science
University of Florida
Gainesville, Florida

I. INTRODUCTION

Iodine is an essential micromineral for all animal species, including humans (Hetzel and Maberly, 1986; Hetzel, 1989). It occurs in plant tissue predominantly as inorganic iodide and is readily absorbed in this form from all segments of the intestinal tract (Barua *et al.*, 1964). Iodine is an integral part of the thyroid hormones thyroxine (tetraiodothyronine) and triiodothyronine, which are essential for normal growth and development in animals. Iodine is not distributed uniformily within the environment, and concentrations of the element in plant material and water are extremely variable. There are vast areas throughout the world where iodine deficiency disorders are a serious problem in both human and domestic animal populations, and supplementation with the element is required.

Few definitive studies of iodine bioavailability have been done since 1973. The current information is primarily from the work of Miller and his associates at the University of Tennessee with dairy cattle. These studies have been well documented by Ammerman and Miller (1972), Miller *et al.* (1975), and Miller (1980), and the general conclusion is that the common supplemental forms of iodine, with the exception of 3,5-diiodosalicylic acid (DIS) for ruminants, are of high bioavailability for animals.

BIOAVAILABILITY OF NUTRIENTS FOR ANIMALS:
AMINO ACIDS, MINERALS, AND VITAMINS

157

II. BIOAVAILABILITY STUDIES

A. Oral Administration

Early studies had shown that either sodium (NaI) or potassium iodide (KI), as supplemental sources of iodine, were effective in maintaining normal thyroid weights in rats fed goitrogenic diets (McClendon, 1927; Remington, 1937; Remington and Remington, 1938). Following these studies, Hixson and Rosner (1957) fed day-old chicks a goitrogenic diet supplemented with either potassium iodide or calcium iodate [$Ca(IO_3)_2 \cdot H_2O$] to 6 weeks of age. Based on maintenance of normal thyroid weight and histological examination of this gland, calcium iodate and potassium iodide were equal as sources of iodine for the chick (Tables I and II). Kuhajek and Andefinger (1970) observed that calcium iodate, pentacalcium orthoperiodate [PCOP; $Ca_5(IO_6)_2$], and sodium iodide were equally effective in maintaining normal thyroid weights when fed at a supplementary dietary iodine concentration of .15 ppm to weanling rats given a goitrogenic diet. Sihombing et al. (1974) and Cromwell et al. (1975) obtained positive responses with potassium iodate (KIO_3) in growing swine. Andrews and Sinclair (1962), in studies with sheep, found that oral administration of potassium iodate to ewes consuming plants with goitrogenic activity was effective in reducing goiter and neonatal mortality in their lambs.

Bioavailable iodine has been defined as that which can be absorbed from the gastrointestinal tract, trapped, and incorporated into thyroactive hormones by the thyroid gland, or otherwise stored in body tissues (Talbot et al., 1976). Several researchers have used uptake of stable or radioactive iodine by the thyroid or other tissue as an indication of bioavailability of an iodine source. Aschbacher et al. (1963) used radioactive iodine to investigate DIS ($C_7H_4I_2O_3$) as a source of iodine for ruminants. Dairy calves were dosed orally with ^{131}I as either [^{131}I]DIS or iodide ($^{131}I^-$). Plasma radioactivity reached greater levels and remained elevated longer for DIS than for iodide. Peak plasma levels of activity for the iodide occurred at 8 to 10 hr post dosing, with less than 1% of the activity being protein-bound. Maximal plasma levels of activity from DIS occurred approximately 24 hr post dosing at which time over 90% of the radioiodine was protein-bound. This was in keeping with an earlier finding by King and Lee (1959) in which unusually high plasma protein-bound iodine levels were observed in cattle receiving DIS. In the study by Aschbacher et al. (1963), urinary radioactivity expressed as a percentage of oral dose was approximately twice as high for DIS as for iodide (83.2 vs 46.1%). When expressed on a similar basis, thyroid uptake of radioiodine averaged 5.5% for DIS and 26.8% for the iodide, yielding a relative bioavailability of 21% for the iodine in DIS. After further research with similar results, Miller et al. (1964) suggested that absorbed DIS is cleared rapidly from the animal body by urinary excretion as intact DIS or as a corresponding salicyluric acid. Rats have a greater capacity than cattle to remove iodine from DIS (Aschbacher and Feil, 1968), which explains the higher bioavailability observed with this species. Based on maintenance of normal thyroid weight, Mittler and Benham (1954) found a relative bioavailability in rats of about 80% for the iodine in DIS when compared with that in potassium iodide. Supplemental dietary DIS given to lactating cows did not influence greatly the metabolism of orally administered ^{125}I-Na. A similar level of iodine given as potassium iodide, however, resulted in a 34% reduction in milk ^{125}I and 38% increase in urinary ^{125}I (Miller et al., 1965). A double tracer technique was used by Aschbacher et al. (1966) to study iodine utilization. Both [^{131}]DIS and iodide (^{125}I$^-$) were given simultaneously as oral doses to pregnant cows. When calculated as mean ratios for radioiodine uptake by maternal thyroid and fetal thyroid, the bioavailability values of iodine in DIS relative to iodide were 13 and 14%, respectively. The results of these studies indicated that the use of absorption information including plasma responses may be misleading in determining the bioavailability of iodine from certain compounds.

Miller et al. (1968) observed that calcium iodate, PCOP and sodium iodide were equal as sources of iodine for cattle. In further studies, Moss and Miller (1970) gave either ^{125}I-labeled calcium iodate or ^{125}I-labeled PCOP in combination with ^{131}I-Na as single doses placed either in the rumen or abomasum of calves. The most rapid absorption of radioiodine from either the rumen or abomasum occurred with sodium iodide but, by 24 hr after dosing, no difference among the iodine sources was found. In vitro studies by the same authors suggested that initial delay in absorption of iodine from PCOP and calcium iodate was caused by the time required for reduction of iodate to iodide, with the time interval being longer for doses placed in the rumen than for those placed in the abomasum. Earlier studies by Barua et al. (1964) indicated the rumen to be a major site of absorption of radioiodine in the form of sodium iodide. Both rats and rabbits have been shown to readily convert orally administered iodate to iodide (Taurog et al., 1966).

Ethylenediamine dihydriodide (EDDI; $C_2H_8N_2 \cdot 2HI$) has been used at relatively high dietary concentrations in the prevention and treatment of soft tissue lumpy jaw and footrot in cattle (Miller and Tillapaugh, 1966; Berg et al., 1984). Based on comparative data from oral doses of ^{125}I-labeled EDDI and ^{131}I-labeled sodium iodide in dairy cows, Miller and Swanson (1973) reported radioiodine from EDDI to be 10% greater in plasma compared to that from sodium iodide. Radioiodine from EDDI was lower in feces and urine suggesting greater retention of iodine from EDDI than occurred from sodium iodide. Milk iodine levels have responded in direct correlation to dietary EDDI (Berg et al., 1988). Preston (1994) administered single oral doses of stable iodine to steers and, based on serum inorganic iodine, found that iodine was absorbed equally from EDDI and potassium iodide and that calcium iodate had a relative bioavailability of 88% when compared to the other two sources.

The predominant sources of iodine used by the animal feed industry are calcium iodate, EDDI, and potassium iodide (Nelson, 1988). Other iodine sources approved for use in the United States in animal feeds are calcium iodobehenate, PCOP, cuprous iodide, potassium iodate, sodium iodate, sodium iodide, th/mol iodide, and DIS (AAFCO, 1994).

B. Injectable Forms

Injectable forms of iodized oils, as well as iodized oils administered orally, have served as effective sources of supplemental iodine in the reduction of endemic goiter in human populations (Hetzel and Maberly, 1986; Hetzel, 1989). Sheep in areas of borderline iodine deficiency in New Zealand were injected intramuscularly with iodized oil or given potassium iodide orally (Myers and Ross, 1959). The two sources of iodine gave equally positive responses as determined by histological examinations of the thyroid. Iodized oil injected once during pregnancy was effective in reducing goiter and neonatal mortality in lambs when the ewes were consuming plants with goitrogenic activity (Andrews and Sinclair, 1962).

III. FACTORS INFLUENCING BIOAVAILABILITY

A. Stability of Compounds

Iodine is unique in that stability of the carrier compound is of importance. Early observations indicated that potassium iodide and sodium iodide can readily lose iodine when mixed with other minerals or when subjected to adverse storage conditions involving moisture, heat, or sunlight. Supplemental iodine is provided frequently to grazing livestock in the United States as iodized salt in the form of blocks or as an iodine compound present in a mineral mixture provided for free-choice consumption. With either practice, the iodine-containing compound is subjected to atmospheric conditions. Iodine can become physically unavailable by leaching or by migration of the iodine compounds from the surface of blocks as a result of absorbed atmospheric moisture. The resulting brine can migrate either inward by capillary action or downward by gravity. Davidson and Watson (1948) showed that potassium iodide was unstable in salt blocks except in dry, dark storage and in further research, Davidson et al. (1951) found that diiododithymol and potassium iodate were relatively stable in salt blocks tested under practical feeding conditions. Shuman and Townsend (1963) tested the physical stability of potassium iodide, calcium iodate, and DIS when added to salt blocks. The salt samples were exposed to high humidity, simulated rainfall, and tested under field conditions. Under these conditions, iodine from potassium iodide and calcium iodate was lost rapidly from the surface layer of the salt, while that as DIS remained in the surface layer. Potassium iodide was highly soluble in water or sodium chloride brine, whereas DIS and calcium iodate were relatively insoluble. It would seem desirable to have an insoluble iodine source for use in mineral mixtures which are exposed to atmospheric conditions that would not be leached by exposure to moisture but would be of high biological availability. Although DIS was the most stable of the iodine compounds tested, its iodine has a very low bioavailability to ruminants.

B. Goitrogenic Substances

Goitrogenic substances present in feed or food are the most important factors influencing iodine bioavailability. Brassica species of plants, such as rape, kale, cabbage, and turnips, contain high concentrations of goitrogens. There are two types of goitrogens, thiocyanates and goitrin (L-5-vinyl-2-thiooxalidone), that originate from these plants (Underwood, 1977). Thiocyanates are converted from cyanogenic glucosides and goitrin from progoitrin. Thiocyanates inhibit the selective concentration of iodine by the thyroid, and their action is reversible by iodine. Goitrin, however, limits hormonogenesis in the gland, presumably through inhibition of thyroid peroxidase, and its action is either not reversible by iodine or is only partly so (Cromwell et al., 1975; Underwood, 1977). Iodine supplementation will alleviate the hypothyroidism and performance reduction caused by feeding high-glucosinolate rapeseed meal to swine, and efficacy of the iodine can be enhanced by dietary copper supplementation (Ludke and Schone, 1988; Schone et al., 1988). The glucosinolate is inactivated by treatment with copper sulfate solution. Moreover, extrusion of rapeseed with barley eliminated its hypothyroidism effect (Maskell et al., 1988). Other feeds, such as soybean, cottonseed, and linseed meals, lentils, and peanuts also contain goitrogenic substances (Sihombing et al., 1974; Miller, 1979; Matovinovic, 1983; NRC, 1988).

C. Other Factors

Perchlorates and rubidium salts were known to interfere with iodine uptake by the thyroid (Underwood, 1977). Bromide, fluoride, cobalt, manganese, and nitrate inhibited normal iodine uptake (Talbot et al., 1976). Likewise, excess calcium intake has been shown to have an antithyroid effect (Taylor, 1954). Selenium is necessary for the conversion of tetraiodothyronine to triiodothyronine through its role in the selenoprotein, 5'-deiodinase (Behne *et al.*, 1992). Thus, selenium deficiency can influence iodine bioavailability. There was also evidence to indicate that protein-calorie malnutrition reduced intestinal iodine absorption and thyroid iodine clearance and radioiodide uptake (Ingenbleek and Beckers, 1973, 1978). Finally, excess iodine intake has been shown to inhibit thyroid activity, presumably by blocking the selective concentration of iodine by the thyroid (Baker and Lindsay, 1968; Nagataki, 1974; Newton and Clawson, 1974; Fish and Swanson, 1983; Kaneko, 1989).

IV. SUMMARY

There has been only limited research on the bioavailability of supplemental dietary sources of iodine. Sodium iodide, potassium iodide, and ethylenediamine dihydriodide are well utilized by animals as sources of iodine. Calcium iodate and pentacalcium orthoperiodate are also of high bioavailability and have been shown to have greater physical stability. Potassium iodide or sodium iodide have usually served as the reference standard when comparative studies were conducted. Diiodosalicyclic acid is a relatively stable compound which is bioavailable to rats but not well utilized by ruminants. Little is known about the bioavailability of iodine from plant material and animal by-products.

Table I. Bioavailability of iodine sources for animals[a]

Source	RV	Standard	Response criterion	Meth cal	Type diet	Added level	Reference
Chickens							
Calcium iodate [Ca(IO$_3$)$_2$·H$_2$O]	95	KI	Thy wt	TP	SP	.59 ppm	Hixson and Rosner (1957)
Cattle							
Ca(IO$_3$)$_2$, (^{125}I)[b]	100	Na ^{131}I	Thy RA	MR	N	NG	Miller et al. (1968)
Ca(IO$_3$)$_2$, (^{125}I)[b]	100	Na ^{131}I	Pla RA	MR	N	NG	Moss and Miller (1970)
Ca(IO$_3$)$_2$	88	KI	Ser I	MR	NG	.2 mg/kg BW	Preston (1994)
Diiodosalicylic acid, (DIS, C$_7$H$_4$I$_2$O$_3$), (^{131}I)[b]	21	Iodide (^{131}I)	Thy RA	MR	N	NG	Aschbacher et al. (1963)
DIS (^{131}I)[b]	13	Iodide (^{125}I)	Maternal thy RA	MR	N	NG	Aschbacher et al. (1966)
DIS (^{131}I)[b]	14	Iodide (^{125}I)	Fetal thy RA	MR	N	NG	Aschbacher et al. (1966)
Ethylenediamine dihydriodide[b] (EDDI, C$_2$H$_8$N$_2$·2HI), (^{125}I)	110	Na ^{131}I	Thy RA	MR	N	NG	Miller and Swanson (1973)
EDDI	100	KI	Ser I	MR	NG	.2 mg/kg BW	Preston (1994)
Pentacalcium orthoperiodate [PCOP, Ca$_5$(IO$_6$)$_2$], (^{125}I)[b]	104	Na ^{131}I	Thy RA	MR	N	NG	Miller et al. (1968)
PCOP (^{125}I)[b]	100	Na ^{131}I	Pla RA	MR	N	NG	Moss and Miller (1970)

Table I. (continued)

Source	RV	Standard	Response criterion	Meth cal	Type diet	Added level	Reference
Rats							
$Ca(IO_3)_2$	87	KI	Thy wt	TP	N	.15 ppm	Kuhajek and Andelfinger (1970)
Cuprous iodide (Cu_2I_2)	104	KI	Thy wt	TP	N	.265 ppm	Mittler and Benham (1954)
Cuprous iodide	110	KI	Thy wt	TP	N	5.25 μg/wk	Mittler and Benham (1954)
DIS	65	KI	Thy wt	TP	N	.265 ppm	Mittler and Benham (1954)
DIS	96	KI	Thy wt	TP	N	5.25 μg/wk	Mittler and Benham (1954)
Diiodothymol $(C_6H_2 \cdot CH_3OIC_3H_2)_2$	54	KI	Thy wt	TP	N	.265 ppm	Mittler and Benham (1954)
Diiodothymol	93	KI	Thy wt	TP	N	5.25 μg/wk	Mittler and Benham (1954)
$Ca_3(IO_6)_2$	92	KI	Thy wt	TP	N	.15 ppm	Kuhajek and Andelfinger (1970)

[a]Abbreviations are found in Appendix I. Chemical formula for a compound given only if provided by the author.
[b]Equal radioactivity as either ^{125}I or ^{131}I in different compounds administered simultaneously in an oral form to the same animal.

Table II. Relative bioavailability of supplemental iodine sources[a]

Source	Poultry	Cattle	Rats
Potassium iodide	100	100	100
Sodium iodide	100	100	100
Calcium iodate	95 (1)	95 (3)	90 (1)
Cuprous iodide	-	-	105 (2)
Diiodosalicylic acid	-	15 (3)	80 (2)
Diiodothymol	-	-	75 (2)
Ethylenediamine dihydriodide	-	105 (2)	-
Pentacalcium orthoperiodate	-	100 (2)	-

[a]Average values rounded to nearest "5" and expressed relative to response obtained with potassium or sodium iodide. Number of studies involved indicated within parentheses.

REFERENCES

Ammerman, C. B. and S. M. Miller. 1972. Biological availability of minor mineral ions: A review. *J. Anim. Sci.* **35**:681.

Andrews, E. D. and D. P. Sinclair. 1962. Goitre and neonatal mortality in lambs. *Proc. N. Z. Soc. Anim. Prod.* **22**:123.

Aschbacher, P. W., R. G. Cragle, E. W. Swanson and J. K. Miller. 1966. Metabolism of oral iodide and 3,5-diiodosalicylic acid in the pregnant cow. *J. Dairy Sci.* **49**:1042.

Aschbacher, P. W. and V. J. Feil. 1968. Metabolism of 3,5-diiodosalicylic acid in cattle and rats. *J. Dairy Sci.* **51**:762.

Aschbacher, P. W., J. K. Miller and R. G. Cragle. 1963. Metabolism of diiodosalicylic acid in dairy calves. *J. Dairy Sci.* **46**:1114.

Association of American Feed Control Officials. 1994. Official publication, pp. 187-201. AAFCO, Atlanta, GA.

Baker, H. J. and J. R. Lindsey. 1968. Equine goiter due to excess dietary iodine. *J. Am. Vet. Med. Assoc.* **153**:1618.

Barua, J., R. G. Cragle and J. K. Miller. 1964. Sites of gastrointestinal-blood passage of iodide and thyroxine in young cattle. *J. Dairy Sci.* **47**:539.

Behne, D., A. Kyriakopoulos, H. Gessner, B. Walzog and H. Meinhold. 1992. Type I iodothyronine deiodinase activity after high selenium intake, and relations between selenium and iodine metabolism in rats. *J. Nutr.* **122**:1542.

Berg, J. N., J. P. Maas, J. A. Paterson, G. F. Krause and L. E. Davis. 1984. Efficacy of ethylenediamine dihydroiodide as an agent to prevent experimentally induced bovine foot rot. *Am. J. Vet. Res.* **45**:1073.

Berg, J. N., D. Padgitt and B. McCarthy. 1988. Iodine concentrations in milk of dairy cattle fed various amounts of iodine as ethylenediamine dihydroiodide. *J. Dairy. Sci.* **71**:3283.

Cromwell, G. L., D. T. H. Sihombing and V. W. Hays. 1975. Effects of iodine level on performance and thyroid traits of growing pigs. *J. Anim. Sci.* **41**:813.

Davidson, W. M., M. M. Finlayson, and C. J. Watson. 1951. The stability of various iodine compounds in salt blocks. *Sci. Agric.* **31**:148.

Davidson, W. M. and C. J. Watson. 1948. The stability of iodine in iodized rock salt. *Sci. Agric.* **28**:1.

Fish, R. E. and E. W. Swanson. 1983. Effects of excessive iodide administered in the dry period on thyroid function and health of dairy cows and their calves in the periparturient period. *J. Anim. Sci.* **56**:162.

Hetzel, B. S. 1989. "The Story of Iodine Deficiency." Oxford Univ. Press, New York.

Hetzel, B. S. and G. F. Maberly. 1986. Iodine. *In* " Trace Elements in Human and Animal Nutrition" (W. Mertz, Ed.), 5th ed., No. 2. p.139. Academic Press, New York.

Hixson, O. F. and L. Rosner. 1957. Calcium iodate as a source of iodine in poultry nutrition. *Poult. Sci.* **36**:712.

Ingenbleek, Y. and C. Beckers. 1973. Evidence for intestinal malabsorption of iodine in protein-calorie malnutrition. *Am. J. Clin. Nutr.* **26**:1323.

Ingenbleek, Y. and C. Beckers. 1978. Thyroidal iodide clearance and radioiodide uptake in protein-calorie malnutrition. *Am. J. Clin. Nutr.* **31**:408.

Kaneko, J. J. 1989. Thyroid function. *In* "Clinical Biochemistry of Domestic Animals" (J. J. Kaneko, Ed.), 4th ed. p. 630. Academic Press, San Diego.

King, W. A. and J. Lee, III. 1959. Source of iodine in salt affects protein-bound iodine content of bovine blood plasma. *J. Dairy Sci.* **42**:2003.

Kuhajek, E. J. and G. F. Andelfinger. 1970. A new source of iodine for salt blocks. *J. Anim. Sci.* **31**:51.

Ludke, H. and F. Schone. 1988. Copper and iodine in pig diets with high glucosinolate rapeseed meal. 1. Performance and thyroid hormone status of growing pigs fed on a diet with rapeseed meal treated with copper sulfate solution or untreated and supplements of iodine, copper, or a quinoxaline derivative. *Anim. Feed Sci. Technol.* **22**:33.

Maskell, I., M. Ellis and R. Smithard. 1988. Nutritive value of pig diets containing extruded or milled full-fat rapeseed. *Anim. Prod.* **46**:522 [Abstract].

Matovinovic, J. 1983. Endemic goiter and cretinism at the dawn of the third millennium. *Annu. Rev. Nutr.* **3**:341.

McClendon, J. F. 1927. The distribution of iodine with special reference to goiter. *Physiol. Rev.* **7**:189.

Miller, E. R. 1980. Bioavailability of minerals. *In* "41st Proceedings of the Minnesota Nutrition Conference" p. 144. Bloomington, MN.

Miller, J. I. and K. Tillapaugh. 1966. Iodide medicated salt for beef cattle. Cornell Feed Service, No. 62. Coop. Ext. Serv., Cornell University, Ithaca, NY.

Miller, J. K., P. W. Aschbacher and E. W. Swanson. 1964. Comparison of the metabolism of sodium iodide and 3,5-diiodosalicylic acid in dairy cattle. *J. Dairy Sci.* **47**:169.

Miller, J. K., B. R. Moss, E. W. Swanson, P. W. Aschbacher and R. G. Cragle. 1968. Calcium iodate and pentacalcium orthoperiodate as sources of supplemental iodine for cattle. *J. Dairy Sci.* **51**:1831.

Miller, J. K. and E. W. Swanson. 1973. Metabolism of ethylenediaminedihydriodide and sodium or potassium iodide by dairy cows. *J. Dairy Sci.* **56**:378.

Miller, J. K., E. W. Swanson and S. M. Hansen. 1965. Effects of feeding potassium iodide, 3,5-diiodosalicylic acid, or L-thyroxine on iodine metabolism of lactating dairy cows. *J. Dairy Sci.* **48**:888.

Miller, J. K., E. W. Swanson and G. E. Spalding. 1975. Iodine absorption, excretion, recycling, and tissue distribution in the dairy cow. *J. Dairy Sci.* **58**:1578.

Miller, W. J. 1979. "Dairy Cattle Feeding and Nutrition." Academic Press, New York.

Mittler, S. and G. H. Benham. 1954. Nutritional availability of iodine from several insoluble iodine compounds. *J. Nutr.* **53**:53.

Moss, B. R. and J. K. Miller. 1970. Metabolism of sodium iodide, calcium iodate, and pentacalcium orthoperiodate initially placed in the bovine rumen or abomasum. *J. Dairy. Sci.* **53**:772.

Myers, B. J. and D. A. Ross. 1959. The effects of iodine and thyroxine administration on the Romney crossbred ewe. *N. Z. J. Agric. Res.* **2**:552.

Nagataki, S. 1974. Effect of excess quantities of iodide. *In* "Handbook of Physiology, III," p. 329. Thyroid American Physiology Society, Washington, DC.

National Research Council (NRC). 1988. "Nutrient Requirements of Swine," 9th ed. National Academy Press, Washington, DC.

Nelson, J. 1988. Bioavailability of trace minerals. *In* "Proceedings of AFIA Nutrition Symposium: Profitable Animal Nutrition for the Future," p. 126. American Feed Industry Association, Arlington, VA.

Newton, G. L. and A. J. Clawson. 1974. Iodine toxicity: Physiological effects of elevated dietary iodine on pigs. *J. Anim. Sci.* **39**:879.

Preston, R. C. 1994. Serum inorganic iodine dynamics in cattle following a single oral dose of several iodine sources. *FASEB J.* **8**:A431 [Abstract].

Remington, R. E. 1937. Improved growth in rats on iodine deficient diets. *J. Nutr.* **13**:223.

Remington, R. E. and J. W. Remington. 1938. The effect of enhanced iodine intake on growth and on the thyroid glands of normal and goitrous rats. *J. Nutr.* **15**:539.

Schone, F., H. Ludke, A. Hennig and G. Jahreis. 1988. Copper and iodine in pig diets with high glucosinolate rapeseed meal. II. Influence of iodine supplements for rations with rapeseed meal untreated or treated with copper ions on performance and thyroid hormone status of growing pigs. *Anim. Feed Sci. Technol.* **22**:45.

Shuman, A. C. and D. P. Townsend. 1963. Evaluation of iodine sources for livestock salt. *J. Anim. Sci.* **22**:72.

Sihombing, D. T. H., G. L. Cromwell and V. W. Hays. 1974. Effects of protein source, goitrogens and iodine level on performance and thyroid status of pigs. *J. Anim. Sci.* **39**:1106.

Talbot, J. M., K. D. Fisher and C. J. Carr. 1976. " A Review of the Effects of Dietary Iodine on Certain Thyroid Disorders." Life Sciences Research Office, Federation of American Society of Experimental Biology, Bethesda, MD.

Taurog, A., E. M. Howells and H. I. Nachimson. 1966. Conversion of iodate to iodide *in vivo* and *in vitro*. *J. Biol. Chem.* **241**:4686.

Taylor, S. 1954. Calcium as a goitrogen. *J. Clin. Endocrinol. Metab.* **14**:1412.

Underwood, E. J. 1977. "Trace Elements in Human and Animal Nutrition," 4th ed. Academic Press, New York.

9

IRON BIOAVAILABILITY

Pamela R. Henry

Department of Animal Science
University of Florida
Gainesville, Florida

Elwyn R. Miller

Department of Animal Science
Michigan State University
East Lansing, Michigan

I. INTRODUCTION

The essentiality of iron has been known since ancient times and its beneficial effect on blood formation was recognized in the 17th century (Underwood, 1956). Practically all of the iron in the animal's body is organic in nature and only a very small percentage is found as free inorganic ions (Georgievskii, 1982). There are two kinds of organic iron, hemal and nonhemal. Hemal iron, which forms part of a porphyrin group, represents 70-75% of total iron and includes hemoglobin, myoglobin, cytochromes, cytochrome oxidase, catalase, and peroxidase. Nonhemal iron includes iron transport and storage forms such as transferrin, ferritin, hemosiderin, and other iron proteinates.

Iron content of the body varies with species, age, sex, nutrition, and state of health and is controlled by adjustment in absorption rate (Finch and Cook, 1984). The body has a limited capacity to excrete iron and considerable recycling of the element occurs, especially as a result of the breakdown of senescent red blood cells. Iron is absorbed mainly from the duodenum after ferric iron is reduced to the ferrous form (Georgievskii, 1982). Iron of plant origin is more readily absorbed than nonhemal iron of animal origin. Iron in nonheme, protein-bound compounds must be released before absorption, whereas iron in heme compounds is absorbed as the heme moiety without release from the bound form (Morris, 1987).

BIOAVAILABILITY OF NUTRIENTS FOR ANIMALS:
AMINO ACIDS, MINERALS, AND VITAMINS
Copyright © 1995 by Academic Press, Inc.

169

Although iron is the most abundant of the trace elements in the animal body, practical deficiency problems in domestic animals are generally limited to nursing pigs and, to a lesser extent, other milk-fed animals. Iron deficiency in grazing animals is generally the result of blood loss from heavy parasite infestation rather than nutritional inadequacy. Iron deficiency is far more prevalent in humans than in livestock, thus, much of the research on bioavailability of the element has concentrated on foods and sources intended for human consumption (Morris, 1987).

II. BIOAVAILABILITY STUDIES

A. Hemoglobin

Attempts to determine bioavailability of iron sources by measuring hemoglobin regeneration date back to the early 20th century (Mitchell and Schmidt, 1926; Waddell *et al.*, 1928; Elvehjem *et al.*, 1929). Interest in iron enrichment of foods for the human population produced numerous studies during the 1970s (Tables I and II). The standard used was generally ferrous sulfate heptahydrate ($FeSO_4 \cdot 7H_2O$) and rats or chicks fed iron-deficient purified diets were used as assay animals. Fritz *et al.* (1970), Pla and Fritz (1970), and others used the formula

$$RBV = 100 \ x \ \frac{mg/kg \ Fe \ as \ FeSO_4 \cdot 7H_2O \ for \ measured \ Hb \ response}{mg/kg \ Fe \ as \ test \ Fe \ source \ for \ equal \ Hb \ response},$$

where RBV is relative bioavailability value or relative availability and Hb is hemoglobin. This approach to bioavailability could essentially be considered that of a standard curve. Supplementation of a basal dried skim milk-corn meal-glucose diet containing about 7 ppm iron with 0, 5, 10, 15, or 20 ppm iron from $FeSO_4 \cdot 7H_2O$ created the standard curve (Pla and Fritz, 1970). Several foods and inorganic iron sources including ferrous and ferric chloride and two ferrous carbonates were added to the basal diet at 20 ppm iron as test sources. Test diets were fed to chicks that had been depleted of iron by feeding the basal diet for 2 weeks. Hemoglobin regeneration was measured after 2 weeks of feeding the test diets. Availability of ferrous chloride was 106% compared with 100% for ferrous sulfate, but that of ferric chloride was 78%. Both ferrous carbonates had very low relative availability estimates at 2 and 7%. Pla and Fritz (1970) also reported that solubility of various iron sources in dilute hydrochloric acid was not a reliable estimate of bioavailability as determined by the above method. Fritz *et al.* (1970) conducted similar experiments with chicks and rats and reported low values for availability of iron from several ferric orthophosphates, ferrous carbonates, and sodium iron pyrophosphates. Somewhat greater values were reported for reduced iron in chicks (41 - 66%) compared with rats (16 - 37%).

Amine *et al.* (1972) used a similar approach but compared slope ratios from the response of hemoglobin to graded concentrations of standard and test sources. These researchers depleted chicks for 3 weeks and fed the iron supplemented test diets for 2 weeks. Based on hemoglobin regeneration with ferrous sulfate set at 100%, bioavailability values were 49, 27, 4, and 2% for reduced iron, ferric orthophosphate, sodium iron pyrophosphate, and ferrous carbonate, respectively.

Pla *et al.* (1973) and Motzok *et al.* (1975) reported that rats were more sensitive in detecting differences among iron sources than were chicks. Fritz *et al.* (1975) introduced the use of a parallel line assay with rats. Weanling rats were depleted of iron stores and final hemoglobin concentrations rather than changes in hemoglobin concentration were used as the response criterion.

In the first half of the 20th century, iron sources were often chosen for food enrichment based on their light color and chemical inertness (failure to induce rancidity in food products) rather than for the bioavailability of their iron (Waddell, 1973). "Reduced iron" was the name applied to all forms of powdered iron used in the United States for food enrichment. The AAFCO (1994) definition of reduced iron is the metallic form of iron obtained by reduction of ferric oxide with hydrogen. A review of the differences among the members of the elemental iron powder family, hydrogen-reduced iron, carbon monoxide-reduced iron, electrolytic iron, and carbonyl iron, is available (Patrick, 1973), but will not be included herein because this form of the element is not used to any great extent by the feed industry for livestock supplementation at the present time.

B. Radioisotopes

Extrinsic and intrinsic radiolabels with ^{59}Fe have been used to study inorganic and nonheme iron bioavailability. The extrinsic label is generally considered a valid measure providing the tracer equilibrates with the nonheme iron pool, although there is a tendency toward slightly greater absorption with the extrinsic label. Extrinsic labeling of milk sources is not valid due to a difference in the binding site, and intrinsic labels must be used in these studies (Gislason *et al.*, 1991, 1992). A stable isotope of iron, ^{54}Fe, has been used to assess bioavailability of iron in humans, but not in domestic animals (Kaltwasser *et al.*, 1991; Hansen *et al.*, 1992).

Ferrous sulfate, ferric chloride, ferrous carbonate, and ferric oxide labeled with ^{59}Fe were given to calves and lambs (Ammerman *et al.*, 1967). Ferrous sulfate and ferric chloride were equal in bioavailability as sources of iron and ferric oxide was unavailable. Absorption of ^{59}Fe from ferrous carbonate was almost as great as that from the sulfate and cloride forms. This high degree of iron absorption from a freshly synthesized carbonate compound may not be representative of that from ferrous carbonate products that have been proposed for animal feeding. Considerable variation has been reported for ferrous carbonates, without any obvious explanation. Consequently, values have been grouped in Table II as "high" or "low" with the majority of researchers reporting results which would be included in the low availability group.

C. Injectable Forms

Iron forms including iron dextran, iron dextrin, and gleptoferron have been effective sources of iron when administered as single intramuscular injections to baby pigs in the first 3 days of life (NRC, 1988).

III. FACTORS INFLUENCING BIOAVAILABILITY

Many of the factors influencing bioavailability of iron were reviewed recently (Johnson et al., 1994).

A. Species

The bioavailability of iron in some feedstuffs can vary for different species. In the cat, a true carnivore, when iron utilization was based on hemoglobin regeneration, iron from beef liver was 350% as available as that from ferrous sulfate compared to 90% in the chick (Chausow and Czarnecki-Maulden, 1988a). Iron in corn gluten meal was 84% available for chicks but only 20% available for cats relative to 100% for ferrous sulfate. The rat is more sensitive to differences in particle size of some iron sources than is the chick.

B. Ascorbic Acid

Ascorbic acid effectively reduced and chelated nonheme iron when consumed with the iron, thus increasing its absorption (Greenberg et al., 1957; van Campen, 1972; Bates et al., 1988; Monsen, 1988). For ferric iron to be soluble in aqueous solutions, the solution pH needs to be less than 4.0 (Conrad and Schade, 1968). Since ascorbic acid at high levels can counteract the cessation of iron absorption induced by increasing pH (Hungerford and Linder, 1983), it is possible that maintenance of a soluble iron complex by ascorbic acid when intestinal lumen content pH increases is the principal mode of action of this antioxidant (Conrad and Schade, 1968), and not its effect on pH.

C. Phytate

Relative to ferrous sulfate, the bioavailability of iron in monoferric phytate, which is the primary form of iron in wheat bran, was 99% in rats (Morris and Ellis, 1982). In the same study, other phytate forms, especially di- or tetraferric phytate, had substantially lower bioavailability.

Sodium phytate reduced iron absorption in humans (Hallberg and Solvell, 1967), whereas in rats the addition of sodium phytate had no effect on iron absorption (Cowan et al., 1966; Hunter, 1981; Morris, 1987). Addition of phytate to the diet of anemic rats enhanced iron bioavailability (Gordon and Chao, 1984). Furthermore, the utilization of iron from wheat bran by rats was high, whereas in humans wheat bran decreased absorption of nonhemal iron. In calves, Bremner and Dalgarno (1973) observed that insoluble iron-phytate complexes contained little biologically available iron. Additions of 6 - 10% wheat bran to the diet of pigs had no inhibitory effects on iron absorption (Frolich, 1982). Furthermore, this research indicated that iron in bran and whole-grain cereal products was as available to pigs as iron from inorganic sources.

D. Protein

Cellular proteins, such as meat, fish, and poultry products, can also enhance iron absorption (Cook and Monsen, 1976). Iron from animal sources is generally more available than iron contained in vegetable foods because of the considerable content of hemal iron (Morris, 1987). Certain amino acids, specifically cysteine (in either its single molecule form or as reduced glutathione), histidine, and lysine, can form tridentate chelates, and by this mechanism improve iron absorption (van Campen, 1972; 1973; Martinez-Torres et al., 1981). Low-protein diets appear to interfere with iron uptake (Coons, 1964; Layrisse et al., 1968), while hematocrit and hemoglobin levels were increased when rat diets contained a higher protein level. Caster and Resurreccion (1982), however, indicated that low protein diets improved iron absorption. Still other research (Beard et al., 1984) has indicated that in iron-deficient rats, iron absorption is unaffected by low protein, and that in high protein/low iron-fed rats, anemia is greater than in rats fed a lower protein level.

Soybean protein also influences iron absorption. Soy protein isolate, when fed to iron-deficient rats in either a pretest meal diet or a test meal diet, decreased total iron retention (Thompson and Erdman, 1984). Hisayasu *et al.* (1992) also reported decreased iron absorption in rats fed soybean protein isolate compared to casein and suggested that the decrease may be due, at least in part, to lectins. Hallberg and Rossander (1982) also observed that soy protein decreased percentage iron absorption in humans when added to a hamburger meal. However, it should be noted that the decrease in percentage absorption availability was related to increased iron intake (Morris, 1987).

Somewhat different results of soy protein effects on iron absorption have been reported in chicks. Aoyagi and Baker (1995) reported that chicks fed a casein-based diet with 5% soy protein concentrate required 85 ppm iron to maximize hemoglobin and serum iron concentration. An earlier study by Southern and Baker (1982) had indicated that the iron requirement was 40 ppm for chicks fed a casein diet without soy products. Thus, because the basal casein-soy concentrate diet of Aoyagi and Baker (1995) contained 47 ppm iron, most of which came from the soy product, yet still required an additional 40 ppm iron from ferrous sulfate to obtain maximal blood hemoglobin, the conclusion was that the iron in soy protein concentrate must be almost entirely unavailable for the chick. Furthermore, they concluded that soy protein concentrate *per se* did not affect the utilization of iron from supplemental ferrous sulfate, which is in agreement with earlier work of Davis *et al.* (1968). Chicks may differ from rats regarding iron metabolism, or alcohol-extracted soy protein concentrate (65% protein) may have minimal effects on inorganic iron utilization, whereas alcohol-extracted soy protein isolate (90% protein) may have considerable capacity to bind inorganic iron that is added to a diet.

E. Pectin

Pectin is an important component of water-soluble dietary fiber and because of its free carboxyl groups can complex with polyvalent cations, including iron, thereby decreasing their availability. However, several pectins were actually found to enhance iron absorption and the efficiency of hemoglobin regeneration in anemic rats (Kim and Atallah, 1992; 1993).

F. Minerals

Increasing dietary calcium and/or phosphorus concentrations decreased iron absorption in chicks (Waddell and Sell, 1964; Sell, 1965) and rats (Amine and Hegsted, 1971; Monsen and Cook, 1976; Kochanowski and McMahan, 1990; Prather and Miller, 1992; Wienk *et al.*, 1993). Studies in rats given various doses of iron with and without added cobalt suggested that cobalt can saturate a common absorptive pathway (Schade *et al.*, 1970). Forth *et al.* (1973) found that a 10-fold excess of cobalt reduced absorption of ^{59}Fe from rat jejunal loops by two-thirds and a 100-fold excess essentially eliminated iron absorption.

In swine, dietary concentrations of 120 to 240 ppm of copper decreased liver iron concentrations by 50 to 60% (Bradley et al., 1983), possibly by impaired absorption of iron. High levels of dietary copper can also cause an iron-deficiency anemia (Gipp et al., 1973; Underwood, 1977). However, physiological levels of copper (up to 5 ppm) may improve iron absorption and utilization in the pig and rat (Lee et al., 1968; Marston et al.,1971; Evans and Abraham, 1973), especially when the animal is in an iron-deficient state.

Excess zinc interferes with iron incorporation into ferritin (Settlemire and Matrone, 1967a). Although the anemia that occurs in rats when dietary zinc levels exceed the animal's requirements are largely due to zinc's antagonistic activity on copper, tissue iron concentrations are also decreased, indicating a direct effect of zinc on iron metabolism (Cox and Harris, 1960; Magee and Matrone, 1960; Story and Gregor, 1987). Furthermore, excess zinc may increase the iron requirement by decreasing the life span of red blood cells (Settlemire and Matrone, 1967b). These rat studies used plethoric levels of zinc (2400 to 6000 ppm) and whether hematopoietic criteria were depressed because of reduction in food intake and thus, iron intake, or because of true antagonism of iron by excess zinc was not easily discernable. With chicks, excess zinc (2000 ppm) has been shown to antagonize iron when the zinc was added to a corn-soybean meal diet containing both phytate and soluble fiber (Bafundo et al., 1984) When a casein-dextrose diet devoid of both phytate and fiber was fed, however, concentrations of excess zinc up to 1500 ppm did not have any effect on iron utilization (Parsons et al., 1989).

Hartman et al. (1955), with young lambs, and Baker and Halpin (1991), with young chicks, reported that excessive dietary manganese decreased hemoglobin. Tissue iron was also depressed in anemic rabbits and pigs when high dietary manganese was fed (Matrone et al., 1959). In rats, high levels of dietary nickel increased the iron content of liver in marginally iron-adequate rats and increased hematopoiesis (Nielsen et al., 1984). Iron absorption was lower in nickel-deficient rats (Morris, 1987).

G. Feed or Food Processing

Heat and pressure processing of ferrous sulfate, sodium ferric pyrophosphate, ferric orthophosphate, or ferric pyrophosphate increased the bioavailability of iron for chicks (Wood et al., 1978). Furthermore, upon sterilization of a milk-based infant formula, the bioavailability of iron from ferric pyrophosphate or sodium iron pyrophosphate was increased (Theurer et al., 1973).

Prolonged warming of meals for humans can also influence iron bioavailability. When meals were kept warm (75°C for 4 hr), the bioavailability of nonheme iron was reduced (Hallberg *et al.*, 1982). This reduction, however, was attributed to a marked loss in ascorbic acid, which, when added to the diet, reversed this reduction in iron utilization

H. Other Factors

Cellulose and oxalate increased the bioavailability of ferrous iron (Gordon and Chao, 1984). However, research by Reinhold *et al.* (1986) indicated that fiber from corn or wheat decreased iron retention. Furthermore, the inclusion of citrate or ascorbic acid may alleviate these negative influences.

Carbohydrates also influenced iron metabolism, especially in copper-deficient rats. Sucrose decreased hemoglobin, tibia iron concentration, and iron absorption, whereas starch had no effect (Johnson and Gratzek, 1986). Amine and Hegsted (1971) also observed that different carbohydrate sources affected iron absorption differently.

Transit time in the small intestine did not affect iron absorption in rats (Fairweather-Tait and Wright, 1991). Iron absorption was lower in riboflavin-deficient rats than in those given sufficient riboflavin (Powers *et al.*, 1988, 1991).

IV. SUMMARY

The importance of iron in human nutrition and the prevalence of iron deficiency among human populations have stimulated research on the bioavailability of iron in potential supplements of the element. Much of the research has been conducted with chicks or rats, and reagent grade ferrous sulfate has been used most frequently as the standard source of iron. Hemoglobin and, in particular, hemoglobin regeneration after iron depletion, has been used as the response criterion in determining iron bioavailability. Hemoglobin response is considered to be the most sensitive indicator of iron utilization. Liver and spleen iron concentrations, as well as radioiron uptake by liver, spleen, or red blood cells, have also been used in iron bioavailability studies. Intrinsic iron labeling with ^{55}Fe or ^{59}Fe has been used in studies with laboratory animals. The citrate, fumarate, and gluconate forms of iron have been found to be equal in bioavailability to that of ferrous sulfate, with the value for tartrate somewhat lower. Iron as ferrous chloride was well utilized, whereas that as ferric chloride was less available. The iron in ferric oxide was essentially unavailable. Results with ferrous carbonate have been inconsistent, and estimated bioavailability of the iron in this compound has varied from low to relatively high. Only limited research has been conducted on bioavailability of iron in feeds and this has been almost entirely with chickens and rats. Estimated relative bioavailabilities have ranged from about 30 to 70% for forages with values for iron in soybeans and in certain grains or grain products being somewhat higher. Interactions with several other nutrients are important in influencing dietary iron utilization.

Table I. Bioavailability of iron sources for animals[a]

Source	RV	Standard	Response criterion	Meth cal	Type diet	Added level, ppm	Reference
Chickens							
Alfalfa meal (340 ppm Fe AD)	65	FeSO$_4$·7H$_2$O	Hb reg	SC	P	10–20	Chausow and Czarnecki-Maulden (1988b)
Beef liver (235 ppm Fe AD)	90	FeSO$_4$·7H$_2$O	Hb reg	SR	P-5 ppm	10, 20	Chausow and Czarnecki-Maulden (1988a)
Beet pulp	26	Ferrous sulfate	Hb reg	SC	P-10 ppm	NG	Fly and Czarnecki-Maulden (1991)
Blood meal (1610 ppm Fe AD)	22	FeSO$_4$·7H$_2$O	Hb reg	SC	P	5–15	Chausow and Czarnecki-Maulden (1988b)
Blood meal	35	FeSO$_4$·7H$_2$O RG	Hb reg	SC[b]	SP	5–20	Pla and Fritz (1970)
Blood meal	35	FeSO$_4$·H$_2$O RG	Hb reg	SC[b]	SP-7 ppm	5–20	Fritz et al. (1970)
Bone meal, steamed	0	FeSO$_4$·7H$_2$O RG	Hb reg	SC	P-5 ppm	5–20	Deming and Czarnecki-Maulden (1989)
Corn fiber, coarse	69	Ferrous sulfate	Hb reg	SC	P-10 ppm	NG	Fly and Czarnecki-Maulden (1991)
Corn germ meal	40	FeSO$_4$·7H$_2$O RG	Hb reg	SC[b]	SP	5–20	Pla and Fritz (1970)
Corn germ	40	FeSO$_4$·7H$_2$O RG	Hb reg	SC[b]	SP-7 ppm	5–20	Fritz et al. (1970)
Corn gluten meal (102 ppm Fe AD)	84	FeSO$_4$·7H$_2$O RG	Hb reg	SC[b]	SP-5 ppm	10, 20	Chausow and Czarnecki-Maulden (1988a)
Corn, ground (100 ppm Fe AD)	20	FeSO$_4$·7H$_2$O	Hb reg	SC	P	10–20	Chausow and Czarnecki-Maulden (1988b)
Egg, yolk	33	FeSO$_4$·7H$_2$O RG	Hb reg	SC[b]	SP-7 ppm	5–20	Fritz et al. (1970)

Feather meal (570 ppm Fe AD)	39	FeSO$_4$·7H$_2$O RG	Hb reg	SC	P	5-15	Chausow and Czarnecki-Maulden (1988b)
Ferric ammonium citrate	107	FeSO$_4$·7H$_2$O RG	Hb reg	SC[b]	SP	5-20	Pla and Fritz (1970)
Ferric ammonium citrate	115	FeSO$_4$·7H$_2$O RG	Hb reg	SC[b]	SP	5-20	Fritz et al. (1970)
Ferric chloride	44	FeSO$_4$·7H$_2$O RG	Hb reg	SC[b]	SP-7 ppm	5-20	Fritz et al. (1970)
Ferric chloride	78	FeSO$_4$·7H$_2$O RG	Hb reg	SC[b]	SP	5-20	Pla and Fritz (1970)
Ferric choline citrate	102	FeSO$_4$·7H$_2$O RG	Hb reg	SC[b]	SP-7 ppm	5-20	Fritz et al. (1970)
Ferric choline citrate	102	FeSO$_4$·7H$_2$O RG	Hb reg	SC[b]	SP	5-20	Pla and Fritz (1970)
Ferric citrate	73	FeSO$_4$·7H$_2$O RG	Hb reg	SC[b]	SP-7 ppm	5-20	Fritz et al. (1970)
Ferric glycerophosphate	93	FeSO$_4$·7H$_2$O RG	Hb reg	SC[b]	SP-7 ppm	5-20	Fritz et al. (1970)
Ferric orthophosphate (.8%) + Rice (FePO$_4$·4H$_2$O)	36	FeSO$_4$·7H$_2$O RG	Hb reg	SR	P<7 ppm	5-40	Amine et al. (1972)
FePO$_4$·4H$_2$O	11	FeSO$_4$·7H$_2$O RG	Hb reg	SR	P<7 ppm	5-40	Amine et al. (1972)
Ferric orthophosphate-1	18	FeSO$_4$·7H$_2$O RG	Hb reg	SC[b]	SP-7 ppm	5-20	Fritz et al. (1970)
Ferric orthophosphate-2	9	FeSO$_4$·7H$_2$O RG	Hb reg	SC[b]	SP-7 ppm	5-20	Fritz et al. (1970)
Ferric orthophosphate-3	12	FeSO$_4$·7H$_2$O RG	Hb reg	SC[b]	SP-7 ppm	5-20	Fritz et al. (1970)
Ferric orthophosphate (FePO$_4$·4H$_2$O)	15	FeSO$_4$·7H$_2$O RG	Hb reg	SR	P<7 ppm	10, 20, 40	Amine et al. (1972)
Ferric orthophosphate (28.6% Fe)	12	FeSO$_4$·7H$_2$O RG	Hb reg	SC[b]	SP-7 ppm	5-20	Pla and Fritz (1971)
Ferric orthophosphate	15	FeSO$_4$·7H$_2$O RG	Hb reg	SC[b]	SP	5-20	Pla and Fritz (1970)
Ferric oxide	4	FeSO$_4$·7H$_2$O RG	Hb reg	SC[b]	SP-7 ppm	5-20	Fritz et al. (1970)
Ferric oxide Fe$_2$O$_3$	17	FeSO$_4$·7H$_2$O	Hb reg	TP	N	2 mg/day	Elvehjem et al. (1929)
Ferric oxide (60% Fe)	67	FeSO$_4$·7H$_2$O	Hb reg	SR	N	10-20	Poitevint (1979)

Table i. (continued)

Source	RV	Standard	Response criterion	Meth cal	Type diet	Added level, ppm	Reference
Ferric pyrophosphate	45	FeSO$_4$·7H$_2$O RG	Hb reg	SC^b	SP	5-20	Pla and Fritz 1970
Ferric pyrophosphate	45	FeSO$_4$·7H$_2$O RG	Hb reg	SC^b	SP-7 ppm	5-20	Fritz et al. (1970)
Ferric sulfate	65	FeSO$_4$·7H$_2$O RG	Hb reg	SC^b	SP-7 ppm	5-20	Fritz et al. (1970)
Ferric sulfate	104	Ferrous sulfate	Hb reg	MR	NG	60, 100	Moore et al. (1988)
Ferric ammonium sulfate	99	FeSO$_4$·7H$_2$O RG	Hb reg	SC^b	SP-7 ppm	5-20	Fritz et al. (1970)
Ferrous carbonate	8	FeSO$_4$·7H$_2$O RG	Hb reg	SR	P<7 ppm	5-40	Amine et al. (1972)
Ferrous carbonate	10	FeSO$_4$·7H$_2$O RG	Hb reg	SR	P<7 ppm	5-40	Amine et al. (1972)
Ferrous carbonate-1	2	FeSO$_4$·7H$_2$O RG	Hb reg	SC^b	SP-7 ppm	5-20	Fritz et al. (1970)
Ferrous carbonate-2	2	FeSO$_4$·7H$_2$O RG	Hb reg	SC^b	SP-7 ppm	5-20	Fritz et al. (1970)
Ferrous carbonate-3	6	FeSO$_4$·7H$_2$O RG	Hb reg	SC^b	SP-7 ppm	5-20	Fritz et al. (1970)
Ferrous carbonate-4	2	FeSO$_4$·7H$_2$O RG	Hb reg	SC^b	SP-7 ppm	5-20	Fritz et al. (1970)
Ferrous carbonate-1	2	FeSO$_4$·7H$_2$O RG	Hb reg	SC^b	SP	5-20	Pla and Fritz (1970)
Ferrous carbonate-2	7	FeSO$_4$·7H$_2$O RG	Hb reg	SC^b	SP	5-20	Pla and Fritz (1970)
Ferrous carbonate-1	2	FeSO$_4$·7H$_2$O RG	Hb reg	SC^b	SP	5-20	Pla and Fritz (1970)
Ferrous carbonate-2	7	FeSO$_4$·7H$_2$O RG	Hb reg	SC^b	SP	5-20	Pla and Fritz (1970)
Ferrous carbonate-3	0	FeSO$_4$·7H$_2$O RG	Hb reg	SC^b	SP	5-20	Pla and Fritz (1970)
Ferrous carbonate-4	2	FeSO$_4$·7H$_2$O RG	Hb reg	SC^b	SP	5-20	Pla and Fritz (1970)
Ferrous carbonate (42% Fe)	88	FeSO$_4$·7H$_2$O	Hb	SR	N	10-20	Poitevint (1979)
Ferrous carbonate ore (38% Fe)	3	FeSO$_4$·7H$_2$O RG	Hb reg	SC^b	SP-7 ppm	5-20	Pla and Fritz (1971)

Source	Value	Form	Response criterion		Level	Reference
Ferrous chloride	98	FeSO$_4$·7H$_2$O RG	Hb reg	SC^b	SP-7 ppm	5-20	Fritz et al. (1970)
Ferrous chloride	106	FeSO$_4$·7H$_2$O RG	Hb reg	SC^b	SP-7 ppm	5-20	Pla and Fritz (1971)
Ferrous EDTA-dihydrogen	99	FeSO$_4$·7H$_2$O	Hb reg	SC^b	SP-7 ppm	5-20	Fritz et al. (1970)
Ferrous fumarate	95	FeSO$_4$·7H$_2$O RG	Hb reg	SC^b	SP-7 ppm	5-20	Fritz et al. (1970)
Ferrous fumarate	102	FeSO$_4$·7H$_2$O RG	Hb reg	SC^b	SP-7 ppm	5-20	Pla and Fritz (1970)
Ferrous gluconate	97	FeSO$_4$·7H$_2$O RG	Hb reg	SC^b	SP-7 ppm	5-20	Fritz et al. (1970)
Ferrous gluconate	97	FeSO$_4$·7H$_2$O RG	Hb reg	SC^b	SP-7 ppm	5-20	Pla and Fritz (1970)
Ferrous sulfate, FG	100	FeSO$_4$·7H$_2$O RG	Hb reg	SC^b	SP-7 ppm	5-20	Fritz et al. (1970)
Ferrous sulfate (FeSO$_4$·H$_2$O) (31%)	103	FeSO$_4$·7H$_2$O RG	Hb reg	SR	N	10-20	Poitevint (1979)
Ferrous sulfate FG (FeSO$_4$·H$_2$O)	102	FeSO$_4$·7H$_2$O RG	Hb reg	SR	P-4 ppm	7.5-22.5	Ammerman et al. (1993)
Ferrous sulfate, anhydrous	100	FeSO$_4$·7H$_2$O RG	Hb reg	SC^b	SP-7 ppm	5-20	Fritz et al. (1970)
Ferrous sulfate, encapsulated	97	FeSO$_4$·7H$_2$O RG	Hb reg	SC^e	SP-7 ppm	5-20	Pla et al. (1973)
Ferrous tartrate	77	FeSO$_4$·7H$_2$O RG	Hb reg	SC^b	SP-7 ppm	5-20	Fritz et al. (1970)
Fishmeal (700 ppm Fe AD)	32	FeSO$_4$·7H$_2$O RG	Hb reg	SC^b	P	5-15	Chausow and Czarnecki-Maulden (1988b)
Fish protein concentrate	22	FeSO$_4$·7H$_2$O RG	Hb reg	SC^b	SP-7 ppm	5-20	Fritz et al. (1970)
Hemoglobin	70	FeSO$_4$·7H$_2$ORG	Hb reg	SR	P<7 ppm	5-40	Amine et al. (1972)
Hemoglobin, bovine	44	FeSO$_4$·7H$_2$O RG	Hb reg	SC^b	SP-7 ppm	5-20	Pla et al. 1973
Iron, reduced (97.0% Fe)	64	FeSO$_4$·7H$_2$O RG	Hb reg	SR	P-7 ppm	5-40	Amine et al. (1972)
Iron, reduced	63	FeSO$_4$·7H$_2$O RG	Hb reg	SR	P<7 ppm	5-40	Amine et al. (1972)
Iron, reduced-1	59	FeSO$_4$·7H$_2$O RG	Hb reg	SC^b	SP-7 ppm	5-20	Fritz et al. (1970)

Table I. (continued)

Source	RV	Standard	Response criterion	Meth cal	Type diet	Added level, ppm	Reference
Iron, reduced-2	41	$FeSO_4 \cdot 7H_2O$ RG	Hb reg	SC[b]	SP-7 ppm	5-20	Fritz et al. (1970)
Iron, reduced-3	66	$FeSO_4 \cdot 7H_2O$ RG	Hb reg	SC[b]	SP-7 ppm	5-20	Fritz et al. (1970)
Iron, reduced-4	43	$FeSO_4 \cdot 7H_2O$ RG	Hb reg	SC[b]	SP-7 ppm	5-20	Fritz et al. (1970)
Iron, reduced (97.0%)	18	$FeSO_4 \cdot 7H_2O$ RG	Hb reg	SC[b]	SP-7 ppm	5-20	Pla and Fritz (1971)
Iron, reduced-1, 90%<10μm	61	$FeSO_4 \cdot 7H_2O$ RG	Hb reg	SC[b]	SP-7 ppm	5-20	Pla et al. (1973)
Iron, reduced-2, 90%<10μm	53	$FeSO_4 \cdot 7H_2O$ RG	Hb reg	SC[b]	SP-7 ppm	5-20	Pla et al. (1973)
Iron, reduced-3, 90%<10μm	60	$FeSO_4 \cdot 7H_2O$ RG	Hb reg	SC[b]	SP-7 ppm	5-20	Pla et al. (1973)
Iron, reduced-4, 90%<10μm	44	$FeSO_4 \cdot 7H_2O$ RG	Hb reg	SC[b]	SP-7 ppm	5-20	Pla et al. (1973)
Iron, reduced-5, 90%<10μm	48	$FeSO_4 \cdot 7H_2O$ RG	Hb reg	SC[b]	SP-7 ppm	5-20	Pla et al. (1973)
Iron, reduced-6, 95%<5μm	51	$FeSO_4 \cdot 7H_2O$ RG	Hb reg	SC[b]	SP-7 ppm	5-20	Pla et al. (1973)
Iron, reduced-7, 40%<10μm; 1%<40μm; electrolytic reduction	46	$FeSO_4 \cdot 7H_2O$ RG	Hb reg	SC[b]	SP-7 ppm	5-20	Pla et al. (1973)
Iron, reduced-8, 3%<10μm; 21%<40μm; hydrogen reduction	44	$FeSO_4 \cdot 7H_2O$ RG	Hb reg	SC[b]	SP-7 ppm	5-20	Pla et al. (1973)
Iron, reduced-9, 35%<32μm; carbon monoxide reduction	42	$FeSO_4 \cdot 7H_2O$ RG	Hb reg	SC[b]	SP-7 ppm	5-20	Pla et al. (1973)
Iron, reduced-9, >32μm	41	$FeSO_4 \cdot 7H_2O$ RG	Hb reg	SC[b]	SP-7 ppm	5-20	Pla et al. (1973)
Iron, reduced-10, 77%<32μm electrolyte reduction	46	$FeSO_4 \cdot 7H_2O$ RG	Hb reg	SC[b]	SP-7 ppm	5-20	Pla et al. (1973)

Iron, reduced-10, >32 μm	59	FeSO$_4$·7H$_2$O RG	Hb reg	SC[b]	SP-7 ppm	5-20	Pla et al. (1973)
Iron, reduced-11, 59%<32μm; hydrogen reduction	56	FeSO$_4$·7H$_2$O RG	Hb reg	SC[b]	SP-7 ppm	5-20	Pla et al. (1973)
Iron, reduced-11, >32μm	49	FeSO$_4$·7H$_2$O RG	Hb reg	SC[b]	SP-7 ppm	5-20	Pla et al. (1973)
Iron, reduced-12, <44μm; electrolyte reduction	66	FeSO$_4$·7H$_2$O RG	Hb reg	SC[b]	SP-7 ppm	5-20	Pla et al. (1973)
Iron, reduced-13, RG; electrolyte reduction	59	FeSO$_4$·7H$_2$O RG	Hb reg	SC[b]	SP-7 ppm	5-20	Pla et al. (1973)
Iron, reduced-14, <149μm; hydrogen reduction	55	FeSO$_4$·7H$_2$O RG	Hb reg	SC[b]	SP-7 ppm	5-20	Pla et al. (1973)
Limestone	52	FeSO$_4$·7H$_2$O RG	Hb reg	SC	P-5 ppm	5-20	Deming and Czarnecki-Maulden (1989)
Limestone, dolomitic	34	FeSO$_4$·7H$_2$O RG	Hb reg	SC	P-5 ppm	5-20	Deming and Czarnecki-Maulden (1989)
Meat and bone meal (575 ppm Fe AD)	48	FeSO$_4$·7H$_2$O RG	Hb reg	SC	P	5-15	Chausow and Czarnecki-Maulden (1988b)
Oat hulls	69	Ferrous sulfate	Hb reg	SC	P-10 ppm	NG	Fly and Czarnecki-Maulden (1991)
Orchardgrass	69	Ferrous sulfate	Hb reg	SC	P-10 ppm	NG	Fly and Czarnecki-Maulden (1991)
Oystershell	10	FeSO$_4$·7H$_2$O RG	Hb reg	SC	P-5 ppm	5-20	Deming and Czarnecki-Maulden (1989)
Phosphate, defluorinated	48	FeSO$_4$·7H$_2$O RG	Hb reg	SR	P-4 ppm	7.5-22.5	Ammerman et al. (1993)
Phosphate, defluorinated	44	FeSO$_4$·7H$_2$O RG	Hb reg	SC	P-5 ppm	5-20	Deming and Czarnecki-Maulden (1989)
Phosphate, dicalcium	55	FeSO$_4$·7H$_2$O RG	Hb reg	SC	P-5 ppm	5-20	Deming and Czarnecki-Maulden (1989)

Table I. (continued)

Source	RV	Standard	Response criterion	Meth cal	Type diet	Added level, ppm	Reference
Phosphate, monocalcium	61	FeSO$_4$·7H$_2$O RG	Hb reg	SC	P-5 ppm	5-20	Deming and Czarnecki-Maulden (1989)
Phosphate, monocalcium/dicalcium	66	FeSO$_4$·7H$_2$O RG	Hb reg	SR	P-4 ppm	7.5-22.5	Ammerman et al. (1993)
Phosphate, soft rock	0	FeSO$_4$·7H$_2$O RG	Hb reg	SC	P-5 ppm	5-20	Deming and Czarnecki-Maulden (1989)
Poultry by-product meal (630 ppm Fe AD)	68	FeSO$_4$·7H$_2$O RG	Hb reg	SC	P	5-15	Chausow and Czarnecki-Maulden (1988b)
Psyllium husk, 5% of diet	0	Ferrous sulfate	Hb reg	SR	P-10 ppm	NG	Fly and Czarnecki-Maulden, (1991)
Rice, bran (120 ppm Fe AD)	77	FeSO$_4$·7H$_2$O	Hb reg	SC	P	10-20	Chausow and Czarnecki-Maulden (1988b)
Sesame seed meal (120 ppm Fe AD)	96	FeSO$_4$·7H$_2$O	Hb reg	SC	P	10-20	Chausow and Czarnecki-Maulden (1988b)
Sodium iron pyrophosphate (14.5% Fe)	30	FeSO$_4$·7H$_2$O RG	Hb reg	SR	P<7 ppm	10,20,40	Amine et al. (1972)
Sodium iron pyrophosphate	14	FeSO$_4$·7H$_2$O RG	Hb reg	SR	P<7 ppm	5-40	Amine et al. (1972)
Sodium iron pyrophosphate	2	FeSO$_4$·7H$_2$O RG	Hb reg	SC[b]	SP-7 ppm	5-20	Fritz et al. (1970)
Sodium iron pyrophosphate	13	FeSO$_4$·7H$_2$O RG	Hb reg	SC[b]	SP-7 ppm	5-20	Fritz et al. (1970)
Sodium iron pyrophosphate (14.5% Fe)	13	FeSO$_4$·7H$_2$O RG	Hb reg	SC[b]	SP-7 ppm	5-20	Pla and Fritz (1971)
Sodium iron pyrophosphate	12	FeSO$_4$·7H$_2$O RG	Hb reg	SC[b]	SP	5-20	Pla and Fritz (1970)
Soybeans (heated to 140°C)	90	FeSO$_4$·7H$_2$O RG	Hb reg	SC[b]	SP-7 ppm	5-20	Pla et al. (1973)

184

Soybeans (heated to 170°C)	77	FeSO$_4$·7H$_2$O RG	Hb reg	SC[b]	SP-7 ppm	5-20	Pla et al. (1973)
Soybean meal (345 ppm Fe AD)	45	FeSO$_4$·7H$_2$O RG	Hb reg	SC	P	10-20	Chausow and Czarnecki-Maulden (1988b)
Soybean hulls	94	Ferrous sulfate	Hb reg	SC	P-10 ppm	NG	Fly and Czarnecki-Maulden (1991)
Soybean protein isolate	97	FeSO$_4$·7H$_2$O RG	Hb reg	SC[b]	P-7 ppm	5-20	Fritz et al. (1970)
Tomato pomace	82	Ferrous sulfate	Hb reg	SC	P-10 ppm	NG	Fly and Czarnecki-Maulden (1991)
Wheat germ	53	FeSO$_4$·7H$_2$O RG	Hb reg	SC[b]	P-7 ppm	5-20	Fritz et al. (1970)
Wheat germ meal	54	FeSO$_4$·7H$_2$O RG	Hb reg	SC[b]	SP	5-20	Pla and Fritz (1970)

Swine

Ferric ammonium citrate	102	Ferrous sulfate	Hb	TP	P-39ppm	88	Harmon et al. (1967)
Ferric choline citrate	144	FeSO$_4$·7H$_2$O	Hb reg	SC	N	50,100	Miller et al. (1981)
Ferric citrate	89	FeSO$_4$·7H$_2$O	Hb	MR	N	176 mg/day	Ullrey et al. (1973)
Ferric citrate	192	FeSO$_4$·7H$_2$O	Liv Fe	MR	N	176 mg/day	Ullrey et al. (1973)
Ferric citrate	190	FeSO$_4$·7H$_2$O	Hb	MR	N	176 mg/day	Ullrey et al. (1973)
Ferric citrate	125	FeSO$_4$·7H$_2$O	Liv Fe	MR	N	176 mg/day	Ullrey et al. (1973)
Ferric copper, cobalt choline citrate	**144**	**FeSO$_4$·7H$_2$O**	**Hb reg**	**SC**	**N**	**50,100**	**Miller et al. (1981)**
Ferric oxide RG Fe$_2$O$_3$	12	FeSO$_4$·7H$_2$O RG	Hb	TP	SP-15 ppm	35-65	Pickett et al. (1961)
Ferric polyphosphate	84.3	FeSO$_4$·7H$_2$O	Hb	TP	P-8 ppm	64-69	Anderson et al. (1974)
Ferrous carbonate (40% Fe)	22	FeSO$_4$·7H$_2$O	Hb	TP	N	NG	Poitevint (1979)
Ferrous carbonate FG-A	97	Ferrous sulfate RG	Hb reg	MR	N-61 ppm	40	Ammerman et al. (1974)

Table I. (continued)

Source	RV	Standard	Response criterion	Meth cal	Type diet	Added level, ppm	Reference
Ferrous carbonate FG-B	87	Ferrous sulfate RG	Hb reg	MR	N-61 ppm	40	Ammerman et al. (1974)
Ferrous carbonate FG-C	101	Ferrous sulfate RG	Hb reg	MR	N-61 ppm	40	Ammerman et al. (1974)
Ferrous carbonate	8	Ferrous sulfate	Hb reg	TP	P-12-34 ppm	36-51	Harmon et al. (1969)
Ferrous carbonate-1	13	$FeSO_4 \cdot 7H_2O$ RG	Hb	TP	SP-15 ppm	35-65	Pickett et al. (1961)
Ferrous carbonate-2	16	$FeSO_4 \cdot 7H_2O$ RG	Hb	TP	SP-15 ppm	35-65	Pickett et al. (1961)
Ferrous sulfate ($FeSO_4 \cdot H_2O$)	87	$FeSO_4 \cdot 7H_2O$	Hb reg	SR	N-56 ppm	50,100	Miller (1978)
Iron EDTA, disodium	90	$FeSO_4 \cdot 7H_2O$	Hb	TP	P-8 ppm	64-68	Anderson et al. (1974)
Iron-methionine	183	Ferrous sulfate	Hb	TP	NG	200 mg	Spears et al. (1992)
Iron-proteinate	123	$FeSO_4 \cdot 7H_2O$	Hb	TP	N	500	Brady et al. (1978)
Iron, reduced catalytic	27	$FeSO_4 \cdot 7H_2O$	Hb	TP	P-8 ppm	64-69	Anderson et al. (1974)
Iron, reduced electrolytic	63	$FeSO_4 \cdot 7H_2O$	Hb	TP	P-8 ppm	64-69	Anderson et al. (1974)
Phosphate, defluorinated	35	Ferrous sulfate	Hb	TP	SP-20 ppm	70-125	Kornegay (1972)
Phosphate, defluorinated	73	Ferrous sulfate	Hb	TP	SP-20 ppm	70-125	Kornegay (1972)
Sodium iron pyrophosphate	29	$FeSO_4 \cdot 7H_2O$	Hb	TP	P-8 ppm	64-69	Anderson et al. (1974)
Cattle							
Ferric citrate	107	$FeSO_4$	Hb	TP	N-10 ppm	30	Bremner and Dalgarno (1973)
Ferric EDTA	93	$FeSO_4$	Hb	TP	N-10 ppm	30	Bremner and Dalgarno (1973)
Ferrous carbonate FG	0	$FeSO_4 \cdot H_2O$ FG	Liv Fe	TP	N-180 ppm	1000	McGuire et al. (1985)
Ferrous carbonate FG	23	$FeSO_4 \cdot H_2O$ FG	Spl Fe	TP	N-180 ppm	1000	McGuire et al. (1985)

			Hb	TP			
Iron phytate (17.7% Fe)	47	FeSO$_4$			N-10 ppm	30	Bremner and Dalgarno (1973)
Rats							
Alfalfa	32	Ferrous chloride	Hb reg	MR	SP-3.1 ppm	.2 mg/day	Raven and Thompson (1959)
Alsike	45	Ferric chloride	Hb reg	MR	SP-3.1 ppm	.2 mg/day	Raven and Thompson (1959)
Clover, red	41	Ferrous chloride	Hb reg	MR	SP-3.1 ppm	.2 mg/day	Raven and Thompson (1959)
Clover, white	30	Ferric chloride	Hb reg	MR	SP-3.1 ppm	.2 mg/day	Raven and Thompson (1959)
Cocksfoot	53	Ferric chloride	Hb reg	MR	SP-1.2 ppm	.2 mg/day	Thompson and Raven (1959)
Ferric ammonium citrate	98	FeSO$_4$·7H$_2$O RG	Hb reg	SC[b]	SP-7 ppm	5-20	Fritz et al. (1970)
Ferric ammonium citrate	80	Ferrous sulfate	Int ^{59}Fe WB	MR	N	SOD-12	Pabon and Lonnerdal (1992)
Ferric citrate	104	Ferrous sulfate	Int ^{59}Fe WB	MR	N	SOD-12	Pabon and Lonnerdal (1992)
Ferric citrate	96	FeSO$_4$·7H$_2$O RG	Hb reg	PL	P-5-10 ppm	6-96	Fritz et al. (1975)
Ferric citrate (16% Fe)	97	FeSO$_4$·7H$_2$O RG	Hb reg	SC[b]	P-5-10 ppm	6-96	Fritz et al. (1975)
Ferric EDTA-sodium	76	Ferrous sulfate	Int lab	MR	N	SOD-12 ppm	Pabon and Lonnerdal (1992)
Ferric glutamate	100	Ferric chloride	Hb reg	MR	N	.5 mg/day	Elvehjem et al. (1933)
Ferric hypophosphite	105	Ferric chloride	Hb reg	MR	N	.5 mg/day	Elvehjem et al. (1933)
Ferric orthophosphate (26.8% Fe)	27	FeSO$_4$·7H$_2$O RG	Hb reg	SR	SP<7 ppm	10,20	Amine et al. (1972)
Ferric orthophosphate-1	12	FeSO$_4$·7H$_2$O RG	Hb reg	SC[b]	SP-7 ppm	5-20	Fritz et al. (1970)
Ferric orthophosphate-2	12	Ferrous sulfate RG (FeSO$_4$·7H$_2$O)	Hb reg	SC[b]	SP-7 ppm	5-20	Fritz et al. (1970)

Table I. (continued)

Source	RV	Standard	Response criterion	Meth cal	Type diet	Added level, ppm	Reference
Ferric orthophosphate-3	30	Ferrous sulfate RG FeSO$_4$·7H$_2$O	Hb reg	SC^b	SP-7 ppm	5-20	Fritz et al. (1970)
Ferric orthophosphate (28.0% Fe)	11	FeSO$_4$·7H$_2$O RG	Hb reg	SC^b	P-5-10 ppm	6-96	Fritz et al. (1975)
Ferric orthophosphate [Fe$_5$H$_8$(NH$_4$)(PO$_4$)$_6$·6H$_2$O]	45	FeSO$_4$·7H$_2$O	Hb reg	SR	P-3 ppm	6,12,24	Kosonen and Mutanen (1992)
Ferric orthophosphate	11	FeSO$_4$·7H$_2$O RG	Hb reg	PL	P-5-10 ppm	6-96	Fritz et al. (1975)
Ferric orthophosphate FG	44	FeSO$_4$·7H$_2$O	Hb reg	PL	P	6-24	Fritz et al. (1974)
Ferric orthophosphate	30	Ferrous sulfate	Hb reg	SR	P-3 ppm	6-24	Forbes et al. (1989)
Ferric oxide	6	FeSO$_4$·7H$_2$O RG	Hb reg	SC^b	SP-7 ppm	5-20	Fritz et al. (1970)
Ferric phosphate FePO$_4$	26	Ferrous sulfate	Int ^{55}Fe WB	MR	SP-35 ppm	SOD	Morris et al. (1987)
Ferric phytate (from wheat bran)	99	Ferrous ammonium sulfate	Hb reg	SR	P	5-20	Morris and Ellis (1976)
Ferric phytate (synthetic)	99	Ferrous ammonium sulfate	Hb reg	SR	P	5-20	Morris and Ellis (1976)
Ferric pyrophosphate	90	Ferrous sulfate	Int ^{59}Fe WB	MR	N	SOD-12 ppm	Pabon and Lonnerdal (1992)
Ferric pyrophosphate	95	Ferric chloride	Hb reg	MR	N	.5 mg/day	Elvehjem et al. (1970)
Ferric sulfate	100	FeSO$_4$·7H$_2$O RG	Hb reg	SC^b	SP-7 ppm	5-20	Fritz et al. (1970)
Ferrous carbonate (38% Fe)	1	FeSO$_4$·7H$_2$O RG	Hb reg	SR	SP-7 ppm	10,20	Amine et al. (1972)
Ferrous carbonate-1	1	FeSO$_4$·7H$_2$O RG	Hb reg	SC^b	SP-7 ppm	5-20	Fritz et al. (1970)
Ferrous carbonate-2	0	FeSO$_4$·7H$_2$O RG	Hb reg	SC^b	SP-7 ppm	5-20	Fritz et al. (1970)

Ferrous carbonate-3	0	FeSO$_4$·7H$_2$O RG	Hb reg	SC[b]	SP-7 ppm	5-20	Fritz et al. (1970)
Ferrous carbonate-4	2	FeSO$_4$·7H$_2$O RG	Hb reg	SC[b]	SP-7 ppm	5-20	Fritz et al. (1970)
Ferrous carbonate	20	Ferrous sulfate	Hb reg	MR	N	.3 mg/day	Nesbit and Elmslie (1960)
Ferrous carbonate	30	Ferrous sulfate	Hb reg	MR	N	.2 mg/day	Nesbit and Elmslie (1960)
Fish protein concentrate	53	FeSO$_4$·7H$_2$O RG	Hb reg	SC[b]	SP-7 ppm	5-20	Fritz et al. (1970)
Glutamic acid parahematin	43	Ferric chloride	Hb reg	MR	N	.5 mg/day	Elvehjem et al. (1933)
Hemoglobin	35	FeSO$_4$·7H$_2$O RG	Hb reg	SR	SP<7 ppm	10,20	Amine et al. (1972)
Iron, elemental	55	Ferrous sulfate	Hb reg	MR	N	.2 mg/day	Nesbit and Elmslie (1960)
Iron phytate (17.7% Fe)	65	Ferric chloride	Hb reg	MR	N	.2 mg/day	Nakamura and Michell (1943)
Iron reduced (97.0% Fe)	49	FeSO$_4$·H$_2$O RG	Hb reg	SR	SP<7 ppm	10,20	Amine et al. (1972)
Iron, reduced-1	34	FeSO$_4$·H$_2$O RG	Hb reg	SC[b]	SP-7 ppm	5-20	Fritz et al. (1970)
Iron, reduced-2	16	FeSO$_4$·H$_2$O RG	Hb reg	SC[b]	SP-7 ppm	5-20	Fritz et al. (1970)
Iron, reduced-3	36	FeSO$_4$·H$_2$O RG	Hb reg	SC[b]	SP-7 ppm	5-20	Fritz et al. (1970)
Iron, reduced-4	37	FeSO$_4$·H$_2$O RG	Hb reg	SC[b]	SP-7 ppm	5-20	Fritz et al. (1970)
Iron, reduced-1, 90%<10μm	15	FeSO$_4$·H$_2$O RG	Hb reg	SC[b]	SP-7 ppm	5-20	Pla et al. (1973)
Iron, reduced-2, 90%<10μm	15	FeSO$_4$·H$_2$O RG	Hb reg	SC[b]	SP-7 ppm	5-20	Pla et al. (1973)
Iron, reduced-3, 90%<10μm	35	FeSO$_4$·ORG	Hb reg	SC[b]	SP-7 ppm	5-20	Pla et al. (1973)
Iron, reduced-4, 90%<10μm	27	FeSO$_4$·H$_2$O RG	Hb reg	SC[b]	SP-7 ppm	5-20	Pla et al. (1973)
Iron, reduced-5, 90%<10μm	24	FeSO$_4$·H$_2$O RG	Hb reg	SC[b]	SP-7 ppm	5-20	Pla et al. (1973)
Iron, reduced-6, 95%<5μm	47	FeSO$_4$·H$_2$O RG	Hb reg	SC[b]	SP-7 ppm	5-20	Pla et al. (1973)
Iron, reduced-9, >32μm	7	FeSO$_4$·H$_2$O RG	Hb reg	SC[b]	SP-7 ppm	5-20	Pla et al. (1973)
Iron, reduced-11 >32μm	20	FeSO$_4$·H$_2$O RG	Hb reg	SC[b]	SP-7 ppm	5-20	Pla et al. (1973)

Table I. (continued)

Source	RV	Standard	Response criterion	Meth cal	Type diet	Added level, ppm	Reference
Iron, reduced, 45μm	84	Ferrous sulfate	Int lab	MR	SP-35 ppm	SOD	Morris et al. (1987)
Iron, reduced 20μm	70	Ferrous sulfate	Int lab	MR	SP-35 ppm	SOD	Morris et al. (1987)
Iron, reduced-RG	96	Ferric chloride	Hb reg	MR	N	.2 mg/day	Nakamura and Mitchell, (1943)
Iron, reduced-9, 35%<32μm; carbron monoxide reduction	19	FeSO₄·7H₂O RG	Hb reg	SC[b]	SP-7 ppm	5-20	Pla et al. (1973)
Iron, reduced-7, 40%<10μm; 1%>40μm; electrolytic reduction	50	FeSO₄·7H₂O RG	Hb reg	SC[b]	SP-7 ppm	5-20	Pla et al. (1973)
Iron, reduced-10, 77%<32μm; electrolytic reduction	35	FeSO₄·7H₂O RG	Hb reg	SC[b]	SP-7 ppm	5-20	Pla et al. (1973)
Iron, reduced-10, 100%>32μm	34	FeSO₄·7H₂O RG	Hb reg	SC[b]	SP-7 ppm	5-20	Pla et al. (1973)
Iron, reduced-12, 100%<44μm; electrolytic reduction	45	FeSO₄·7H₂O RG	Hb reg	SC[b]	SP-7 ppm	5-20	Pla et al. (1973)
Iron, reduced-13, RG; electrolytic reduction	34	FeSO₄·7H₂O RG	Hb reg	SC[b]	SP-7 ppm	5-20	Pla et al. (1973)
Iron, reduced, electrolytic	72	Ferrous sulfate	Hb reg	SR	P-3 ppm	6-24	Forbes et al. (1989)
Iron, reduced-8, 3%<10μm; 21%>40μm; hydrogen reduction	32	FeSO₄·7H₂O RG	Hb reg	SC[b]	SP-7 ppm	5-20	Pla et al. (1973)

190

Description	No.	Iron compound	Method				Reference
Iron, reduced-11, 59%<32μm; hydrogen reduction	23	FeSO$_4$·7H$_2$O RG	Hb reg	SC[b]	SP-7 ppm	5-20	Pla et al. (1973)
Iron, reduced-14, 100%<149μm; hydrogen reduction	18	FeSO$_4$·7H$_2$O RG	Hb reg	SC[b]	SP-7 ppm	5-20	Pla et al. (1973)
Iron, reduced-hydrogen reduction	30	FeSO$_4$·7H$_2$O RG	Hb reg	SC[b]	P-5-10 ppm	6-96	Fritz et al. (1975)
Iron, reduced-hydrogen reduction	27	FeSO$_4$·7H$_2$O RG	Hb reg	PL	P-5-10 ppm	6-96	Fritz et al. (1975)
Iron, reduced 7-10μm, electrolytic reduction	64	FeSO$_4$·7H$_2$O RG	Hb reg	PL	P	6-24	Fritz et al. (1974)
Iron, reduced 27-40μm, electrolytic reduction	38	FeSO$_4$·7H$_2$O RG	Hb reg	PL	P	6-24	Fritz et al. (1974)
Milk, cow	14	FeSO$_4$·7H$_2$O	Hb reg	SC	N-12.7 ppm	8-24	Park et al. (1986)
Milk, goat	54	FeSO$_4$·7H$_2$O	Hb reg	SC	N-12.7 ppm	8-24	Park et al. (1986)
Potato	69	Ferrous sulfate	^{59}Fe liv	MR	SP	SOD-79 μg	Fairweather-Tait (1983)
Ryegrass, perennial	46	Ferric chloride	Hb reg	MR	SP-1.2 ppm	.2 mg/day	Thompson and Raven (1959)
Sodium iron pyrophosphate	4	FeSO$_4$·H$_2$O RG	Hb reg	SR	SP<7 ppm	10,20	Amine et al. (1972)
Sodium iron pyrophosphate	11	FeSO$_4$·H$_2$O RG	Hb reg	SC[b]	SP-7 ppm	5-20	Fritz et al. (1970)
Sodium iron pyrophosphate	19	FeSO$_4$·H$_2$O RG	Hb reg	SC[b]	SP-7 ppm	5-20	Fritz et al. (1970)
Sodium iron pyrophosphate	42	Ferric chloride	Hb reg	TP	N	.25 mg/day	Freeman and Burrill (1945)
Sodium iron pyrophosphate [Na$_8$Fe$_4$(P$_2$O$_7$)$_5$·6H$_2$O]	102	Ferric chloride	Hb reg	MR	N	.2 mg/day	Nakamura and Mitchell (1943)
Soybeans - mature	109	FeCl$_3$	Int lab	MR	P-13 ppm	SOD-15-50 μg	Welch and van Campen (1975)
Soybeans - immature	60	FeCl$_3$	Int lab	MR	P-13 ppm	SOD-15-50 μg	Welch and van Campen (1975)

Table I. (continued)

Source	RV	Standard	Response criterion	Meth cal	Type diet	Added level, ppm	Reference
Soy protein isolate	61	$FeSO_4 \cdot 7H_2O$	Hb reg	SR	P	6-30	Steinke and Hopkins (1978)
Timothy	73	Ferric chloride	Hb reg	MR	SP-1.2 ppm	.2 mg/day	Thompso. and Raven (1959)
Trefoil	34	Ferric chloride	Hb reg	MR	SP-3.1ppm	.2mg/day	Raven and Thompson (1959)
Wheat bran	95	$FeSO_4 \cdot 7H_2O$	True abs	MR	P	SOD-30 ppm	Buchowski and Mahoney) (1992)
Mice							
Ferrous chloride ($FeCl_2$)	103	$FeSO_4$	^{59}Fe ret	MR	N	NG	Kwock et al. (1984)
Ferric citrate	74	$FeSO_4$	^{59}Fe ret	MR	N	NG	Kwock et al. (1984)
Ferric EDTA	81	$FeSO_4$	^{59}Fe ret	MR	N	NG	Kwock et al. (1984)
Ferric lactobionate	145	$FeSO_4$	^{59}Fe ret	MR	N	NG	Kwock et al. (1984)
Ferric nitrilotriacetate	103	$FeSO_4$	^{59}Fe ret	MR	N	NG	Kwock et al. (1984)

[a] Abbreviations can be found in Appendix I. Chemical formula for a compound given only if provided by the author; RG indicates reagent grade, FG indicates feed grade.

[b] RV = 100 x (ppm Fe from standard / ppm from test source to give equal curative effect).

Table II. Relative bioavailability of supplemental iron sources[a]

Source	Poultry	Swine	Cattle	Sheep	Rats
Ferrous sulfate heptahydrate	100	100	100	100	100
Ferric ammonium citrate	110 (2)	100 (1)	-	-	90 (2)
Ferric chloride	60 (2)	-	-	91 (1)	-
Ferric choline citrate	100 (2)	145 (1)	-	-	-
Ferric citrate	75 (1)	150 (4)	110 (1)	-	100 (3)
Ferric EDTA	-	-	95 (1)	-	75 (1)
Ferric glycerophosphate	95 (1)	-	-	-	-
Ferric orthophosphate	10 (7)	-	-	-	20 (8)
Ferric oxide	10 (2)	10 (1)	-	5 (1)	5 (1)
Ferric phytate	-	-	45 (1)	-	100 (2)
Ferric polyphosphate	-	85 (1)	-	-	-
Ferric pyrophosphate	45 (2)	-	-	-	95 (2)
Ferric sulfate	85 (2)	-	-	-	100 (1)
Ferrous ammonium sulfate	100 (1)	-	-	-	-
Ferrous carbonate-low[b]	5 (11)	15 (2)	10 (2)	-	5 (7)
Ferrous carbonate-high[b]	90 (1)	95 (3)	-	85 (1)	-
Ferrous chloride	100 (2)	-	-	-	-
Ferrous EDTA	100 (1)	90 (1)	-	-	-
Ferrous fumarate	100 (2)	-	-	-	-
Ferrous gluconate	100 (2)	-	-	-	-
Ferrous sulfate, anhydrous	100 (1)	-	-	-	-
Ferrous sulfate monohydrate	100 (3)	85 (1)	-	-	-
Ferrous tartate	75 (1)	-	-	-	-
Iron methionine	-	185 (1)	-	-	-
Iron proteinate	-	125 (1)	-	-	-
Iron, reduced	50 (24)	45 (2)	-	-	40 (30)
Sodium iron pyrophosphate	15 (6)	-	-	-	20 (4)

Table II. (continued)

[a]Average values rounded to nearest "5" and expressed relative to response obtained with ferrous sulfate heptahydrate. Number of studies or samples involved indicated within parentheses.

[b]Most ferrous carbonates have been reported to be low in iron bioavailability, however, several were found to be of high availability and they are listed separately.

REFERENCES

Amine, E. K. and D. M. Hegsted. 1971. Effect of diet on iron absorption in iron-deficient rats. *J. Nutr.* **101**:927.

Amine, E. K., R. Neff and D. M. Hegsted. 1972. Biological estimation of available iron using chicks or rats. *J. Agric. Food Chem.* **20**:246.

Ammerman, C. B., J. M. Wing, B. G. Dunavant, W. K. Robertson, J. P. Feaster and L. R. Arrington. 1967. Utilization of inorganic iron by ruminants as influenced by form of iron and iron status of the animal. *J. Anim. Sci.* **26**:404.

Ammerman, C. B., J. F. Standish, C.E. Holt, R.H. Houser, S.M. Miller and G.E. Combs. 1974. Ferrous carbonates as sources of iron for weanling pigs and rats. *J. Anim. Sci.* **38**:52.

Ammerman, C. B., P. R. Henry, R. D. Miles and R. C. Littell. 1993. Feed grade phosphates and iron sulfates as sources of iron for animals. *In* "Trace Elements in Man and Animals - TEMA 8" (M. Anke, D. Meissner and C. F. Mills, Eds.). Verlag Media Touristik, Gersdorf, Germany.

Anderson, T. A., L. J. Filer, Jr., S. J. Fomon, D. W. Andersen, T. L. Nixt, R. R. Rogers, R. L. Jensen and S. E. Nelson. 1974. Bioavailability of different sources of dietary iron fed to Pitman-Moore miniature pigs. *J. Nutr.* **104**:619.

Aoyagi, S. and D. H. Baker. 1995. Iron requirement of chicks fed a semipurified diet based on casein and soy protein concentrate. *Poult. Sci.* **74**:412.

Association of American Feed Control Official (AAFCO). 1994. Official publication, p. 192. AAFCO, Atlanta, GA.

Bafundo, K. W., D. H. Baker and P. R. Fitzgerald. 1984. The iron-zinc interrelationship in the chick as influenced by *Eimeria acervulina* infection. *J. Nutr.* **114**:1306.

Baker, D. H. and K. M. Halpin. 1991. Manganese and iron interrelationship in the chick. *Poult. Sci.* **70**:146.

Bates, C. J., T. D. Cowen and H. Tsuchiya. 1988. Growth, ascorbic acid and iron contents of tissues of young guinea-pigs whose dams received high or low levels of dietary ascorbic acid or Fe during pregnancy and suckling. *Br. J. Nutr.* **60**:487.

Beard, J. L., H. A. Huebers and C. A. Finch. 1984. Protein depletion and iron deficiency in rats. *J. Nutr.* **114**:1396.

Bradley, B. D., G. Graber, R. J. Condon and L. T. Frobish. 1983. Effects of graded levels of dietary copper on copper and iron concentrations in swine tissues. *J. Anim. Sci.* **56**:625.

Brady, P. S., P. K. Ku, D. E. Ullrey and E. R. Miller. 1978. Evaluation of an amino acid-iron chelate hematinic for the baby pig. *J. Anim. Sci.* **47**:1135.

Bremner, I. and A. C. Dalgarno. 1973. Iron metabolism in the veal calf. The availability of different iron compounds. *Br. J. Nutr.* **29**:229.

Buchowski, M. S. and A. W. Mahoney. 1992. Intestinal ^{59}Fe distribution and absorption in rats with different iron status and given wheat bran or ferrous sulfate as dietary iron sources. *Nutr. Res.* **12**:1479.

Caster, W. O. and A. V. A. Resurreccion. 1982. Influence of copper, zinc, and protein on biological response to dietary iron. *In* "Nutritional Bioavailability of Iron" (C. Kies, Ed.). p.97. American Chemical Society, Washington, DC.

Chausow, D. G. and G. L. Czarnecki-Maulden. 1988a. The relative bioavailability of plant and animal sources of iron to the cat and chick. *Nutr. Res.* **8**:1041.

Chausow, D. G. and G. L. Czarnecki-Mauldin. 1988b. The relative bioavailability of iron from feedstuffs of plant and animal origin to the chick. *Nutr. Res.* **8**:175.

Conrad, M. E. and S. G. Schade. 1968. Ascorbic acid chelates in iron absorption: A role for hydrochloric acid and bile. *Gastroenterology* **55**:35.

Cook, J. D. and E. R. Monsen. 1976. Food iron absorption in human subjects: III. Comparison of the effect of animal proteins on non-heme iron absorption. *Am. J. Clin. Nutr.* **29**:859.

Coons, C. M. 1964. Iron metabolism. *Annu. Rev. Biochem.* **33**:459.

Cowan, J. W., M. Esfahani, J. P. Salji and S. A. Azzam. 1966. Effect of phytate on iron absorption in the rat. *J. Nutr.* **90**:423.

Cox, D. H. and D. L. Harris. 1960. Effect of excess dietary zinc on iron and copper in the rat. *J. Nutr.* **70**:514.

Davis, P. N., L. C. Norris and F. H. Kratzer. 1968. Iron utilization and metabolism in the chick. *J. Nutr.* **94**:407.

Deming, J. G. and G. L. Czarnecki-Maulden. 1989. Iron bioavailability in calcium and phosphorus sources. *J. Anim. Sci.* **67**(Suppl. 1):253 [Abstract].

Elvehjem, C. A., E. B. Hart and A. R. Kemmerer. 1929. The relation of iron and copper to hemoglobin synthesis in the chick. *J. Biol. Chem.* **84**:131.

Elvehjem, C. A., E. B. Hart and W. C. Sherman. 1933. The availability of iron from different sources for hemoglobin formation. *J. Biol. Chem.* **103**:61.

Evans, J. L. and P. A. Abraham. 1973. Anemia, iron storage and ceruloplasmin in copper nutrition in the growing rat. *J. Nutr.* **103**:196.

Fairweather-Tait, S. J. 1983. Studies on the availability of iron in potatoes. *Br. J. Nutr.* **50**:15.

Fairweather-Tait, S. J. and J. A. Wright. 1991. Small intestinal transit time and iron absorption. *Nutr. Res.* **11**:1465.

Finch, C. A. and J. D. Cook. 1984. Iron deficiency. *Am. J. Clin. Nutr.* **39**:471.

Fly, A. D. and G. L. Czarnecki-Mauldin. 1991. Iron bioavailability in diets containing isolated or intact sources of hemicellulose (HC). *FASEB J.* **5**:A589 [Abstract].

Forbes, G. L., C. E. Adams, M. J. Arnaud, C. O. Chichester, J. D. Cook, B. N. Harrison, R. F. Hurrell, S. G. Kahn, E. R. Morris, J. T. Tanner and P. Whittaker. 1989. Comparison of *in vitro*, animal, and clinical determinations of iron bioavailability: International nutritional anemia consultative group task force report on iron bioavailability. *Am. J. Clin. Nutr.* **49**:225.

Forth, W., H. Hubers, E. Hubers and W. Rummel. 1973. Does a transfer system for iron exist in the mucosal cells of the small intestine? *In* "Trace Elements in Environmental Health - VI" (D. D. Hemphill, Ed.), p.121. University of Missouri Press, Columbia, MO.

Freeman, S. and M. W. Burrill. 1945. Comparative effectiveness of various iron compounds in promoting iron retention and hemoglobin regeneration by anemic rats. *J. Nutr.* **30**:293.

Fritz, J. C., G. W. Pla, T. Roberts, J. W. Boehne and E. L. Hove. 1970. Biological availability in animals of iron from common dietary sources. *J. Agric. Food Chem.* **18**:647.

Fritz, J. C., G. W. Pla, B. N. Harrison and G. A. Clark. 1974. Collaborative study of the rat hemoglobin repletion test for bioavailability of iron. *J. Assoc. Off. Anal. Chem.* **57**:513.

Fritz, J. C., G. W. Pla, B. N. Harrison and G. A. Clark. 1975. Estimation of the bioavailability of iron. *J. Assoc. Off. Anal. Chem.* **58**:902.

Frolich, W. 1982. Bioavailability of iron from bran in pigs. *In* "Nutritional Bioavailability of Iron" (C. Kies, Ed.), p.163. Amererican Chemical Society, Washington, DC.

Georgievskii, V.I. 1982. The physiological role of microelements. *In* "Mineral Nutrition of Animals" (V. I. Georgievskii, B. N. Annenkov and V. T. Samokhin, Eds.) p. 171. Butterworths, London, UK.

Gipp, W. F., W. G. Pond, J. Tasker, D. van Campen, L. Krook and W. J. Visek. 1973. Influence of level of dietary copper on weight gain, hematology and liver copper and iron storage of young pigs. *J. Nutr.* **103**:713.

Gislason, J., B. Jones, B. Lonnerdal and L. Hambraeus. 1992. Iron absorption differs in piglets fed extrinsically and intrinsically ^{59}Fe-labeled sow's milk. *J. Nutr.* **122**:1287.

Gislason, J., B. Jones, B. Lonnerdal and L. Hambraeus. 1991. Intrinsic labeling of milk iron: Effect of iron status on isotope transfer into goat milk. *J. Nutr. Biochem.* **2**:375.

Gordon, D. T. and L. S. Chao. 1984. Relationship of components in wheat bran and spinach to iron bioavailability in the anemic rat. *J. Nutr.* **114**:526.

Greenberg, S. M., R. G. Tucker, A. E. Heming, J. K. Mathues. 1957. Iron absorption and metabolism. I. Interrelationship of ascorbic acid and vitamin E. *J. Nutr.* **63**:19.

Hallberg, L. and L. Rossander. 1982. Effect of soy protein on nonheme iron absportion in man. *Am. J. Clin. Nutr.* **36**:514.

Hallberg, L. and L. Solvell. 1967. Absorption of hemoglobin iron in man. *Acta Med. Scand.* **181**:335.

Hallberg, L., L. Rossander, H. Persson and E. Svahn. 1982. Deleterious effects of prolonged warming of meals on ascorbic acid content and iron absorption. *Am. J. Clin. Nutr.* **36**:846.

Hansen, C., E. Werner and J. P. Kaltwasser. 1992. Measurement of iron bioavailability by means of stable ^{54}Fe and mass spectrometry. *Phys. Med. Biol.* **37**:1349.

Harmon, B. G., D. E. Becker and A. H. Jensen. 1967. Efficacy of ferric ammonium citrate in preventing anemia in young swine. *J. Anim. Sci.* **26**:1051.

Harmon, B. G., D. E. Hoge, A. H. Jensen and D. H. Baker. 1969. Efficacy of ferrous carbonate as a hematinic for young swine. *J. Anim. Sci.* **29**:706.

Hartman, R. H., G. Matrone and G. H. Wise. 1955. Effect of high dietary manganese on hemoglobin formation. *J. Nutr.* **57**:429.

Hisayasu, S., H. Orimo, S. Migita, Y. Ikeda, K. Satoh, S. Shinjo (Kanda), Y. Hirai and Y. Yoshino. 1992. Soybean protein isolate and soybean lectin inhibit iron absorption in rats. *J. Nutr.* **122**:1190.

Hungerford, D. M., Jr. and M. C. Linder. 1983. Interactions of pH and ascorbate in intestinal iron absorption. *J. Nutr.* **113**:2615.

Hunter, J. E. 1981. Iron availability and absorption in rats fed sodium phytate. *J. Nutr.* **111**:841.

Johnson, M. A., J. G. Fischer, B. A. Bowman and E. W. Gunter. 1994. Iron nutriture in elderly individuals. *FASEB J.* **8**:609.

Johnson, M. A. and J. M . Gratzek. 1986. Influence of sucrose and starch on the development of anemia in copper- and iron-deficient rats. *J. Nutr* . **116**:2443.

Kaltwasser, J. P., C. Hansen, Y. Oebike and E. Werner. 1991. Assessment of iron availability using stable ^{54}Fe. *Eur. J. Clin. Invest.* **21**:436.

Kim, M. and M. T. Atallah. 1992. Structure of dietary pectin, iron bioavailability and hemoglobin repletion in anemic rats. *J. Nutr.* **122**:2298.

Kim, M. and M. T. Atallah. 1993. Intestinal solubility and absorption of ferrous iron in growing rats are affected by different dietary pectins. *J. Nutr.* **123**:117.

Kochanowski, B. A. and C. L. McMahan. 1990. Inhibition of iron absorption by calcium in rats and dogs: Effects of mineral separation by time and enteric coating. *Nutr. Res.* **10**:219.

Kornegay. E.T. 1972. Availability of iron contained in deflourinated phosphate. *J. Anim. Sci.* **34**:569.

Kosonen, T. and M. Mutanen. 1992. Relative bioavailability of iron in carbonyl iron and complex ferric orthophosphate to rat. *Int. J. Vit. Nutr. Res.* **62**:60.

Kwock, R. O., C. L. Keen, J. Hegenauer, P. Saltman, L. S. Hurley and B. Lonnerdal. 1984. Retention and distribution of iron added to cow's milk and human milk as various salts and chelates. *J. Nutr.* **114**:1454.

Layrisse, M., C. Martinez-Torres and M. Roche. 1968. Effect of interaction of various foods on iron absorption. *Am. J. Clin. Nutr.* **21**:1175.

Lee, G. R., S. Nacht, J. N. Lukens and G. E. Cartwright. 1968. Iron metabolism in copper-deficient swine. *J. Clin. Invest.* **47**:2058.

Magee, A. C. and G. Matrone. 1960. Studies on the growth, copper metabolism and iron metabolism of rats fed high levels of zinc. *J. Nutr.* **72**:233.

Marston, H. R., S. H. Allen and S. L. Swaby. 1971. Iron metabolism in copper-deficient rats. *Br. J. Nutr.* **25**:15.

Martinez-Torres, C., E. Romano and M. Layrisse. 1981. Effect of cysteine on iron absorption in man. *Am. J. Clin. Nutr.* **34**:322.

Matrone, G., R. H. Hartman and A. J. Clawson. 1959. Studies of manganese-iron antagonism in the nutrition of rabbits and baby pigs. *J. Nutr.* **67**:309.

McGuire, S. O., W. J. Miller, R. P. Gentry, M. W. Neathery, S. Y. Ho and D. M. Blackmon. 1985. Influence of high dietary iron as ferrous carbonate and ferrous sulfate on iron metabolism in young calves. *J. Dairy Sci.* **68**:2621.

Miller, E. R. 1978. Biological availability of iron in iron supplements. *Feedstuffs* **50**(35):20.

Miller, E. R., M. J. Parsons, D. E. Ullrey and P. K. Ku. 1981. Bioavailability of iron from ferric choline citrate and a ferric copper cobalt choline citrate complex for young pigs. *J. Anim. Sci.* **52**:783.

Mitchell, H. S. and L. Schmidt. 1926. The relation of iron from various sources to nutritional anemia. *J. Biol. Chem.* **70**:471.

Monsen, E. R. 1988. Iron nutrition and absorption: Dietary factors which impact iron bioavailability. *J. Am. Diet. Assoc.* **88**:786.

Monsen, E. R. and J. D. Cook. 1976. Food iron absorption in human subjects IV. The effects of calcium and phosphate salts on the absorption of nonheme iron. *Am. J. Clin. Nutr.* **29**:1142.

Moore, J. R., J. P. Hitchcock and L. C. Miller. 1988. Effect of nickel level, iron level and iron form on performance, hematological and mineral parameters of broiler chicks. *J. Anim. Sci.* **66**(Suppl. 1):326 [Abstract].

Morris, E. R. 1987. Iron. *In* "Trace Element in Human and Animal Nutrition" (W. Mertz, Ed.), Vol. 1, 5th ed. Academic Press, New York.

Morris, E. R. and R. Ellis. 1976. Isolation of monoferric phytate from wheat bran and its biological value as an iron source to the rat. *J. Nutr.* **106**:753.

Morris, E. R. and R. Ellis. 1982. Phytate, wheat bran, and bioavailability of dietary iron. *In* "Nutritional Bioavailability of Iron" (C. Kies, Ed.), p.121. American Chemical Society, Washington, DC.

Morris, E. R., A. D. Hill and J. T. Tanner. 1987. Assessment of bioavailability of iron fortification compounds using a rat model. *Fed. Proc.* **46**:912 [Abstract].

Motzok, I., M. D. Pennell, M. I. Davies and H. U. Ross. 1975. Effect of particle size on the biological availability of reduced iron. *J. Assoc. Off. Anal. Chem.* **58**:99.

Nakamura, F. I. and H. H. Mitchell. 1943. The utilization for hemoglobin regeneration of the iron in salts used in the enrichment of flour and bread. *J. Nutr.* **25**:39.

National Research Council (NRC). 1988. "Nutrient Requirements of Domestic Animals. Nutrient Requirements of Swine," 9th revised ed. National Academy of Sciences, Washington, DC.

Nesbit, A. H. and W. P . Elmslie. 1960. Biological availability to the rat of iron and copper from various compounds. *Trans. Illinois State Acad. Sci.* **53**:101.

Nielsen, F. H., T. R. Shuler, T. G. McLeod and T. J. Zimmerman. 1984. Nickel influences iron metabolism through physiologic, pharmacologic, and toxicologic mechanisms in the rat. *J. Nutr.* **114**:1280.

Pabon, M. L. and B. Lonnerdal. 1992. Distribution of iron and its bioavailability from iron-fortified milk and formula. *Nutr. Res.* **12**:975.

Park, Y. W., A. W. Mahoney and D. G. Hendricks. 1986. Bioavailability of iron in goat milk compared with cow milk fed to anemic rats. *J. Dairy Sci.* **69**:2608.

Parsons, C. M., D. H. Baker and C. C. Welch. 1989. Effect of excess zinc on iron utilization by chicks fed a diet devoid of phytate and fiber. *Nutr. Res.* **9**:227.

Patrick, J. Jr. 1973. Considerations of the effect of physical properties on the bioavailability of elemental iron powders. *In* "The Bioavailability of Iron Sources and Their Utilization in Food Enrichment" (J. Waddell, Ed.), p. 77. Life Science Research Office, Bethesda, MD.

Pickett, R. A., M. P. Plumlee and W. M. Beeson. 1961. Availability of dietary iron in different compounds for young pigs. *J. Anim. Sci.* **20**:946 [Abstract].

Pla, G. W., B. N. Harrison and J. C. Fritz. 1973. Comparison of chicks and rats as test animals for studying bioavailability of iron, with special reference to use of reduced iron in enriched bread. *J. Assoc. Off. Anal. Chem.* **56**:1369.

Pla, G. W. and J. C. Fritz. 1970. Availability of iron. *J. Assoc. Off. Anal. Chem.* **53**:791.

Pla, G. W. and J. C. Fritz. 1971. Collaborative study of the hemoglobin repletion test in chicks and rats for measuring availability of iron. *J. Assoc. Off. Anal. Chem.* **54**:13.

Poitevint, A. L. 1979. Determination of the true biological availability of ferrous carbonate. *Feedstuffs* **51**(3):31.

Powers, H. J., L. T. Weaver, S. Austin, A. J. A. Wright and S. J. Fairweather-Tait. 1991. Riboflavin deficiency in the rat: Effects on iron utilization and loss. *Br. J. Nutr.* **65**:487.

Powers, H. J., A. J. A. Wright and S. J. Fairweather-Tait. 1988. The effect of riboflavin deficiency in rats on the absorption and distribution of iron. *Br. J. Nutr.* **59**:381.

Prather, T. A. and D. D. Miller. 1992. Calcium carbonate depresses iron bioavailability of rats more than calcium sulfate or sodium carbonate. *J. Nutr.* **122**:327.

Raven, A. M. and A. Thompson. 1959. The availability of iron in certain grass, clover and herb species. Part II. Alsike, broad red clover, Kent wild white clover, trefoil and lucerne. *J. Agric. Sci.* **53**:224.

Reinhold, J. G., J. G. Estrada, P. M. Garcia and P. Garzon. 1986. Retention of iron by rat intestine in vivo as affected by dietary fiber, ascorbate and citrate. *J. Nutr.* **116**:1007.

Schade, S. G., B. F. Felsher, B. E. Glader and M. E. Conrad. 1970. Effect of cobalt upon iron absorption. *Proc. Soc. Exp. Biol. Med.* **134**:741.

Sell, J. L. 1965. Utilization of iron by the chick as influenced by dietary calcium and phosphorus. *Poult. Sci.* **44**:550.

Settlemire, C.T . and G. Matrone. 1967a. *In vivo* interference of zinc with ferritin iron in the rat. *J. Nutr.* **92**:153.

Settlemire, C. T. and G. Matrone. 1967b. *In vivo* effect of zinc on iron turnover in rats and life span of the erythrocyte. *J. Nutr.* **92**:159.

Southern, L. L. and D. H. Baker. 1982. Iron status of chicks as affected by *Eimeria acervulina* infection and by variable iron ingestion. *J. Nutr.* **112**:2353.

Spears, J. W., W. D. Schoenherr, E. B. Kegley, W. L. Flowers and H. D. Alhusen. 1992. Efficacy of iron methionine as a source of iron for nursing pigs. *J. Anim. Sci.* **70**(Suppl. 1):243 [Abstract]

Steinke, F. H. and D. T. Hopkins. 1978. Biological availability of the rat of intrinsic and extrinsic iron with soybean protein isolates. *J. Nutr.* **108**:481.

Story, M. L. and J. L. Greger. 1987. Iron, zinc and copper interactions: Chronic *versus* acute responses in rats. *J. Nutr.* **117**:1434.

Theurer, R. C.. W. H. Martin, J. F. Wallander and H. P. Sarett. 1973. Effect of processing on availability of iron salts in liquid infant formula products. Experimental milk-based formulas. *J. Agric. Food Chem.* **21**:482.

Thompson, D. B. and J. W. Erdman, Jr. 1984. The effect of soy protein isolate in the diet on retention by the rat of iron from radiolabeled test meals. *J. Nutr.* **114**:307.

Thompson, A. and A. M. Raven. 1959. The availabilioty of iron in certain grass, clover and herb species. I. Perennial ryegrass, cocksfoot and timothy. *J. Agric. Sci.* **52**:177

Ullrey, D. E., E. R. Miller, J. P. Hitchcock, P. K. Ku, R. L. Covert, J. Hegenauer and P. Saltman. 1973. Oral ferric citrate vs ferrous sulfate for prevention of baby pig anemia. *Michigan Agric. Exp. Sta. Rep.* **232**:34.

Underwood, E. J. 1956. "Trace Elements in Human and Animal Nutrition". Academic Press, New York.

Underwood. E. J. 1977. " Trace Elements in Human and Animal Nutrition," 4th ed. Academic Press, New York.

van Campen, D. 1973. Enhancement of iron absorption from ligated segments of rat intestine by histidine, cysteine, and lysine: Effects of removing ionizing groups and of stereoisomerism. *J. Nutr.* **103**:139.

van Campen, D. 1972. Effect of histidine and ascorbic acid on the absorption and retention of ^{59}Fe by iron-depleted rats. *J. Nutr.* **102**:165.

Waddell, D. G. and J. L. Sell. 1964. Effects of dietary calcium and phosphorus on the utilization of dietary iron by the chick. *Poult. Sci.* **43**:1249.

Waddell, J. 1973. "The Bioavailability of Iron Sources and their Utilization in Food Enrichment. " Life Science Research Office, Bethesda, MD.

Waddell. J., H. Steenbock, C. A. Elvehjem, E. B. Hart and B. M. Riising. 1928. Iron in nutrition. V. The availability of the rat for studies in anemia. *J. Biol. Chem.* **77**:769.

Welch, R. M. and D. R. van Campen. 1975. Iron availability to rats from soybeans. *J. Nutr.* **105**:253.

Wienk, K. J. H., J. J. M . Marx, A. G. Lemmens, E. J. Brink, R. van der Meer and A. C. Beynen. 1993. Calcium carbonate decreases iron bioavailability in rats as based on five different measures. *In* "Trace Elements in Man and Animals - TEMA 8" (M. Anke, D. Meissner and C.F. Mills, Eds.), p. 638. Verlag Media Touristik, Gersdorf, Germany.

Wood, R. J., P. E. Stake, J. H. Eiseman, R. L. Shippee, K. E. Wolski and U. Koehn. 1978. Effects of heat and pressure processing on the relative biological value of selected dietary supplemental inorganic iron salts as determined by chick hemoglobin repletion assay. *J. Nutr.* **108**:1477.

10
MAGNESIUM BIOAVAILABILITY

Pamela R. Henry

Department of Animal Science
University of Florida
Gainesville, Florida

Sharon A. Benz

Food and Drug Administration
Rockville, Maryland

I. INTRODUCTION

Magnesium has been recognized as an essential dietary element for about 70 years, and the element's role in hypomagnesemic tetany, also known as grass tetany, has been known since the early 1930s. Magnesium is a structural component of the skeletal system and plays a major role in nerve excitation and muscle contraction. Numerous enzymes involved in carbohydrate, protein, and lipid metabolism require magnesium. Signs of deficiency include reduced serum, cerebrospinal, and urinary magnesium concentrations, neuromuscular hyperirritability, profuse salivation, convulsions, tetany, soft tissue calcification, and death (Mayo et al., 1959; O'Dell et al., 1960; Rook and Storry, 1962; Meyer and Scholz, 1972; Ammerman and Henry, 1983).

Information concerning magnesium metabolism and bioavailability is limited compared with certain other macroelements. The reasons for this are perhaps threefold: (1) natural feed ingredients are relatively high in magnesium and most practical diets, therefore, contain sufficient levels to promote optimal performance under most production situations; (2) the concentration of magnesium in natural feeds makes it necessary to use purified dietary ingredients for requirement studies and this can be a serious impediment to research especially with ruminants; and (3) the only radiotracer of magnesium suitable for biological experiments (^{28}Mg) is expensive and has a half-life of only 21.3 hr, which seriously limits its use in research.

Reviews of various aspects of magnesium in animal nutrition include those of Mayland and Grunes, (1979), Sell and Fontenot (1980), Fontenot *et al.* (1983), and Itokawa and Durlach (1989). This review will emphsize the bioavailability of magnesium sources and will not consider their effect on buffering capacity and milk fat production.

With regard to human nutrition, healthy persons consuming varied diets are considered to receive adequate magnesium. Excellent sources of magnesium for the human diet include nuts, legumes, and unmilled grains (NRC, 1989). Removal of the germ and outer layers from cereal grains, however, results in a loss of about 80% of the magnesium. Green vegetables are good sources of the element for humans, whereas fish, meat, and milk contain relatively low concentrations of magnesium.

II. BIOAVAILABILITY STUDIES

A. *In Vitro* Estimates of Bioavailability

The solubility of magnesium compounds in various solutions has been used by several researchers to predict bioavailability of supplemental sources. Solubility may be influenced by the origin of the material, temperature of calcination, particle size, and contamination with other elements (Beede *et al.*, 1989). Studies using hydrochloric acid (HCl) at a pH below 3 as the solvent may be indicative of solubility and availability for monogastric animals, but results may tend to overestimate availability for ruminants where a significant quantity of magnesium is absorbed from the rumen at a pH that frequently may be closer to 6 or 7 (van Ravenswaay *et al.*, 1989).

In vitro rates of dissolution determined by pH-stat titration for 28 min at pH 3 were not particularly useful in predicting ruminal magnesium concentration from three magnesium oxides (MgO; Noller *et al.*, 1987), and Jensen *et al.* (1986) indicated that dissolution rates should be determined at pH 6 to 7 for more useful information concerning utilization of products by ruminants. More recently, Xin *et al.* (1989) reported that solubility of MgO at pH 5.6 to 5.7 was related to particle size and indicative of availability of magnesium sources, with smaller particles being more available. Solubility of three MgO sources at pH 6.8 was related to ruminal fluid magnesium concentration and apparent absorption of magnesium (Aaes, 1986). At 24 hr, the percentages of dissolved magnesium were approximately 25, 45, and 78 for three calcined magnesite sources.

After 24-hr *in vitro* incubation in ruminal fluid with three MgO products, the magnesium concentration in the fluid was greater from the MgO product ground to pass a 20-mesh screen than from the original 12 x 40 prilled product (Jesse *et al.*, 1981). Lough *et al.* (1990) reported more rapid solubilization of magnesium from a magnesium-proteinate than from MgO in ruminal fluid during *in vitro* culture.

Beede *et al.* (1989) developed a two stage *in vitro* ruminal + abomasal system to determine solubility of magnesium sources. Ruminal fluid was collected from fistulated cows and transferred to tubes to simulate ruminal digestion and a solution of hydrochloric acid and pepsin, that had a pH less than 2, was used to simulate the abomasal environment. Solubility averaged 14% in the ruminal phase and 45% in the abomasal stage. Solubility in both stages as a percentage of total magnesium in the source ranged from 37% for a MgO to 81% for a magnesium phosphate.

B. *In Vivo* Estimates of Bioavailability

The solubility of magnesium from forages has been examined by feeding ruminally fistulated animals various forages and collecting ruminal fluid for magnesium analysis or by measuring disappearance of magnesium from forages incubated in dacron bags in the rumen (Moseley and Griffiths, 1984; van Eys and Reid, 1987). Either of these methods identified the more soluble sources of magnesium, but neither accounted for the actual amount of soluble magnesium that was absorbed by the host or by ruminal microflora.

Ruminal fluid from animals fed a high-magnesium Italian ryegrass (*Lolium multiflorum*) contained a greater concentration of soluble magnesium than those fed a low-magnesium ryegrass (Moseley and Griffiths, 1984). Two tetany-prone orchardgrass (*Dactylis glomeratus*) hays were compared with a nontetany-prone bromegrass (*Bromus inermis*) hay (Grings and Males, 1987). The magnesium concentrations in hays were .19, .14, and .10%, respectively, and resulted in soluble ruminal magnesium concentrations of 2.01, 1.41, and .99 mM, respectively.

Disappearance of magnesium from Kentucky 31 tall fescue, Kenhy fescue, and red clover-tall fescue samples collected at six stages of maturity and incubated in dacron bags in the rumen averaged about 75% after 3 hr and 93% after 48 hr (van Eys and Reid, 1987). The rate of magnesium disappearance based on potentially degradable, slowly solubilizing fraction disappearing between 3 and 48 hr averaged 8.6%/hr. The disappearances of magnesium after a 72-hr incubation in dacron bags in the rumen averaged 95, 99, 98, 97, 88, and 93% for "Florida 77" alfalfa (*Medicago sativa*), "Florigraze" rhizoma peanut (*Arachis glabrata*), "Mott" dwarf elephantgrass (*Pennisetum purpureum*), "Tifton 78" bermudagrass (*Cynodon dactylon*), "Pensacola" bahiagrass (*Paspalum notatum*), and "Floralta" limpograss (*Hemarthria altissima*), respectively (Emanuele and Staples, 1990). The same six forages were studied with a mobile dacron bag technique in which bags were incubated in the rumen for 24 hr, removed and subjected to *in vitro* HCl and pepsin digestion for 1 hr

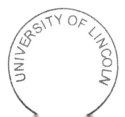

to simulate abomasal digestion, reinserted through a duodenal cannula, and recovered in feces (Emanuele et al., 1991). Magnesium release in the rumen was 96, 98, 95, 96, 88, and 93% for respective forages, whereas values after acid and pepsin digestion were about 1% greater. Thus, little additional mineral release occurred with acid and pepsin digestion. In this study, bahiagrass and limpograss bound magnesium in the lower intestinal tract. In another study, considerable magnesium was released from Glyricidia maculata and corn silage during a 6-hr incubation in ruminal fluid, while essentially no magnesium was released from rice straw in similar circumstances (Ibrahim et al., 1990).

Unlike certain other macroelements, growth response in animals has not been utilized to any great extent to determine bioavailability of magnesium in feedstuffs or supplemental sources (Table I). McGillivray and Smidt (1975) reported that reagent grade $MgSO_4 \cdot 7H_2O$, MgO, and $MgCO_3$ added to a purified diet (210 ppm magnesium) at 100, 200, and 300 ppm resulted in better growth of chicks than did $MgCl_2 \cdot 6H_2O$, but the authors did not provide data. There was no difference in growth of rats fed low-magnesium diets supplemented with various magnesium sources (Cook, 1973; Ranhotra et al., 1976; Forbes et al., 1979).

Serum magnesium concentrations have been used as a criterion of availability (Huffman et al., 1941; McConaghy et al., 1963; Fishwick and Hemingway, 1973; Amos et al., 1975; Thompson and Reid, 1981; Reid et al., 1984). Many researchers, however, do not consider serum concentrations of magnesium as particularly sensitive to changes in dietary intake, especially if basal diets are adequate in the element. Rook and Storry (1962) indicated that serum magnesium values above the renal threshold were a poor index of changes in absorption, and a significant response might well be found only when magnesium intake was marginal. In hypomagnesemic animals, serum magnesium may be an indicator of bioavailability of magnesium in various drenches and enemas used to treat hypomagnesemia. Allcroft and Burns (1968) found that serum magnesium concentrations were increased more by drenching hypomagnesemic cows with calcined magnesite than with dolomite at an equivalent amount of magnesium. Serum magnesium increased when cattle or sheep were given enemas with $MgCl_2 \cdot 6H_2O$ or $MgSO_4 \cdot 7H_2O$ (Bell et al., 1978). Plasma magnesium concentration increased more rapidly in calves given 30 g $MgCl_2 \cdot 6H_2O$ in water rectally than in those given a similar quantity orally (Bacon et al., 1990).

Generally, urinary magnesium concentrations are considered to provide more accurate information than serum magnesium concerning the element's status in animals (Rook and Balch, 1958; Kemp et al., 1961; Storry and Rook, 1963; Chicco et al., 1972; Kemp and Geurink, 1978; Thomas et al., 1984; Alexander, 1985; Sutherland et al., 1986; Littledike and Goff, 1987; Xin et al., 1989; van Ravenswaay et al., 1989; 1992). Several researchers have estimated magnesium bioavailability in terms of urinary magnesium excretion above the renal threshold (Table I). Storry and Rook (1963) supplemented a low-magnesium (200 ppm) diet composed of paper pulp and corn gluten with several magnesium sources and reported availability values for dairy cows based on urinary magnesium excretion. Jesse *et al.* (1981) measured urinary magnesium excretion of dairy cows for 1 or 2 days following a single 100 g MgO load to estimate availability of various sources of differing particle sizes. Urinary magnesium excretion by sheep on the fourth and fifth day following a change to practical diets containing 1400 ppm added magnesium was used to estimate relative availability of supplemental magnesium sources (van Ravenswaay *et al.*, 1989; 1992). Generally, good correlations have been reported between magnesium absorption and urinary excretion of the element.

Apparent absorption, and to a far lesser extent, true absorption of magnesium in feedstuffs have been determined especially for ruminants (Table II), and these values have been used to estimate relative bioavailability among sources (Tables I and III). Apparent magnesium absorption of a diet containing purified ingredients was 42% for lactating sows (Harmon *et al.*, 1976) and ranged from 16 to 35% in younger pigs (Bartley *et al.*, 1961). Absorption of magnesium from various practical diets by swine ranged from about 20 to 60% (Partridge, 1978). Guenter and Sell (1974) developed a procedure using a combination of comparative balance and ^{28}Mg isotope dilution techniques to estimate the "true" availability of magnesium in feedstuffs for chickens. True availabilities were 57, 54, 83, 42, and 60% for $MgSO_4 \cdot 7H_2O$, barley, oats, rice, and soybean meal, respectively. Apparent absorption of magnesium in milk by dairy calves ranged from 30 to 87% (Raven and Robinson, 1959). Net retention of milk magnesium declined from 45 to 25% of intake as calves increased in age from 2 to 9 weeks. Apparent absorption values ranged from 9 to 54% for ruminants consuming mixed concentrate and roughage diets, although most values were between 15 and 30% (Forbes *et al.*, 1916; 1917; 1918; 1929; Monroe, 1924; Miller *et al.*, 1924; 1925; Monroe and Perkins, 1925; Rook *et al.*, 1958; Pfeffer *et al.*, 1970; House and Mayland, 1976a; Poe *et al.*, 1985; McLean *et al.*, 1985; Kirk *et al.*, 1985; Teller and Godeau, 1987; Chester-Jones *et al.*, 1989; Jackson *et al.*, 1989).

Information concerning availability of magnesium in fresh forages and hays is presented in Table II. Apparent absorption of magnesium in grass-legume mixed pastures or hays ranged from 8 to 29% in cattle and sheep. Apparent absorption by ruminants fed fresh grasses or grass hays ranged from -4 to 66% with the majority of values from about 10 to 38%. Similar measures for legumes ranged from 5 to 40%, with the majority from about 20 to 36%.

Apparent magnesium absorption in horses fed mixed diets ranged from 44 to 61%. Horses fed grasses with various concentrations of oxalates had apparent magnesium absorption values which ranged from -8 to 46% (Table II). Other studies by

McKenzie *et al.* (1981) indicated that oxalate does not affect magnesium absorption by the horse.

Investigators, including Hintz and Schryver (1973) and Blaney *et al.* (1981), have estimated true absorption of magnesium from forages by horses in which calculations were based on an endogenous fecal magnesium excretion of 2.2 mg/kg BW daily (Hintz and Schryver, 1973) and Blaney *et al.* (1982) estimated true absorption in cattle based on an endogenous fecal excretion of 3.0 mg/kg BW daily (ARC, 1980). Dietary magnesium intake in these studies varied from about two to six times the requirement. Such estimates are only realistic if dietary intake of the element is at or below requirement (see Chapter 4).

Apparent absorption values have also been used to estimate the relative bioavailability of supplemental magnesium sources for several species of animals. In some studies, especially with ruminants, double collections were made during the balance trials. The absorption of magnesium from ingredients in the basal diet was calculated during the first collection period, following which supplemental sources of magesium were added to the diet and second collections made. The apparent absorption of magnesium from the sources was then calculated by difference. Magnesium from supplemental magnesium sulfate, basic carbonate, lactate, citrate, acetate, phosphate, chloride, oxide, and trisilicate was all well absorbed by rats (Table II). Magnesium from dolomitic limestone was only absorbed by steers at 28% of that from MgO (Gerken and Fontenot, 1967) but at 55% by sheep (Rahnema and Fontenot, 1983). Dolomitic limestone magnesium was also less well absorbed by steers than that from magnesium oxide or basic carbonate (Moore *et al.*, 1971). Magnesium hydroxide [$Mg(OH)_2$] was not as well absorbed by sheep as that in the sulfate or oxide (Bouwman, 1978). However, two recent reports in which $Mg(OH)_2$ was supplemented to diets for cattle at .2 or .3% magnesium indicated that $Mg(OH)_2$ was as well utilized as MgO based on serum magnesium and apparent magnesium absorption (Emery *et al.*, 1986; Davenport *et al.*, 1987; Cronrath and Kincaid, 1988). Magnesium basic carbonate, which has been described by Ammerman *et al.* (1972) as $(MgCO_3)_4 \cdot Mg(OH)_2 \cdot nH_2O$ was well absorbed by ruminants, whereas the natural magnesium carbonate, magnesite, was utilized to a very limited extent by ruminants (Ammerman *et al.*, 1972; Bouwman, 1978; van Ravenswaay *et al.*, 1989). Considerable variation has been shown in the utilization of magnesium oxides. In general, magnesium in smaller size particles was more available than that in larger particles (Wilson, 1981; Jesse *et al.*, 1981; van Ravenswaay *et al.*, 1989), and the larger particles may tend to settle and remain in the bottom of the rumen (Noller *et al.*, 1986; 1987). Temperature of calcination will also affect availability of MgO sources with "dead-burnt" products being of lower value (Wilson, 1981; Bouwman, 1978). Calcination of magnesite at 800, 900, or 1100°C increased apparent absorption of magnesium by a factor of three compared with unprocessed magnesite

(Wilson, 1981). Some MgO sources of brine origin have been shown to be lower in availability than some other types of MgO (Wilson, 1981; van Ravenswaay et al., 1989), probably due to a difference in processing rather than source. Relative bioavailability values for magnesium oxides compared to sulfate ranged from 21 to 117% with an average of about 75%. Because of this variability it was difficult and erroneous to assign a single value to the oxide relative to sulfate to attempt to convert bioavailability estimates from studies in which the oxide was used as a standard. Consequently, values presented in Table III represent only the studies in which magnesium sulfate was used as the standard and do not include the studies in which magnesium oxide was used. Due to the extreme variability in origin, composition and availability of magnesium oxide sources, their use as standards should be considered cautiously.

In lactating cows, an estimate of apparent availability of magnesium from various diets has been calculated based on the ratio of urinary + milk magnesium excretion to urinary + milk + fecal excretion expressed as a percentage. Using this method, Rook and Balch (1958) reported a value of 11% for orchardgrass and values for perennial ryegrass and white clover mixed pasture were reported to be 11 and 16% by Field (1970) and Moate et al. (1987), respectively. Wilson (1981) studied the utilization of numerous magnesium sources in sheep and dairy cows and developed a technique for availability calculations that used the ratio of magnesium to a chromium marker in supplements and in feces (Table II).

The response of sheep and cattle to supplemental magnesium from magnesium alloy pellets has varied considerably. In some experiments, significant differences were found in either serum magnesium concentration or incidence of clinical cases of tetany in cattle or sheep administered pellets (Davey, 1968; Davey and Gilbert, 1969; Ritchie et al., 1962; Ritchie and Hemingway, 1968; House and Mayland, 1976a). Even in these studies, however, efficacy was not always demonstrated. In several other studies, no benefit from pellets was observed (Foot et al., 1969; Kemp and Todd, 1970; Stuedemann et al., 1984).

III. FACTORS INFLUENCING BIOAVAILABILITY

A. Dietary Factors

Many factors have been found that influence the absorption and, consequently, bioavailability, of magnesium. Papers from a symposium summarized many aspects of the soil-plant-animal interrelationships regarding magnesium metabolism and hypomagnesemic tetany (Mayland and Wilkinson, 1989; Fontenot et al., 1989;

Sleper et al., 1989; Greene et al., 1989; Robinson et al., 1989; Grunes and Welch, 1989). Littledike and Goff (1987) discussed the interrelationships among magnesium, calcium, phosphorus, vitamin D, and parathyroid hormone and indicated that there was no strong evidence to indicate that any single hormone or vitamin was concerned principally and directly with magnesium homeostasis or metabolism. However, their interactions along with other animal factors and physiological conditions make magnesium homeostasis extremely dynamic and complex.

Addition of high dietary levels of animal fat or hydrogenated whole oil decreased magnesium utilization, but butterfat had no effect (Breirem, 1967; Kemp et al., 1966). Citric acid decreased serum magnesium concentration in calves (Burt and Thomas, 1961) and rats fed citric acid had lower serum magnesium than rats fed tricarballylic acid (a nonmetabolizable ruminal fermentation product of trans-aconitic acid) but it did not differ from pair-fed control rats not given citric acid (Schwartz et al., 1988). Rats given tricarballylic acid excreted more magnesium in urine than pair-fed control rats. In other studies citric acid or trans-aconitic acid alone had little effect on magnesium utilization, but in combination with KCl, urinary magnesium excretion and serum magnesium were lower and observed clinical cases of tetany were greater (Bohman, 1969; House and van Campen, 1971).

Supplementation of ruminants with various sources of readily fermentable carbohydrates has improved magnesium utilization (House and Mayland, 1976b; Madsen et al., 1976; Boling et al., 1979; Giduck and Fontenot, 1987).

Incidence of hypomagnesemic tetany in ruminants is generally most severe when young, rapidly growing, lush pastures are being grazed. Elevated dietary nitrogen has generally been reported to decrease magnesium absorption and retention in ruminants, with little difference due to the form of nitrogen (Stillings et al., 1964; L'Estrange et al., 1967; Moore et al., 1972; Henry and Smith, 1976; Henry et al., 1977; Care et al., 1984; Gabel and Martens, 1986; Teller and Godeau, 1987; Martens et al., 1988). Protein source (isolated soy, casein, formalin-treated casein, lyophilized beef, soybean meal, and corn gluten meal), however, had no effect on magnesium availability in rats, sheep, or steers (Garces and Evans, 1971; Grace and Macrae, 1972; Lo et al., 1980; Boila and Phillips, 1988).

The adverse effect of potassium on magnesium absorption and serum magnesium concentrations is very well documented (Suttle and Field, 1969; House and van Campen, 1971; Newton et al., 1972; Tomas and Potter, 1976; Macgregor and Armstrong, 1979; Greene et al., 1983a,b; Bohman et al., 1983; Wylie et al., 1985; Poe et al., 1985; Greene et al., 1986a; Martens et al., 1988; Bunting and Boling, 1988; Yano et al., 1988; Johnson and Powley, 1990). The decrease in magnesium absorption in the rumen in response to potassium appears to be due to a decrease in unidirectional magnesium absorption rather than an increase in secretion of magnesium into the rumen (Beardsworth et al., 1987; Grace et al., 1988). Sodium-deficient diets resulted in increased ruminal potassium concentration and, consequently, decreased magnesium absorption (Martens *et al.*, 1987). Increasing ruminal sodium concentration at a constant level of potassium had no effect on magnesium absorption (Martens *et al.*, 1988). Further work indicated that there are two mechanisms for transepithelial movement of magnesium. The electrogenic pathway uses the potential difference of the apical membrane as the driving force for the uptake of magnesium and potassium conductance in the membrane and the potassium gradient across this membrane contributes to the potential difference and thus must be considered as "potassium sensitive" (Leonhard *et al.*, 1989). High sodium in the presence of high potassium further reduced magnesium absorption in sheep (Poe *et al.*, 1985) and cattle (Grace, 1988).

Dietary monensin increased magnesium absorption and retention in ruminants (Kirk *et al.*, 1985; Greene *et al.*, 1986a; 1988b). Infusion of water into the rumen decreased magnesium apparent absorption in cattle (Teller and Godeau, 1987), but Suttle and Field (1966; 1967) observed either no effect on magnesium absorption in sheep or a slight increase when sheep were infused with water to simulate water intake on young, lush pastures.

Dietary fluoride (100 ppm) was found to increase plasma magnesium without affecting the rate of release of magnesium in the bone of guinea pigs (O'Dell *et al.*, 1973). Boron fed to sheep at 200 mg/day increased magnesium retention (Brown *et al.*, 1989). Aluminum fed to sheep at 2000 ppm as the citrate but not sulfate or chloride, decreased serum magnesium but had no effect on magnesium absorption or urinary excretion (Allen and Fontenot, 1984). Whereas, Kappel *et al.* (1983) reported no decrease in serum magnesium concentrations associated with high ruminal aluminum concentrations.

Excessive dietary phosphorus accentuated signs of magnesium deficiency in guinea pigs (O'Dell *et al.*, 1960) and decreased apparent magnesium absorption in horses (Hintz and Schryver, 1972) but improved magnesium retention in lactating sows without affecting serum magnesium concentration (Harmon *et al.*, 1976). Dietary phosphorus increased various levels of plasma magnesium (Chicco *et al.*, 1973a), but form of phosphorus (organic *vs* inorganic) had no effect on magnesium absorption or retention (Dutton and Fontenot, 1967). Oral supplementation of already hypomagnesemic cattle with Na_2HPO_4 or Na_2SO_4 precipitated tetany, possibly by decreasing serum calcium (Dishington, 1965; Dishington and Tollersrud, 1967). Feeding high dietary calcium decreased serum and bone magnesium concentrations in sheep (Chicco *et al.*, 1973b) and tended to increase fecal magnesium excretion over time (Shiga, 1988). Calcium also decreased magnesium absorption in rats (Behar, 1975).

B. Animal Factors

It is generally accepted that absorption of magnesium from the intestinal tract and tubular reabsorption of magnesium in the kidney are lower in older animals than in younger animals (Smith, 1958; Hemingway *et al.*, 1963; Chicco *et al.*, 1973b; Deetz *et al.*, 1982; Shiga *et al.*, 1985). Grace (1972) reported no effect of pregnancy or lactation on plasma magnesium concentration in sheep or young cattle. In mature cattle, pregnancy increased serum magnesium until about 3 weeks prior to parturition, and lactation caused a decrease about 3 weeks after parturition. On days during which hens lay eggs, magnesium absorption was greater and urinary magnesium excretion lower than on nonlaying days (Taylor and Kirkley, 1967).

Apparent absorption of magnesium as a percentage of intake was similar for Angus *vs* Simmental cows (Chavez *et al.*, 1988). Brahman cows and Brahman x British cows absorbed more magnesium than Jersey, Holstein, and Hereford but not Angus cows (Greene *et al.*, 1986b). Field *et al.* (1986) found little difference among sheep with regard to efficiency of magnesium absorption with Blackface, East Friesland, Finnish Landrace, Suffolk, and Texel breeds.

Availability of magnesium from tall fescue and fescue-red clover herbage was greater in mature wethers than dry cows, with weaned calves being intermediate (van Eys *et al.*, 1980).

IV. SUMMARY

Standard magnesium sources used in comparative assay studies have generally been either magnesium sulfate or magnesium oxide with some use of magnesium phosphate. Magnesium sulfate is a highly soluble, uniform product and is considered the standard of choice. Magnesium oxides, especially feed grade products, are considerably more variable in parent material, processing, solubility, and in their absorption by animals. Only limited testing has been conducted with magnesium phosphate. Most studies with animals in which the bioavailability of magnesium in supplemental sources has been estimated have involved either apparent absorption or urinary excretion as the criterion. Magnesium in the sulfate, acetate, and chloride forms was equal in bioavailability for ruminants. In a limited number of studies in which magnesium sulfate served as the standard, magnesium phosphate and magnesium basic carbonate had relative utilization values of about 90 and 85%, respectively. Magnesium in the form of magnesite, which is a natural magnesium carbonate, was absorbed to only a very limited extent. Magnesium oxide has been the supplemental source of the element which has been assayed most frequently. The relative values obtained have been extremely variable with an average value of about 75%. In a limited number of studies, the value for magnesium as magnesium hydroxide relative to that for the sulfate form was about 60%.

The apparent absorption of magnesium from several forages has been determined primarily with sheep. Absorption values within plant species are quite variable and average values ranged from about 20 to 45%. Apparent absorption of magnesium in alfalfa by the guinea pig as determined in one study was more than twice that observed with sheep. Very few true absorption values for magnesium in either feeds or supplements have been obtained because of the difficulty in determining metabolic fecal excretion levels for the element.

Table I. Relative bioavailability of magnesium sources for animals[a]

Source	RV	Standard	Response criterion	Meth cal	Type diet	Added level	Reference
Chickens							
Barley	95	Magnesium sulfate ($MgSO_4 \cdot 7H_2O$)	True abs	MR	P-22 ppm	300 ppm	Guenter and Sell (1974)
Beans	89	$MgSO_4 \cdot 7H_2O$	True abs	MR	P-22 ppm	300 ppm	Guenter and Sell (1974)
Beef, rib steak	73	$MgSO_4 \cdot 7H_2O$	True abs	MR	P-22 ppm	300 ppm	Guenter and Sell (1974)
Egg, whole	99	$MgSO_4 \cdot 7H_2O$	True abs	MR	P-22 ppm	300 ppm	Guenter and Sell (1974)
Milk, skim	108	$MgSO_4 \cdot 7H_2O$	True abs	MR	P-22 ppm	300 ppm	Guenter and Sell (1974)
Oats	144	$MgSO_4 \cdot 7H_2O$	True abs	MR	P-22 ppm	300 ppm	Guenter and Sell (1974)
Peas	84	$MgSO_4 \cdot 7H_2O$	True abs	MR	P-22 ppm	300 ppm	Guenter and Sell (1974)
Rice	74	$MgSO_4 \cdot 7H_2O$	True abs	MR	P-22 ppm	300 ppm	Guenter and Sell (1974)
Soybean meal	105	$MgSO_4 \cdot 7H_2O$	True abs	MR	P-22 ppm	300 ppm	Guenter and Sell (1974)
Japanese quail							
Soybean, protein	80	$MgSO_4$	Tibia Mg	SR	P-16 ppm	116-325 ppm	Spivey-Fox et al. (1976)
Cattle							
Limestone, dolomitic	53	Magnesium oxide (MgO)	App abs	MR	N	9.0 g/day	Gerken and Fontenot (1967)
Limestone, dolomitic	28	MgO	App abs[b]	MR	N	9.0 g/day	Gerken and Fontenot (1967)
Limestone, dolomitic	71	Magnesium oxide	App abs	MR	N-800 ppm	.9 g/day	Moore et al. (1971)
Magnesium acetate	109	$MgSO_4$	Ser Mg	MR	N	36 mg/kg BW	Thomas (1959)
Magnesium acetate	106	$MgSO_4$	Ser Mg	MR	N	36 mg/kg BW	Thomas (1959)

Magnesium acetate	107	MgO	Ur Mg exc	MR	N-200 ppm	13-20 g/day	Storry and Rook (1963)
Magnesium acetate	110	MgO	Ser Mg	MR	N	22 g/day	Rogers and Poole (1976)
Magnesium basic carbonate	102	MgSO$_4$	Ser Mg	MR	N	36 mg/kg BW	Thomas (1959)
Magnesium basic carbonate	95	Magnesium oxide	App abs	MR	N-800 ppm	.9 g/day	Moore et al. (1971)
Magnesium chloride	90	MgO	Ur Mg exc	MR	N-200 ppm	13-20 g/day	Storry and Rook (1963)
Magnesium chloride (MgCl$_2$)	96	MgO	Ser Mg	MR	N	8.5-9.6 g/day	Kendall (1975)
Magnesium citrate	147	MgO	Ur Mg exc	MR	N-200 ppm	13-20 g/day	Storry and Rook (1963)
Magnesium hydroxide [Mg(OH)$_2$]	100	MgO	Ur Mg exc	MR	N-.19%	.2%	Davenport et al. (1990)
Mg(OH)$_2$	101	MgO	App abs	MR	N-.19%	.2%	Davenport et al. (1990)
Magnesium lactate	97	MgO	Ur Mg exc	MR	N-200 ppm	13-20 g/day	Storry and Rook (1963)
Magnesium nitrate	97	MgO	Ur Mg exc	MR	N-200 ppm	13-20 g/day	Storry and Rook (1963)
Magnesium oxide (12x40)	13	Magnesium oxide (-200)	Ur Mg exc[c]	MR	N	35-50 g/day	Jesse et al. (1981)
Magnesium oxide (30x100)	23	Magnesium oxide (-200)	Ur Mg exc[c]	MR	N	35-50 g/day	Jesse et al. (1981)
Magnesium oxide (-20)	62	Magnesium oxide (-200)	Ur Mg exc[c]	MR	N	35-50 g/day	Jesse et al. (1981)
Magnesium oxide	140	MgSO$_4$	Ur Mg exc	MR	N	11.9 g/day	Grings and Males (1988)
Magnesium oxide - low reactivity	62	Magnesium oxide - high reactivity	Ur Mg exc	MR	N	76 g MgO/day	Wheeler et al. (1985)
Magnesium oxide - low reactivity	85	Magnesium oxide - high reactivity	Ur Mg exc	MR	N	.4% MgO	Xin et al. (1989)

Table I. (continued)

Source	RV	Standard	Response criterion	Meth cal	Type diet	Added level	Reference
Sheep							
Calcium magnesium phosphate	94	MgO	App abs	MR	N-1.1 g/day	.57 g/day	Fishwick and Hemingway (1973)
Calcium magnesium phosphate	85[b]	MgO	App abs[b]	MR	N-1.1 g/day	.57 g/day	Fishwick and Hemingway (1973)
Limestone, dolomitic	55	MgO	App abs	MR	N-1.1 g/day	1.1 g/day	Rahnema and Fontenot (1983)
Limestone, dolomitic	26	MgO	App abs[b]	MR	N-1.1 g/day	1.1 g/day	Rahnema and Fontenot (1983)
Magnesite	29	$MgSO_4$	Ur Mg exc[b]	MR	N-.13%	.3-.4%	Araujo (1976)
Magnesite	25	$MgSO_4$ RG	App abs[b]	MR	P-210 ppm	600 ppm	Bouwman (1978)
Magnesite	18	$MgSO_4$ RG	App abs[b]	MR	P-250 ppm	800 ppm	Ammerman et al. (1972)
Magnesite	0	$MgSO_4$ RG	Ur Mg exc[b]	MR	N-.13%	.1-.3%	van Ravenswaay et al. (1992)
Magnesium basic carbonate $[(MgCO_3)_4 \cdot Mg(OH)_2 \cdot nH_2O]$	93	$MgSO_4$ RG	App abs[b]	MR	P-250 ppm	800 ppm	Ammerman et al. (1972)
Magnesium basic carbonate RG	78	$MgSO_4$	Ur Mg exc[b]	MR		.3-.4%	Araujo (1976)
$MgCl_2$	118	$MgSO_4$	Ur Mg exc	MR	N	2 g	Naito (1981)
Magnesium citrate RG	176	Magnesium oxide FG	App abs	MR	N-.12%	.23%	Hurley et al. (1987)
$Mg(OH)_2$ RG	155	Magnesium oxide FG	App abs	MR	N-.12%	.23%	Hurley et al. (1987)

Mg(OH)$_2$	67	MgSO$_4$	Ur Mg exc[b]	MR	N-.13%	.3-4%	Araujo (1976)
Magnesium hydroxide-granular	65	MgSO$_4$ RG	App abs[b]	MR	P-210 ppm	600 ppm	Bouwman (1978)
Magnesium hydroxide	54	MgSO$_4$ RG	App abs[b]	MR	P-210 ppm	600 ppm	Bouwman (1978)
Magnesium-mica	133	Magnesium oxide FG	App abs	MR	N-.12%	.23%	Hurley et al. (1987)
Magnesium-mica	91	MgSO$_4$	App abs	MR	SP	.24%	Jackson et al. (1989)
Magnesium-mica	117	MgSO$_4$	App abs	MR	SP	.24%	Jackson et al. (1989)
MgO	94	MgSO$_4$ RG	App abs[b]	MR	P-250 ppm	800 ppm	Ammerman et al. (1972)
MgO FG	52	MgSO$_4$	Ur Mg exc[b]	MR	N-.13%	.3-4%	Araujo (1976)
Magnesium oxide FG	110	MgSO$_4$ RG	App abs[b]	MR	P-210 ppm	600 ppm	Bouwman (1978)
Magnesium oxide FG	93	MgSO$_4$ RG	App abs[b]	MR	P-162 ppm	600 ppm	Bouwman (1978)
Magnesium oxide FG	43	MgSO$_4$ RG	App abs[b]	MR	P-162 ppm	600 ppm	Bouwman (1978)
Magnesium oxide	76	Magnesium oxide FG	App abs[b]	MR	P-135 ppm	600 ppm	Bouwman (1978)
Magnesium oxide	83	Magnesium oxide FG	App abs[b]	MR	P-135 ppm	600 ppm	Bouwman (1978)
MgO	82	MgSO4	Ur Mg exc	MR	N	2 g	Naito (1981)
Magnesium oxide 75-150 μm	71	Magnesium oxide <75 μm	App abs[b]	MR	N-.23%	981 mg/day	Wilson (1981)
Magnesium oxide 150-250 μm	91	Magnesium oxide <75 μm	App abs[b]	MR	N-.23%	1017 mg/day	Wilson (1981)
Magnesium oxide 250-500 μm	73	Magnesium oxide <75 μm	App abs[b]	MR	N-.23%	1038 mg/day	Wilson (1981)

Table I. (continued)

Source	RV	Standard	Response criterion	Meth cal	Type diet	Added level	Reference
Magnesium oxide 500-1000 μm	12	Magnesium oxide <75 μm	App abs[b]	MR	N-.23%	1022 mg/day	Wilson (1981)
Magnesium oxide	29	Magnesium phosphate	App abs	MR	NG	4 g/day	Hemingway (1986)
Magnesium oxide	59	Magnesium phosphate	App abs	MR	NG	4 g/day	Hemingway (1986)
Magnesium oxide	76	Magnesium phosphate	App abs	MR	NG	4 g/day	Hemingway (1986)
Magnesium oxide	26	Magnesium phosphate	App abs	MR	NG	4 g/day	Hemingway (1986)
Magnesium oxide	86	MgSO$_4$ RG	Ur Mg exc	MR	N-.13%	.14%	van Ravenswaay et al. (1992)
Magnesium oxide	78	MgSO$_4$ RG	Ur Mg exc	MR	N-.13%	.14%	van Ravenswaay et al. (1992)
Magnesium oxide	77	MgSO$_4$ RG	Ur Mg exc	MR	N-.13%	.14%	van Ravenswaay et al. (1992)
Magnesium oxide FG	85	MgSO$_4$ RG	Ur Mg exc	MR	N-.13%	.14%	van Ravenswaay et al. (1992)
Magnesium oxide FG	78	MgSO$_4$ RG	Ur Mg exc	MR	N-.13%	.14%	van Ravenswaay et al. (1992)
Magnesium oxide FG	82	MgSO$_4$ RG	Ur Mg exc	MR	N-.13%	.14%	van Ravenswaay et al. (1992)
Magnesium oxide FG	58	MgSO$_4$ RG	App abs	MR	P-200 ppm	600 ppm	van Ravenswaay et al. (1989)
Magnesium oxide FG	21	MgSO$_4$ RG	App abs	MR	P-200 ppm	600 ppm	van Ravenswaay et al. (1989)
Magnesium oxide FG	89	MgSO$_4$ RG	App abs	MR	P-200 ppm	600 ppm	van Ravenswaay et al. (1989)
Magnesium oxide FG	70	MgSO$_4$ RG	Ur Mg exc	SR	N-.14%	.14%	van Ravenswaay et al. (1989)
Magnesium oxide FG	29	MgSO$_4$ RG	Ur Mg exc	SR	N-.14%	.14%	van Ravenswaay et al. (1989)
Magnesium oxide FG	91	MgSO$_4$ RG	Ur Mg exc	SR	N-.14%	.14%	van Ravenswaay et al. (1989)

Magnesium phosphate	87	Magnesium oxide	App abs	MR	N-1.4 g/day	2.66 g/day	Hemingway and McLaughlin (1979)
Magnesium phosphate	80	Magnesium oxide	App abs[b]	MR	P-162 ppm	600	Bouwman (1978)
Magnesium phosphate <.5 mm	97	Magnesium phosphate .5-2.0 mm	App abs	MR	NG	4.0 g/day	Hemingway (1986)
Magnesium phosphate	75	Magnesium oxide	App abs[b]	MR	N-1.1 g/day	1.87 g/day	Fishwick and Hemingway (1973)
Magnesium polysaccharide	69	Magnesium oxide	App abs	MR	N	.17-.18%	Greene et al. (1988a)
Magnesium sulfate FG	106	$MgSO_4$ RG	App abs[b]	MR	P-162 ppm	600 ppm	Bouwman (1978)

Rats

Magnesium acetate	104	$MgSO_4$ RG	App abs	MR	P-40 ppm	150 ppm	Ranhotra et al. (1976)
Magnesium carbonate RG	122	$MgSO_4 \cdot 7H_2O$ RG	App abs	MR	P-16 ppm	200, 400 ppm	Cook (1973)
Magnesium carbonate	103	$MgSO_4$	App abs	MR	P-40 ppm	150 ppm	Ranhotra et al. (1976)
Magnesium chloride	100	$MgSO_4$	App abs	MR	P-40 ppm	150 ppm	Ranhotra et al. (1976)
$MgCl_2 \cdot 6H_2O$ RG	114	$MgSO_4 \cdot 7H_2O$	App abs	MR	P-16 ppm	200, 400 ppm	Cook (1973)
Magnesium citrate	101	Magnesium sulfate	App abs	MR	P-40	150 ppm	Ranhotra et al. (1976)
Magnesium lactate	103	Magnesium sulfate	App abs	MR	P-40	150 ppm	Ranhotra et al. (1976)
Magnesium oxide	100	$MgSO_4$	App abs	MR	P-40 ppm	150 ppm	Ranhotra et al. (1976)
Magnesium oxide	109	$MgSO_4 \cdot 7H_2O$	App abs	MR	P-16 ppm	200, 400 ppm	Cook (1973)
Magnesium phosphate	97	Magnesium carbonate	App abs	MR	SP-200 ppm	.12%	Meintzer and Steenbock (1955)
Magnesium phosphate	102	$MgSO_4$	App abs	MR	P-40 ppm	150 ppm	Ranhotra et al. (1976)

Table I. (continued)

Source	RV	Standard	Response criterion	Meth cal	Type diet	Added level	Reference
Magnesium phosphate	101	$MgSO_4 \cdot 7H_2O$ RG	App abs	MR	P-16 ppm	200, 400 ppm	Cook (1973)
Magnesium silicate $(Mg_2Si_3O_8)$	102	$MgSO_4 \cdot 7H_2O$ RG	App abs	MR	P-16 ppm	200, 400 ppm	Cook (1973)
Soybean flour	106	Casein	Tibia Mg	SR	P	50-650 ppm	Forbes et al. (1979)
Wheat flour	99	$MgSO_4$	App abs	MR	P-40 ppm	150 ppm	Ranhotra et al. (1976)

[a] Abbreviations can be found in Appendix I. Chemical formula for a compound given only if provided by the author; RG indicates reagent grade, FG indicates feed grade.

[b] Source alone, corrected for amount contributed from basal diet.

[c] Urinary magnesium excretion (g/day) above baseline for 2 days following a 100 g MgO load.

218

Table II. Apparent and true absorption of magnesium in feedstuffs by animals[a]

Source	Value, %[b]	Response criterion	Total Mg level	Reference
Cattle				
Alfalfa	5	App abs	11.8 g/day	Rook and Campling (1962)
Alfalfa, hay	11	App abs	16 g/day	Forbes et al. (1929)
Alfalfa, silage	18	App abs	11.7 g/day	Rook and Campling (1962)
Barley straw	0	App abs	1.8 g/day	Rook and Campling (1962)
Buffel grass (Cenchrus ciliaris)	9	App abs	14.3 mg/kg BW	Blaney et al. (1982)
Clover, red	19	App abs	18.1 g/day	Rook and Campling (1962)
Fescue, meadow	21	App abs	8.8 g/day	Rook and Campling (1962)
Fescue, tall	-4	App abs	7.2 g/day	Rook and Campling (1962)
Kale, narrow stem	27	App abs	12.0 g/day	Rook and Campling (1962)
Milk, whole	68	App abs	12-13 mg/dL	Smith (1958)
Milk, whole	14	App abs	12-13 mg/dL	Smith (1958)
Milk, whole, spray dried[c]	87	App abs	.670 g/day	Raven and Robinson (1959)
Milk, whole, spray dried + 10% butterfat[c]	76	App abs	.625 g/day	Raven and Robinson (1959)
Milk, separated, spray dried[c]	30	App abs	.812 g/day	Raven and Robinson (1959)
Milk, separated, spray dried + unhydrogenated palm oil[c]	76	App abs	.656 g/day	Raven and Robinson (1959)
Orchardgrass	27	App abs	8.4 g/day	Rook and Campling (1962)
Orchardgrass	18	App abs	14.7 g/day	Rook and Balch (1958)

219

Table II. (continued)

Source	Value, %[b]	Response criterion	Total Mg level	Reference
Orchardgrass	27	App abs	8.4 g/day	Rook and Campling (1962)
Orchardgrass	18	App abs	14.7 g/day	Rook and Balch (1958)
Orchardgrass + ryegrass, early growth	18	App abs	10.4 g/day	Rook and Balch (1958)
Orchardgrass + ryegrass, late growth	18	App abs	12.5 g/day	Rook and Balch (1958)
Orchardgrass, hay	33	App abs	7.75 g/day	Rook and Campling (1962)
Ryegrass	15	App abs	7.88 g/day	Rook and Campling (1962)
Ryegrass, perennial (*Lolium perenne*)	19	App abs	9.55 g/day	Rook and Campling (1962)
Ryegrass, perennial + clover, white (*Trifolium repens*)	40	App abs	25 g/day	Moate et al. (1987)
Ryegrass + clover	20	App abs	32 g/day	Hutton et al. (1965)
Ryegrass + clover, hay	21	App abs	8.4 g/day	Rook and Campling (1962)
Setaria grass (*Setaria sphacelata var. sericea*)	10	App abs	15.3 mg/kg BW	Blaney et al. (1982)
Spear + bluegrass (*Aristada spp.* + *Brothriochloa spp.*)	12	App abs	17.8 mg/kg BW	Blaney et al. (1982)
Timothy, hay	17	App abs	5.05 g/day	Rook and Campling (1962)
Wheaten grass (*Triticum aestivum*)	15	App abs	14.1 mg/kg BW	Blaney et al. (1982)
Sheep				
Alfalfa + clover, red	10	App abs	.26%	Reid et al. (1987)
Alfalfa, hay (*Medicago satimva L.*)	34	App abs	.29%	Reid et al. (1978)
Alfalfa, hay	27	App abs	.36%	Reid et al. (1978)
Alfalfa, hay	28	App abs	.41%	Reid et al. (1978)

Feed	No.	Absorption	Value	Reference
Alfalfa, hay	35	App abs	.29%	Reid et al. (1978)
Alfalfa, hay	35	App abs	.29%	Reid et al. (1978)
Alfalfa, hay fert. 112 kg Mg/ha	44	App abs	.31%	Reid et al. (1978)
Alfalfa, hay fert. 112 kg Mg/ha	40	App abs	.31%	Reid et al. (1978)
Alfalfa, hay fert. 112 kg Mg/ha	31	App abs	.37%	Reid et al. (1978)
Alfalfa, hay fert. 224 kg Mg/ha	29	App abs	.36%	Reid et al. (1978)
Alfalfa, hay fert. 448 kg Mg/ha	31	App abs	.41%	Reid et al. (1978)
Alfalfa, hay 1st cutting	35	App abs	2.64 g/day	Reid et al. (1979)
Alfalfa, hay 2nd cutting	29	App abs	2.79 g/day	Reid et al. (1979)
Alfalfa, hay 1st cutting	33	App abs	1.15 g/day	Reid et al. (1979)
Alfalfa, hay 2nd cutting	25	App abs	1.61 g/day	Reid et al. (1979)
Alfalfa, hay 3rd cutting	36	App abs	2.87 g/day	Reid et al. (1979)
Alfalfa, hay 1st cutting	32	App abs	2.55 g/day	Reid et al. (1979)
Alfalfa, hay 2nd cutting	25	App abs	2.53 g/day	Reid et al. (1979)
Alfalfa, ensiled	27	App abs	1.3 g/day	Ivan et al. (1983)
Alfalfa, ensiled with formic acid	24	App abs	1.28 g/day	Ivan et al. (1983)
Alfalfa, pelleted	29	App abs	3.18 g/day	Hjerpe (1968)
Alfalfa, pelleted	31	True abs	3.18 g/day	Hjerpe (1968)
Bluegrass, Kentucky, hay (Poa pratensis L.)	34	App abs	.10%	Reid et al. (1978)
Bluegrass, Kentucky, hay	31	App abs	.21%	Reid et al. (1978)
Bluegrass, Kentucky, hay fert. 112 kg Mg/ha	38	App abs	.12%	Reid et al. (1978)
Bluegrass, Kentucky, hay fert. 112 kg Mg/ha	37	App abs	.27%	Reid et al. (1978)

Table II. (continued)

Source	Value, %[b]	Response criterion	Total Mg level	Reference
Bromegrass, smooth, prebloom (*Bromusinermis Leyss.*)	23	App abs	.53 g/day	Powell *et al.*, 1978
Bromegrass, smooth, full bloom	33	App abs	.33 g/day	Powell *et al.* (1978)
Bromegrass, smooth, immature	31	App abs	.66 g/day	Powell *et al.* (1978)
Bromegrass, smooth, early bloom	46	App abs	.37 g/day	Powell *et al.* (1978)
Bromegrass, smooth	53	App abs	1.26 g/day	Grings and Males (1987)
Bromegrass, hay	9	App abs	.16%	Reid *et al.* (1978)
Bromegrass, hay	24	App abs	5.5 g/day	Harmon and Britton (1983)
Bromegrass, hay fert. 112 kg Mg/ha	5	App abs	.14%	Reid *et al.* (1978)
Clover, red, hay (*Trifolium pratense L.*)	33	App abs	.23%	Reid *et al.* (1978)
Clover, red, hay fert. 112 kg Mg/ha	32	App abs	.28%	Reid *et al.* (1978)
Clover, white (*Trifolium repens*)	18	App abs	1.27 g/day	Grace *et al.* (1974)
Clover, white	29	App abs	2.04 g/day	Grace *et al.* (1974)
Clover, white	40	App abs	2.6 g/day	Joyce and Rattray (1970)
Corn, ensiled	41	App abs	1.1 g/day	Ivan *et al.* (1983)
Corn, ensiled with urea	42	App abs	1.2 g/day	Ivan *et al.* (1983)
Fescue, tall, prebloom (*Festuca arundinacea Schreb.*)	27	App abs	1.18 g/day	Powell *et al.* (1978)
Fescue, tall, full bloom	25	App abs	1.38 g/day	Powell *et al.* (1978)
Fescue, tall, immature	23	App abs	1.03 g/day	Powell *et al.* (1978)
Fescue, tall, early bloom	42	App abs	.62 g/day	Powell *et al.* (1978)

Fescue, tall, hay	31	App abs	.20%	Reid et al. (1978)
Fescue, tall, hay	26	App abs	.28%	Reid et al. (1978)
Fescue, tall, hay	19	App abs	.18%	Reid et al. (1978)
Fescue, tall, hay, fert. 112 kg Mg/ha	27	App abs	.18%	Reid et al. (1978)
Fescue, tall, hay, fert. 112 kg Mg/ha	30	App abs	.23%	Reid et al. (1978)
Fescue, tall, hay, fert. 112 kg Mg/ha	21	App abs	.30%	Reid et al. (1978)
Fescue x ryegrass hybrid, early	14	App abs	1.71 g/day	Rosero et al. (1980)
Fescue x ryegrass hybrid, late	35	App abs	2.25 g/day	Rosero et al. (1980)
Guineagrass , 28 days regrowth (*Panicum maximum*)	25	App abs	.16%	Perdomo et al. (1977)
Guineagrass, 42 day regrowth	45	App abs	.17%	Perdomo et al. (1977)
Guineagrass, 56 days regrowth	57	App abs	.16%	Perdomo et al. (1977)
Oatgrass, tall (*Arrhenatherum elatium L. Presl.*)	30	App abs	.13%	Reid et al. (1978)
Oatgrass, tall, fert. 112 kg Mg/ha	24	App abs	.16%	Reid et al. (1978)
Orchardgrass, early (*Dactylis glomerata L.*)	27	App abs	1.81 g/day	Rosero et al. (1980)
Orchardgrass, late	23	App abs	1.69 g/day	Rosero et al. (1980)
Orchardgrass	25	App abs	.22%	Thompson and Reid (1981)
Orchardgrass, 2.4% N	18	App abs	1.13 g/day	Stillings et al. (1964)
Orchardgrass, 3.7% N	12	App abs	1.51 g/day	Stillings et al. (1964)
Orchardgrass, 2.1% N	18	App abs	1.33 g/day	Stillings et al. (1964)
Orchardgrass, 4.1% N	11	App abs	1.86 g/day	Stillings et al. (1964)
Orchardgrass	26	App abs	.5-3.0 g/day	Shockey et al. (1984)
Orchardgrass	36	App abs	2.25 g/day	Grings and Males (1987)

Table II. (continued)

Source	Value, %[b]	Response criterion	Total Mg level	Reference
Orchardgrass	53	App abs	1.85 g/day	Grings and Males (1987)
Orchardgrass, 1st cutting	19	App abs	1.5 g/day	Giduck and Fontenot (1987)
Orchardgrass, prebloom	42	App abs	.76 g/day	Powell et al. (1978)
Orchardgrass, full bloom	43	App abs	.93 g/day	Powell et al. (1978)
Orchardgrass, immature	40	App abs	1.14 g/day	Powell et al. (1978)
Orchardgrass, early bloom	48	App abs	.6 g/day	Powell et al. (1978)
Orchardgrass, fert. 390 kg Mg/ha	37	App abs	.29%	Thompson and Reid (1981)
Orchardgrass, hay	10	App abs	.12%	Reid et al. (1978)
Orchardgrass, hay	32	App abs	.16%	Reid et al. (1978)
Orchardgrass, hay	22	App abs	.12%	Reid et al. (1978)
Orchardgrass, hay	45	App abs	.13%	Reid et al. (1978)
Orchardgrass, hay, fert. 112 kg Mg/ha	32	App abs	.15%	Reid et al. (1978)
Orchardgrass, hay, fert. 112 kg Mg/ha	24	App abs	.19%	Reid et al. (1978)
Orchardgrass, hay, fert. 112 kg Mg/ha	30	App abs	.13%	Reid et al.(1978)
Orchardgrass, hay, fert. 112 kg Mg/ha	44	App abs	.18%	Reid et al. (1978)
Pangola, 28 days regrowth (Digitaria decumbens)	41	App abs	.06%	Perdomo et al. (1977)
Pangola, 42 days regrowth	32	App abs	.05%	Perdomo et al. (1977)
Pangola, 56 days regrowth	66	App abs	.06%	Perdomo et al. (1977)
Ryegrass, Italian (Lolium multiflorum)	33	App abs	1.21 g/day	Moseley and Griffiths (1984)
Ryegrass, Italian	40	App abs	2.22 g/day	Moseley and Griffiths (1984)

Ryegrass, perennial (*Lolium perenne* L.)	20	App abs	1.1 g/day	Grace *et al.* (1974)
Ryegrass, perennial	30	App abs	1.76 g/day	Grace *et al.* (1974)
Ryegrass, perennial	34	App abs	1.8 g/day	Joyce and Rattray (1970)
Ryegrass, perennial, prebloom	28	App abs	.77 g/day	Powell *et al.* (1978)
Ryegrass, perennial, full bloom	45	App abs	.85 g/day	Powell *et al.* (1978)
Ryegrass, perennial, immature	35	App abs	1.2 g/day	Powell *et al.* (1978)
Ryegrass, perennial, early bloom	45	App abs	.63 g/day	Powell *et al.* (1978)
Ryegrass, perennial + orchardgrass	15	App abs	1.06 g/day	Field *et al.* (1958)
Ryegrass, perennial + orchardgrass	7	App abs	.31%	Reid *et al.* (1987)
Ryegrass, perennial + clover, white	13	App abs[d]	2.97 g/day	Field (1967)
Ryegrass, perennial + clover, white	39	App abs	2.2 g/day	Joyce and Rattray, (1970)
Ryegrass, short rotation (*Lolium multiflorum* x *perenne*)	16	App abs	1.15 g/day	Grace *et al.* (1974)
Ryegrass, short rotation	27	App abs	1.84 g/day	Grace *et al.* (1974)
Sheepgrass, 28 days regrowth (*Brachiaria decumbens*)	62	App abs	.14%	Perdomo *et al.* (1977)
Sheepgrass, 42 days regrowth	46	App abs	.13%	Perdomo *et al.* (1977)
Sheepgrass, 56 days regrowth	65	App abs	.14%	Perdomo *et al.* (1977)
Timothy, hay	26	App abs	.13%	Reid *et al.* (1978)
Timothy, hay	11	App abs	.07%	Reid *et al.* (1978)
Timothy, hay, fert. 112 kg Mg/ha	25	App abs	.09%	Reid *et al.* (1974)
Timothy, hay, fert. 112 kg Mg/ha	34	App abs	.17%	Reid *et al.* (1978)
Timothy, hay, fert. 390 kg Mg/ha	27	App abs	1.14 g/day	Reid *et al.* (1984)

Table II. (continued)

Source	Value, %[b]	Response criterion	Total Mg level	Reference
Goats				
Orchardgrass, 1st cutting	17	App abs	NG	Reid et al. (1974)
Orchardgrass, regrowth	29	App abs	NG	Reid et al. (1974)
Alfalfa, pelleted	61	App abs	70 mg/kg BW	Hintz and Schryver (1972)
Alfalfa hay + oats	52	App abs	17 mg/kg BW	Hintz et al. (1984)
Buffel grass (Cenchrus ciliaris)	15	App abs	44 mg/kg BW	Blaney et al. (1981)
Buffel grass	3	App abs	18 mg/kg BW	Blaney et al. (1981)
Buffel grass	9	App abs	15 mg/kg BW	Blaney et al. (1981)
Buffel grass	-8	App abs	20 mg/kg BW	Blaney et al. 1981
Flinders grass (Iseilema spp.)	22	App abs	11 mg/kg BW	Blaney et al. (1981)
Kikuyu grass (Pennisetum clandestinum)	-3	App abs	37 mg/kg BW	Blaney et al. (1981)
Oat, chaff (Arena sativa)	44	App abs	20 mg/kg BW	Blaney et al. (1981)
Pangola grass (Digitaria decumbens)	21	App abs	31 mg/kg BW	Blaney et al. (1981)
Panic grass, green (Panicum maximum var. trichoglume)	13	App abs	35 mg/kg BW	Blaney et al. (1981)
Paragrass (Brachiaria mulica)	13	App abs	33 mg/kg BW	Blaney et al. (1981)
Rhodes grass (Chloris gayana)	46	App abs	54 mg/kg BW	Blaney et al. (1981)
Setaria grass (Setaria sphaceleta var. sericea)	26	App abs	21 mg/kg BW	Blaney et al. (1981)
Setaria grass	6	App abs	28 mg/kg BW	Blaney et al. (1981)

Guinea Pigs

Alfalfa, hay	76	App abs	.29%	Reid et al. (1978)
Alfalfa, hay, fert. 112 kg Mg/ha	80	App abs	.31%	Reid et al. (1978)
Alfalfa, hay, fert. 224 kg Mg/ha	81	App abs	.36%	Reid et al. (1978)
Alfalfa, hay, fert. 448 kg Mg/ha	89	App abs	.41%	Reid et al. (1978)

[a]Abbreviations can be found in Appendix I.
[b]Absorption value expressed as percentage of intake and the source represented 100% of the diet.
[c]Reconstituted before feeding.
[d]Grazing sheep, intake estimated, feces collected and analyzed.

Table III. Relative bioavailability of supplemental magnesium sources[a]

	Species	
Source	Cattle	Sheep
Magnesium sulfate	100	100
Magnesite	-	25 (2)
Magnesium acetate	110 (2)	-
Magnesium basic carbonate	100 (1)	85 (2)
Magnesium chloride	-	120 (1)
Magnesium hydoxide	-	60 (3)
Magnesium oxide	-	75 (18)
Magnesium mica	-	90 (1)

[a]Average values rounded to nearest "5" and expressed relative to response obtained with magnesium sulfate. Number of studies or samples involved indicated within parentheses.

REFERENCES

Aaes, O. 1986. The influence of the feed composition on availability of magnesium in dairy cows. *In* "Proceedings of the Boliden Kemi Conference on Magnesium for Ruminants," pp. 1-11. Helsingborg, Sweden.

Alexander, A. M. 1985. Magnesium status of dairy cows. *N. Z. Vet. J.* **33**:171.

Allcroft, R. and K. N. Burns. 1968. Hypomagnesaemia in cattle. *N. Z. Vet. J.* **16**:109.

Allen, V. G. and J. P. Fontenot. 1984. Influence of aluminum as sulfate, chloride and citrate on magnesium and calcium metabolism in sheep. *J. Anim. Sci.* **59**:798.

Ammerman, C. B., C. F. Chicco, P. E. Loggins and L. R. Arrington. 1972. Availability of different inorganic salts of magnesium to sheep. *J. Anim. Sci.* **34**:122.

Ammerman, C. B. and P. R. Henry. 1983. Dietary magnesium requirements in ruminants and nonruminants. *In* "Role of Magnesium in Animal Nutrition" (J. P. Fontenot, G. E. Bunce, K. E. Webb, Jr., and V. G. Allen, Eds.), pp. 93-106. Proceedings of the John Lee Pratt International Symposium, Blacksburg, VA.

Amos, R. L., G. J. Crissman, R. F. Keefer and D. J. Horvath. 1975. Serum magnesium levels of ewes grazing orchardgrass topdressed with dolomite or calcite. *J. Anim. Sci.* **41**:198.

Araujo, E. C. 1976. Biological availability of inorganic sources of magnesium to sheep. M. S. Thesis. University of Florida, Gainesville.

ARC. 1980. "The Nutrient Requirements of Ruminant Livestock." Commonwealth Agricultural Bureaux, Slough, U.K.

Bacon, J. A., M. C. Bell, J. K. Miller, N. Ramsey and F. J. Mueller. 1990. Effect of magnesium administration route on plasma minerals in Holstein calves receiving either adequate of insufficient magnesium in their diets. J. Dairy Sci. 73:470.

Bartley, J. C., E. F. Reber, J. W. Yusken and H. W. Norton. 1961. Magnesium balance study in pigs three to five weeks of age. J. Anim. Sci. 20:137.

Beardsworth, L. J., P. M. Beardsworth and A. D. Care. 1987. The effect of increased potassium concentration on the absorption of magnesium from the reticulo-rumen of conscious sheep. J. Physiol. 386:89P.

Beede, D. K., E. M. Hirchert, D. S. Lough, W. K. Sanchez and C. Wang. 1989. Solubility of magnesium from feed grade sources in an in vitro ruminal + abomasal system. In Proceedings of the 26th Florida Dairy Production Conference, pp 47-54. University of Florida, Gainesville.

Behar, J. 1975. Effect of calcium on magnesium absorption. Am. J. Physiol. 229:1590.

Bell, M. C., J. A. Oluokun, N. Ramsey and G. E. Beckman. 1978. Magnesium treatment of cows for grass tetany. Feedstuffs 50(6):24.

Blaney, B. J., R. J. W. Gartner and T. A. Head. 1982. The effects of oxalate in tropical grasses on calcium, phosphorus and magnesium availability to cattle. J. Agric. Sci. Camb. 99:533.

Blaney, B. J., R. J. W. Gartner and R. A. McKenzie. 1981. The effects of oxalate in some tropical grasses on the availability to horses of calcium, phosphorous and magnesium. J. Agric. Sci. Camb. 97:507.

Bohman, V. R., F. P. Horn, B. A. Stewart, A. C. Mathers and D. L. Grunes. 1983. Wheat pasture parsoning. 1. An evaluation of cereal pastures as related to tetany in beef cows. J. Anim. Sci. 57:1352.

Bohman, V. R., A. L. Lesperance, G. D. Harding and D. L. Grunes. 1969. Induction of experimental tetany in cattle. J. Anim. Sci. 29:99.

Boila, R. J. and G. D. Phillips. 1988. Effects of faunation, protein source and surgical modification of the intestinal tract upon flows of calcium, phosphorus and magnesium in the digestive tract of sheep. Can. J. Anim. Sci. 68:853.

Boling, J. A., T. O. Okolo, N. Gay and N. W. Bradley. 1979. Effect of magnesium and energy supplementation on blood constituents of fall-calving beef cows. J. Anim. Sci. 48:1209.

Bouwman, G. W. 1978. The utilization of dietary magnesium by ruminants. Ph.D. Dissertation, University of Florida, Gainesville.

Breirem, K. 1967. The effect of various fats on serum-magnesium in young calves. Reprint 309, Agric. Coll. Norway, Inst. Anim. Nutr.

Brown, T. F., M. E. McCormick, D. R. Morris and L. K. Zeringue. 1989. Effects of dietary boron on mineral balance in sheep. Nutr. Res. 9:503.

Bunting, L. D. and J. A. Boling. 1988. Magnesium and nitrogen metabolism in lambs fed or abomasally infused with a high level of potassium. Int. J. Vit. Nutr. Res. 58:93.

Burt, A. W. A. and D. C. Thomas. 1961. Dietary citrate and hypomagnesaemia in the ruminant. Nature 192:1193.

Care, A. D., R. C. Brown, A. R. Farrar and D. W. Pickard. 1984. Magnesium absorption from the digestive tract of sheep. Q. J. Exp. Physiol. 69:577.

Chavez, E., J. C. Laurenz, L. W. Greene, F. M. Byers and G. T. Schelling. 1988. Apparent absorption of phosphorus, calcium, magnesium and copper in two herds of cows. J. Anim. Sci. 66(Suppl. 1):463 [Abstract].

Chester-Jones, H., J. P. Fontenot, H. P. Veit and K. E. Webb, Jr. 1989. Physiological effects of feeding high levels of magnesium to sheep. *J. Anim. Sci.* **67**:1070.

Chicco, C. F., C. B. Ammerman, J. P. Feaster and B. G. Dunavant. 1973b. Nutritional interrelationships of dietary calcium, phosphorus and magnesium in sheep. *J. Anim. Sci.* **36**:986.

Chicco, C. F., C. B. Ammerman, W. G. Hillis and L. R. Arrington. 1972. Utilization of dietary magnesium by sheep. *J. Physiol.* **222**:1469.

Chicco, C. F., C. B. Ammerman and P. E. Loggins. 1973a. Effect of age and dietary magnesium on voluntary feed intake and plasma magnesium in ruminants. *J. Dairy Sci.* **56**:822.

Cook, D. A. 1973. Availability of magnesium: Balance studies in rats with various inorganic magnesium salts. *J. Nutr.* **103**:1365.

Cronrath, J. D. and R. L. Kincaid. 1988. Magnesium hydroxide and calcined magnesite-limestone as magnesium sources for cattle. *J. Dairy Sci.* **71** (Suppl. 1):155 [Abstract].

Davenport, G. M., J. A. Boling, L. D. Bunting and N. Gay. 1987. Bioavailability of magnesium in beef cattle fed different sources of magnesium. *J. Anim. Sci.* **65**(Suppl. 1):490 [Abstract].

Davenport, G. M., J. A. Boling, and N. Gay. 1990. Bioavailability of magnesium in beef cattle fed magnesium oxide or magnesium hydroxide. *J. Anim. Sci.* **68**:3765.

Davey, L. A. 1968. Magnesium alloy bullets for grazing sheep. *Vet. Rec.* **82**:142.

Davey, L. A. and G. A. Gilbert. 1969. Magnesium bullets. *Vet. Rec.* **85**:194.

Deetz, L. E., R. E. Tucker, G. E. Mitchell, Jr. and R. M. DeGregorio. 1982. Renal function and magnesium clearance in young and old cows given potassium chloride and sodium citrate. *J. Anim. Sci.* **55**:680.

Dishington, I. W. 1965. Changes in serum magnesium levels of ruminants, as influenced by abrupt changes in the composition of the diet. Effect of oral administration of various inorganic and organic compounds on the serum-magnesium level. *Acta Vet. Scand.* **6**:150.

Dishington, I. W. and S. Tollersrud. 1967. Hypomagnesaemia and hypomagnesaemic tetany induced in lactating cows by changing the diet. *Acta Vet. Scand.* **8**:14.

Dutton, J. E. and J. P. Fontenot. 1967. Effect of dietary organic phosphorus on magnesium metabolism in sheep. *J. Anim. Sci.* **26**:1409.

Emanuele, S. M. and C. R. Staples. 1990. Ruminal release of minerals from six forage species. *J. Anim. Sci.* **68**:2052.

Emanuele, S. M., C. R. Staples and C. J. Wilcox. 1991. Extent and site of mineral release from six forage species incubated in mobile dacron bags. *J. Anim. Sci.* **69**:801.

Emery, R. S., J. Luoma, J. Liesman, J. W. Thomas, H. A. Tucker and L. T. Chapin. 1986. Effect of serum magnesium and feed intake on serum growth hormone concentrations. *J. Dairy Sci.* **69**:1148.

Field, A. C. 1967. Studies on magnesium in ruminant nutrition. 7. Excretion of magnesium, calcium, potassium and faecal dry matter by grazing sheep. *Br. J. Nutr.* **21**:631.

Field, A. C. 1970. Studies on magnesium in ruminant nutrition. 10. Effect of lactation on the excretion of magnesium and faecal dry matter by grazing monozygotic twin cows. *Br. J. Nutr.* **24**:71.

Field, A. C., J. W. McCallum and E. J. Butler. 1958. Studies on magnesium in ruminant nutrition. Balance experiments on sheep with herbage from fields associated with lactation tetany and from control pastures. *Br. J. Nutr.* **12**:433.

Field, A. C., J. A. Woolliams and C. Woolliams. 1986. The effect of breed of sire on the urinary excretion of phosphorus and magnesium in lambs. *Anim. Prod.* **42**:349.

Fishwick, G. and R. G. Hemingway. 1973. Magnesium phosphates as dietary supplements for growing sheep. *J. Agric. Sci. Camb.* **81**:441.

Fontenot, J. P., V. G. Allen, G. E. Bunce and J. P. Goff. 1989. Factors influencing magnesium absorption and metabolism in ruminants. *J. Anim. Sci.* **67**:3445.

Fontenot, J. P., G. E. Bunce, K. E. Webb, Jr. and V. G. Allen, Eds. 1983. " Role of Magnesium in Animal Nutrition." Proceedings of the John Lee Pratt International Symposium, Blacksburg, VA.

Foot, A. S., J. Connell, R. A. Allcroft and M. K. Lloyd. 1969. Magnesium bullets. *Vet. Rec.* **84**:467.

Forbes, E. B., F. M. Beegle, C. M. Fritz, L. E. Morgan and S. N. Rhue. 1916. The mineral metabolism of the milch cow. First paper. *Ohio Agric. Exp. Stat. Bull.* **295**: 323.

Forbes, E. B., F. M. Beegle, C. M. Fritz, L. E. Morgan and S. N. Rhue. 1917. The mineral metabolism of the milch cow. Second paper. *Ohio Agric. Exp. Stat. Bull.* **308**:451.

Forbes, E. B., R. B. French and T. V. Letonoff. 1929. The mineral metabolism of the beef steer. *J. Nutr.* **1**:201.

Forbes, E. B., J. O. Halverson, L. E. Morgan, J. A. Schulz, C. E. Mangels, S. N. Rhue and G. W. Burke. 1918. The mineral metabolism of the milch cow. Third paper. *Ohio Agric. Exp. Stat. Bull.* **300**: 91.

Forbes, R. M., K. E. Weingartner, H. M. Parker, R. R. Bell and J. W. Erdman, Jr. 1979. Bioavailability to rats of zinc, magnesium and calcium in casein-, egg- and soy protein- containing diets. *J. Nutr.* **109**:1652.

Gabel, G. and H. Martens. 1986. The effect of ammonia on magnesium metabolism in sheep. *J. Anim. Physiol. Anim. Nutr.* **55**:278.

Garces, M. A. and J. L. Evans. 1971. Calcium and magnesium absorption in growing cattle as influenced by age of animal and source of dietary nitrogen. *J. Anim. Sci.* **32**:789.

Gerken, H. J., Jr. and J. P. Fontenot. 1967. Availability and utilization of magnesium from dolomitic limestone and magnesium oxide in steers. *J. Anim. Sci.* **26**:1404.

Giduck, S. A. and J. P . Fontenot. 1987. Utilization of magnesium and other macrominerals in sheep supplemented with different readily-fermentable carbohydrates. *J. Anim. Sci.* **65**:1667.

Grace, N. D. 1988. Effect of varying sodium and potassium intakes on sodium, potassium, and magnesium contents of the ruminoreticulum and apparent absorption of magnesium in non-lactating dairy cattle. *N.Z. J. Agric. Res.* **31**:401.

Grace, N. D. 1972. Grass tetany. III. Observations on plasma magnesium levels in grazing ruminants during pregnancy and lactation. *N.Z. J. Agric. Res.* **15**:79.

Grace, N. D., I. W. Caple and A. D. Care. 1988. Studies in sheep on the absorption of magnesium from a low molecular weight fraction of the reticulo-rumen contents. *Br. J. Nutr.* **59**:93.

Grace, N. D. and J. C. Macrae. 1972. Influence of feeding regimen and protein supplementation on the sites of net absorption of magnesium in sheep. *Br. J. Nutr.* **27**:51.

Grace, N. D., M. J. Ulyatt and J. C. Macrae. 1974. Quantitative digestion of fresh herbage by sheep. III. The movement of Mg, Ca, P, K and Na in the digestive tract. *J. Agric. Sci. Camb.* **82**:321.

Greene, L. W., J. F. Baker and P. F. Hardt. 1989. Use of animal breeds and breeding to overcome the incidence of grass tetany: A review. *J. Anim. Sci.* **67**:3463.

Greene, L. W., J. P. Fontenot and K. E. Webb, Jr. 1983a. Site of magnesium and other macromineral absorption in steers fed high levels of potassium. *J. Anim. Sci.* **57**:503.

Greene, L. W., L. A. Hurley, N. K. Chirase, P. F. Hardt, F. M. Byers and G. T. Schelling. 1988a. Site and level of apparent magnesium absorption in lambs fed a polysaccharide complex of magnesium or magnesium oxide. *J. Anim. Sci.* **67**(Suppl. 1):31 [Abstract].

Greene, L. W., B. J. May, G. T. Schelling and F. M. Byers. 1988b. Site and extent of apparent magnesium and calcium absorption in steers fed monensin. *J. Anim. Sci.* **66**:2987.

Greene, L. W., G. T. Schelling and F. M. Byers. 1986a. Effects of dietary monensin and potassium on apparent absorption of magnesium and other macroelements in sheep. *J. Anim. Sci.* **63**:1960.

Greene, L. W., J. C. Solis, F. M. Byers and G. T. Schelling. 1986b. Apparent and true digestibility of magnesium in mature cows of five breeds and their crosses. *J. Anim. Sci.* **63**:189.

Greene, L. W., K. E. Webb, Jr. and J. P. Fontenot. 1983b. Effect of potassium level on site of absorption of magnesium and other macroelements in sheep. *J. Anim. Sci.* **56**:1214.

Grings, E. E. and J. R. Males. 1987. Macromineral absorption in sheep fed tetany-prone and non-tetany prone hays. *J. Anim. Sci.* **65**:821.

Grings, E. E. and J. R. Males. 1988. Performance, blood and ruminal characteristics of cows receiving monensin and a magnesium supplement. *J. Anim. Sci.* **66**:566.

Grunes, D. L. and R. M. Welch. 1989. Plant contents of magnesium, calcium and potassium in relation to ruminant nutrition. *J. Anim. Sci.* **67**:3485.

Guenter, W. and J. L. Sell. 1974. A method for determining "true" availability of magnesium from foodstuffs using chickens. *J. Nutr.* **104**:1446.

Harmon, D. L. and R. A. Britton. 1983. Balance and urinary excretion of calcium, magnesium and phosphorus in response to high concentrate feeding and lactate infusion in lambs. *J. Anim. Sci.* **57**:1306.

Harmon, B. G., C. T. Liu, A. H. Jensen and D. H. Baker. 1976. Dietary magnesium levels for sows during gestation and lactation. *J. Anim. Sci.* **42**:860.

Hemingway, R. G. 1986. The evaluation of magnesium phosphates and oxides as supplements for ruminants. *In* "Proceedings of the 1985 Boliden Kemi Conference on Magnesium for Ruminants." Boliden Kemi, Helsingborg, Sweden.

Hemingway, R. G. and A. M. McLaughlin. 1979. Retention by sheep of magnesium, phosphorus and fluoring from magnesium and calcium phosphates. *Br. Vet. J.* **135**:411.

Hemingway, R. G., N. S. Ritchie, A. R. Rutherford and G. M. Jolly. 1963. Effects of potassium fertilizers, age of ewe, and small magnesium supplementation on blood magnesium and calcium levels of lactating ewes. *J. Agric. Sci.* **60**:307.

Henry, P. R. and W. H. Smith. 1976. Magnesium and urea effect on hypomagnesemia. *J. Anim. Sci.* **43**:325 [Abstract].

Henry, P. R., W. H. Smith and M. D. Cunningham. 1977. Effect of histamine and ammonia on hypomagnesemia in ruminants. *J. Anim. Sci.* **44**:276.

Hintz, H. F. and H. F. Schryver. 1972. Magnesium metabolism in the horse. *J. Anim. Sci.* **35**:755.

Hintz, H. F. and H. F. Schryver. 1973. Magnesium, calcium and phosphorus metabolism in ponies fed varying levels of magnesium. *J. Anim. Sci.* **37**:927.

Hintz, H. F., H. F. Schryver, J. Doty, C. Lakin and R. A. Zimmerman. 1984. Oxalic acid content of alfalfa hays and its influence on the availability of calcium, phosphorus and magnesium to ponies. *J. Anim. Sci.* **58**:939.

Hjerpe, C. A. 1968. Experiments with herbage from a field associated with hypomagnesemic tetany in beef cattle. *Cornell Vet.* **58**:193.

House, W. A. and H. F. Mayland. 1976a. Magnesium and calcium utilization in sheep treated with magnesium alloy rumen bullets or fed magnesium sulfate. *J. Anim. Sci.* **42**:506.

House, W. A. and H. F. Mayland. 1976b. Magnesium utilization in wethers fed diets with varying ratios of nitrogen to readily fermentable carbohydrate. *J. Anim. Sci.* **43**:842.

House, W. A. and D. van Campen. 1971. Magnesium metabolism of sheep fed different levels of potassium and citric acid. *J. Nutr.* **101**:1483.

Huffman, C. F., C. L. Conley, C. C. Lightfoot and C. W. Duncan. 1941. Magnesium studies in calves. II. The effect of magnesium salts and various natural feeds upon the magnesium content of the blood plasma. *J. Nutr.* **22**:609.

Hurley, L. A., L. W. Greene, G. T. Schelling and F. M. Byers. 1987. Magnesium and calcium balanced in lambs fed different sources of magnesium. *J. Anim. Sci.* **65**(Suppl. 1):489 [Abstract].

Hutton, J. B., K. E. Jury and E. B. Davies. 1965. Studies of the nutritive value of New Zealand dairy pastures. IV. The intake and utilization of magnesium in pasture herbage by lactating dairy cattle. *N. Z. J. Agric. Res.* **8**:479.

Ibrahim, M. N. M ., A. van der Kamp, G. Zemmelink and S. Tamminga. 1990. Solubility of mineral elements present in ruminant feeds. *J. Agric. Sci. Camb.* **114**:265.

Itokawa, Y. and J. Durlach, eds. 1989. 'Magnesium in Health and Disease. Fifth International Symposium". Libbey, London.

Ivan, M., M. Ihnat and D. M. Veira. 1983. Solubility and flow of calcium, magnesium and phosphorus in the digestive tract of sheep given maize or alfalfa silages. *Anim. Feed Sci. Technol.* **9**:131.

Jackson, K. E., R. E. Tucker and G. E. Mitchell, Jr. 1989. Bioavailability of magnesium and potassium in lambs fed different magnesium sources. *Nutr. Rep. Int.* **39**:493.

Jensen, A., O. Aaes and H. E. Lundager Madsen. 1986. The reactivity of magnesium oxide in relation to its use as a feed additive. *Acta Agric. Scand.* **36**:217.

Jesse, B. W., J. W. Thomas and R. S. Emery. 1981. Availability of magnesium from magnesium oxide particles of differing sizes and surfaces. *J. Dairy Sci.* **64**:197.

Johnson, C. L. and G. Powley. 1990. Magnesium metabolism in lactating goats fed on grass diets differing in mineral content. *J. Agric. Sci. Camb.* **114**:133.

Joyce, J. P. and P. V. Rattray. 1970. Nutritive value of white clover and perennial ryegrass. III. Intake and utilisation of calcium, phosphorus and magnesium. *N. Z. Agric. Res.* **13**:800.

Kappel, L. C., H. Youngberg, R. H. Ingraham, F. G. Hembry, D .L. Robinson and J. H. Cherney. 1983. Effects of dietary aluminum on magnesium status of cows. *Am. J. Vet. Res.* **44**:770.

Kemp, A., W. B. Deijs, O. J. Hemkes and A. J. H. van Es. 1961. Hypomagnesaemia in milking cows: Intake and utilization of magnesium from herbage by lactating cows. *Neth. J. Agric. Sci.* **9**:134.

Kemp, A., W. B. Deijs and E. Kluvers. 1966. Influence of higher fatty acids on the availability of magnesium in milking cows. *Neth. J. Agric. Sci.* **14**:290.

Kemp, A. and J. H. Geurink. 1978. Grassland farming and minerals in cattle. *Neth. J. Agric. Sci.* **26**:161.

Kemp, A. and J. R. Todd. 1970. Prevention of hypomagnesaemia in cows: The use of magnesium alloy bullets. *Vet. Rec.* **86**:463.

Kendall, J. D. 1975. Extra magnesium cuts grass tetany in trials. *Feedstuffs* **8**:14.

Kirk, D. J., L. W. Greene, G. T. Schelling and F. M. Byers. 1985. Effects of monensin on Mg, Ca, P and Zn metabolism and tissue concentrations in lambs. *J. Anim. Sci.* **60**:1485.

Leonhard, S., H. Martens and G. Gabel. 1989. New aspects of magnesium transport in ruminants. *Acta Vet. Scand. Suppl.* **86**:146.

L'Estrange, J. L. , J. B. Owen and D. Wilman. 1967. Effects of a high level of nitrogenous fertilizer and date of cutting on the availability of the magnesium and calcium of herbage to sheep. *J. Agric. Sci. Camb.* **68**:173.

Littledike, E. T. and J. Goff. 1987. Interactions of calcium, phosphorus, magnesium and vitamin D that influence their status in domestic meat animals. *J. Anim. Sci.* **65**:1727.

Lo, G. S., F. H. Steinke and D. T. Hopkins. 1980. Effect of isolated soybean protein on magnesium bioavailability. *J. Nutr.* **110**:829.

Lough, D. S., D. K. Beede and C. J. Wilcox. 1990. Lactational responses to and in vitro ruminal solubility of magnesium oxide or magnesium chelate. *J. Dairy Sci.* **73**:413.

Macgregor, R. C. and D. G. Armstrong. 1979. The effect of increasing potassium intake on absorption of magnesium by sheep. *Proc. Nutr. Soc.* **38**:66A.

Madsen, F. C., D. E. Lentz, J. K. Miller, D. Lowrey-Harnden and S. L. Hansard. 1976. Dietary carbohydrate effects upon magnesium metabolism in sheep. *J. Anim. Sci.* **42**:1316.

Martens, H., G. Heggemann and K. Regier. 1988. Studies on the effect of K, Na, NH_4^+, VFA and CO_2 on the net absorption of magnesium from the temporarily isolated rumen of heifers. *J. Vet. Med. A* **35**:73.

Martens, H., O. W. Kubel, G. Gabel and H. Honig. 1987. Effects of low sodium intake on magnesium metabolism of sheep. *J. Agric. Sci. Camb.* **108**:237.

Mayland, H. F. and D. L. Grunes. 1979. Soil-climate-plant relationships in the etiology of grass tetany. *In* "Grass Tetany" (V.V. Rendig and D.L. Grunes, Eds.), pp. 123-175. Am. Soc. Agron., Madison, WI.

Mayland, H. F. and S. R. Wilkinson. 1989. Soil factors affecting magnesium availability in plant-animal systems: A review. *J. Anim. Sci.* **67**:3437.

Mayo, R. H., M. P. Plumlee and W. M. Beeson. 1959. Magnesium requirement of the pig. *J. Anim. Sci.* **18**:264.

McConaghy, S., J. S. V. McAllister, J. R. Todd, J. E. F. Rankin and J. Kerr. 1963. The effects of magnesium compounds and of fertilizers on the mineral composition of herbage and on the incidence of hypomagnesaemia in dairy cows. *J. Agric. Sci.* **60**:313.

McGillivray, J. J. and M. J. Smidt. 1975. Biological evaluation of magnesium sources. *Poult. Sci.* **54**:1792. [Abstract].

McKenzie, P. A., B. J. Blancy and R. J. W. Gartner. 1981. The effect of dietary oxalate on calcium, phosphorus and magnesium balances in horses. *J. Agric. Sci. Camb.* **97**:69.

McLean, A. F., W. Buchan and D. Scott. 1985. The effect of potassium and magnesium infusion on plasma Mg concentration and Mg balance in ewes. *Br. J. Nutr.* **54**:713.

Meintzer, R. B. and H. Steenbock. 1955. Vitamin D and magnesium absorption. *J. Nutr.* **56**:285.

Meyer, H. and H. Scholz. 1972. Pathogenesis of hypomagnesemic tetany: I. Relationship between Mg content of blood and cerebrospinal fluid of sheep. *Dtsch. Tieraerztl. Wochenschr.* **80**:541.

Miller, H. G., P. M. Brandt and R. C. Jones. 1924. Mineral metabolism studies with dairy cattle. *Am. J. Physiol.* **69**:169.

Miller, H. G., W. W. Yates, R. C. Jones and P. M. Brandt. 1925. Mineral metabolism studies with dairy cows. Mineral equilibrium after prolonged lactation. *Am. J. Physiol.* **72**:647.

Moate, P. J., K. M. Schneider, D. D. Leaver and D. C. Morris. 1987. Effect of 1,25 dihydroxyvitamin D_3 on the calcium and magnesium metabolism of lactating cows. *Aust. Vet. J.* **64**:73.

Monroe, C. F. 1924. The metabolism of calcium, magnesium, phosphorus and sulfur in dairy cows fed high and low protein rations. *J. Dairy Sci.* **7**:58.

Monroe, C. F. and A. E. Perkins. 1925. The mineral metabolism of dairy cows as affected by distilled water and previous feeding. *J. Dairy Sci.* **8**:293.

Moore, W. F., J. P. Fontenot and R. E. Tucker. 1971. Relative effects of different supplemental magnesium sources on apparent digestibility in steers. *J. Anim. Sci.* **33**:502.

Moore, W. F., J. P. Fontenot and K. E. Webb, Jr. 1972. Effect of form and level of nitrogen on magnesium utilization. *J. Anim. Sci.* **35**:1046.

Moseley, G. and D. W. Griffiths. 1984. The mineral metabolism of sheep fed high- and low-magnesium selections of Italian ryegrass. *Grass Forage Sci.* **39**:195.

National Reasearch Council. 1989. "Recommended Dietary Allowances," 10th ed. National Academy Press, Washington, DC.

Naito, Y. 1981. Clinico-pharmacological studies of magnesium compounds to hypomagnesemia in ruminants. *Iwate Daigaku Nogaku* **15**:206.

Newton, G. L., J. P. Fontenot, R. E. Tucker and C. E. Polan. 1972. Effects of high dietary potassium intake on the metabolism of magnesium by sheep. *J. Anim. Sci.* **35**:440.

Noller, C. H., L. J. Wheeler and J. A. Patterson. 1986. Retention of supplemental magnesium oxide in the rumen and implication in balance studies. *J. Anim. Sci.* **63**(Suppl. 1):405 [Abstract].

Noller, C. H., L. J. Wheeler and J. A. Patterson. 1987. Effect of particle size of magnesium oxide on ruminal magnesium concentrations and pH. *J. Dairy Sci.* **70**(Suppl. 1):200 [Abstract].

O'Dell, B. L., E. R. Morris and W. O. Regan. 1960. Magnesium requirement of guinea pigs and rats. Effect of calcium and phosphorus and symptoms of magnesium deficiency. *J. Nutr.* **70**:103.

O'Dell, B. L., R. I. Moroni and W. O. Regan. 1973. Interaction of dietary fluoride and magnesium in guinea pigs. *J. Nutr.* **103**:841.

Partridge, I. G. 1978. Studies on digestion and absorption in the intestines of growing pigs. 3. Net movements of mineral nutrients in the digestive tract. *Br. J. Nutr.* **39**:527.

Perdomo, J. T., R. L. Shirley and C. F. Chicco. 1977. Availability of nutrient minerals in four tropical forages fed freshly chopped to sheep. *J. Anim. Sci.* **45**:1114.

Pfeffer, E., A. Thompson and D. G. Armstrong. 1970. Studies on intestinal digestion in the sheep. 3. Net movement of certain inorganic elements in the digestive tract on rations containing different proportions of hay and rolled barley. *Br. J. Nutr.* **24**:197.

Poe, J. H., L. W. Greene, G. T. Schelling, F. M. Byers and W. C. Ellis. 1985. Effects of dietary potassium and sodium on magnesium utilization in sheep. *J. Anim. Sci.* **60**:578.

Powell, K., R. L. Reid and J. A. Balasko. 1978. Performance of lambs on perennial ryegrass, smooth bromegrass, orchardgrass and tall fescue pastures. II. Mineral utilization, in vitro digestibility and chemical composition of herbage. *J. Anim. Sci.* **46**:1503.

Rahnema, S. H. and J. P. Fontenot. 1983. Effect of supplemented magnesium from magnesium oxide or dolomitic limestone upon digestion and absorption of minerals in sheep. *J. Anim. Sci.* **57**:1545.

Ranhotra, G. S., R. J. Loewe and L. V. Puyat. 1976. Bioavailability of magnesium from wheat flour and various organic and inorganic salts. *Cereal Chem.* **53**:770.

Raven, A. M. and K. L. Robinson. 1959. Studies of the nutrition of the young calf. 2. The nutritive value of unhydrogenated palm oil, unhydrogenated palm-kernel oil, and butterfat, as additions to a milk diet. *Br. J. Nutr.* **13**:178.

Reid, R. L., B. S. Baker and L. C. Vona. 1984. Effects of magnesium sulfate supplementation and fertilization on quality and mineral utilizatiion of timothy hays by sheep. *J. Anim. Sci.* **59**:1403.

Reid, R. L., K. Daniel and J. D. Bubar. 1974. Mineral relationships in sheep and goats maintained on orchardgrass fertilized with different levels of nitrogen, or nitrogen with micro-elements, over a five year period. In "Proceedings of the XII International Grasslands Congress Moscow, USSR" (V.G. Iglovikov and A.P. Movsissyants, Eds.), Vol 3, Pt. 1:426.

Reid, R. L., G. A. Jung, I. J. Roemig and R. E. Kocher. 1978. Mineral utilization by lambs and guinea pigs fed Mg-fertilized grass and legume hays. *Agron. J.* **70**:9.

Reid, R. L., G. A. Jung, C. H. Wolf and R. E. Kocher. 1979. Effects of magnesium fertilization on mineral utilization and nutritional quality of alfalfa for lambs. *J. Anim. Sci.* **48**:1191.

Reid, R. L., W. C. Templeton, Jr., T. S. Ranney and W. V. Thayne. 1987. Digestibility, intake and mineral utilization of combinations of grasses and legumes by lambs. *J. Anim. Sci.* **64**:1725.

Ritchie, N. S. and R. G. Hemingway. 1968. Magnesium alloy bullets for dairy cattle. *Vet. Rec.* **82**:87.

Ritchie, N. S., R. G. Hemingway, J. S. S. Inglis and R. M. Peacock. 1962. Experimental production of hypomagnesaemia in ewes and its control by small magnesium supplements. *J. Agric. Sci.* **58**:399.

Robinson, D. L., L. C. Kappel and J. A. Boling. 1989. Management practices to overcome the incidence of grass tetany. *J. Anim. Sci.* **67**:3470.

Rogers, P. A. M. and D. B. R. Poole. 1976. Control of hypomagnesaemia in cows: A comparison of magnesium acetate in the water supply with magnesium oxide in the feed. *Irish Vet. J.* **30**:129.

Rook, J. A. F. and C. C. Balch. 1958. Magnesium metabolism in the dairy cow. II. Metabolism during spring grazing season. *J. Agric. Sci.* **51**:199.

Rook, J. A. F., C. C. Balch and C. Line. 1958. Magnesium metabolism in the dairy cow. I. Metabolism on stall rations. *J. Agric. Sci.* **51**:189.

Rook, J. A. F. and R. C. Campling. 1962. Magnesium metabolism in the dairy cow. IV. The availability of the magnesium in various feedingstuffs. *J. Agric. Sci.* **59**:225.

Rook, J. A. F. and J. E. Storry. 1962. Magnesium in the nutrition of farm animals. *Nutr. Abstr. Rev.* **32**:1055.

Rosero, O. R., R. E. Tucker, G. E. Mitchell, Jr. and G. T. Schelling. 1980. Mineral utilization in sheep fed spring forages of different species, maturity and nitrogen fertility. *J. Anim. Sci.* **50**:128.

Schwartz, R., M. Topley and J. B. Russell. 1988. Effect of tricarballylic acid, a nonmetabolizable rumen fermentation product of trans-aconitic acid, on Mg, Ca and Zn utilization of rats. *J. Nutr.* **118**:183.

Sell, J. L. and J. P. Fontenot. 1980. "Magnesium in Animal Nutrition." National Feed Ingredients Association, West Des Moines, IA.

Shiga, A. 1988. Effects of calcium carbonate supplementation on Ca, Mg and P metabolism in ewes. *Jap. J. Vet. Sci.* **50**:175.

Shiga, A., K. Abe, S. Hamamoto, M. Keino, K. Tsukamoto and O. Fujio. 1985. Effects of age, milking and season on magnesium, calcium and inorganic phosphorus metabolisms in cows. *Jap. J. Vet. Sci.* **47**:275.

Shockey, W. L., H. R. Conrad and R. L. Reid. 1984. Relationship between magnesium intake and fecal magnesium excretion of ruminants. *J. Dairy Sci.* **67**:2594.

Sleper, D. A., K. P. Vogel, K. H. Asay and H. F. Mayland. 1989. Using plant breeding and genetics to overcome the incidence of grass tetany. *J. Anim. Sci.* **67**:3456.

Smith, R. H. 1958. Calcium and magnesium metabolism in calves. 2. Effect of dietary vitamin D and ultraviolet irradiation on milk-fed calves. *Biochem. J.* **70**:201.

Spivey-Fox, M. R., B. E. Fry, Jr., J. E. Rothlein and R. P. Hamilton. 1976. Magnesium bioassay in Japanese quail. *Fed. Proc.* **35**:744 [Abstract].

Stillings, B. R., J. W. Bratzler, L. F. Marriott and R. C. Miller. 1964. Utilization of magnesium and other minerals by ruminants consuming low and high nitrogen-containing forages and vitamin D. *J. Anim. Sci.* **23**:1148.

Storry, J. E. and J. A. F. Rook. 1963. Magnesium metabolism in the dairy cow. V. Experimental observations with a purified diet low in magnesium. *J. Agric. Sci.* **61**:167.

Stuedemann, J. A., S. R. Wilkinson and R. S. Lowrey. 1984. Efficacy of a large magnesium alloy rumen bolus in the prevention of hypomagnesemic tetany in cows. *Am. J. Vet. Res.* **45**:698.

Sutherland, R. J., K. C. Bell, K. D. McSporran and G. W. Carthew. 1986. A comparative study of diagnostic tests for the assessment of herd magnesium status in cattle. *N. Z. Vet. J.* **34**:133.

Suttle, N. F. and A. C. Field. 1966. Studies on magnesium in ruminant nutrition. 6. Effect of intake of water on the metabolism of magnesium, calcium, sodium, potassium, and phosphorus in sheep. *Br. J. Nutr.* **20**:609.

Suttle, N. F. and A. C. Field. 1967. Studies on magnesium in ruminant nutrition. 8. Effect of increased intakes of potassium and water on the metabolism of magnesium, phosphorus, sodium, potassium and calcium in sheep. *Br. J. Nutr.* **21**:631.

Suttle, N. F. and A. C. Field. 1969. Studies on magnesium in ruminant nutrition. 9. Effect of potassium and magnesium intakes on development of hypomagnesaemia in sheep. *Br. J. Nutr.* **23**:81.

Taylor, T. G. and J. Kirkley. 1967. The absorption and excretion of minerals by laying hens in relation to egg shell formation. *Br. Poult. Sci.* **8**:289.

Teller, E. and J. M. Godeau. 1987. Some observation about magnesium absorption in cattle. *J. Anim. Physiol. Anim. Nutr.* **57**:16.

Thomas, J. W. 1959. Magnesium nutrition of the calf. *In* "Proceedings of the Symposium on Magnesium and Agriculture," pp. 131-152. West Virginia University, Morgantown, WV.

Thomas, J. W., R. S. Emery, J. K. Breaux and J. S. Liesman. 1984. Response of milking cows fed a high concentrate, low roughage diet plus sodium bicarbonate, magnesium oxide, or magnesium hydroxide. *J. Dairy Sci.* **67**:2532.

Thompson, J. K. and R. L. Reid. 1981. Mineral status of beef cows and sheep on spring pasture fertilized with kieserite. *J. Anim. Sci.* **52**:969.

Tomas, F. M. and B. J. Potter. 1976. The effect and site of action of potassium upon magnesium absorption in sheep. *Aust. J. Agric. Res.* **27**:873.

van Eys, J. E., G. Madata and R. L. Reid. 1980. Comparative utilization of fescue and fescue-clover herbage by beef cows, calves and sheep. *J. Anim. Sci.* **51**(Suppl. 1):250 [Abstract].

van Eys, J. E. and R. L. Reid. 1987. Ruminal solubility of nitrogen and minerals from fescue and fescue-red clover herbage. *J. Anim. Sci.* **65**:1101.

van Ravenswaay,R. O., P. R. Henry, C. B. Ammerman and R. C. Littell. 1989. Comparison of methods to determine relative bioavailability of magnesium in magnesium oxides for ruminants. *J. Dairy Sci.* **72**:2968.

van Ravenswaay, R. O., P. R. Henry, C. B. Ammerman and R. C. Littell. 1992. Relative bioavailability of magnesium sources for ruminants as measured by urinary magnesium excretion. *Anim. Feed Sci. Technol.* **39**:13.

Wheeler, L. J., C. H. Noller and J. A. Patterson. 1985. Rate of dissolution of magnesium oxide and concentration of magnesium in urine and blood of cattle. *J. Anim. Sci.* **61**(Suppl. 1):465 [Abstract].

Wilson, C. L. 1981. Magnesium supplementation of ruminant diets. Ph.D. Dissertation, University of Glasgow.

Wylie, M. J., J. P. Fontenot and L. W. Greene. 1985. Absorption of magnesium and other macrominerals in sheep infused with potassium in different parts of the digestive tract. *J. Anim. Sci.* **61**:1219.

Xin, Z., W. B. Tucker and R. W. Henken. 1989. Effect of reactivity rate and particle size of magnesium oxide on magnesium availability, acid-base balance, mineral metabolism, and milking performance of dairy cows. *J. Dairy Sci.* **72**:462.

Yano, F., K. Horiuchi and R. Kawashima. 1988. Effect of potassium infusion into the rumen on magnesium absorption from the rumen wall of sheep. *Mem. Coll. Agric., Kyoto Univ.* **131**:13.

11

MANGANESE BIOAVAILABILITY

Pamela R. Henry

Department of Animal Science
University of Florida
Gainesville, Florida

I. INTRODUCTION

Manganese was recognized as an essential dietary nutrient for growth and reproduction in rats and mice in the early 1930s (Kemmerer *et al.*, 1931; Orent and McCollum, 1931) and its role with regard to prevention of perosis in chicks was reported 5 years later (Wilgus *et al.*, 1936). Since that time, manganese has been shown to be an essential element for all species of domestic livestock and laboratory animals, as well as for humans (Underwood, 1977).

High concentrate diets based predominantly on cereal grains and soybean meal are likely to be deficient in the element for all species of poultry and for finishing sheep and cattle. Signs of manganese deficiency include impaired growth, skeletal abnormalities, abnormal male and female reproductive function, ataxia in newborns, impaired carbohydrate and lipid metabolism, and impaired mucopolysaccharide synthesis. The biochemical and physiological roles of manganese have been reviewed by Hurley and Keen (1987).

II. BIOAVAILABILITY STUDIES

A. *In Vitro* Estimates of Bioavailability

Solubility in various solutions that mimic physiological conditions has been used to predict bioavailability of inorganic manganese sources. Bandemer *et al.* (1940) reported that decreasing the particle size of rhodochrosite (a natural manganese carbonate ore) from that which was retained by a U.S. No. 100 (150 μm) screen to that which passed a No. 300 (~50 μm) screen increased the solubility of manganese

BIOAVAILABILITY OF NUTRIENTS FOR ANIMALS:
AMINO ACIDS, MINERALS, AND VITAMINS

in .1 N HCl from 26 to 82%, nonetheless, the ore failed to prevent perosis in chicks compared with a precipitated manganese carbonate. The precipitated carbonate prevented perosis when fed to chicks at 30 ppm manganese, but the rhodochrosite was ineffective at manganese concentrations up to 125 ppm. After testing the solubility of manganese oxide sources (.1 g source in 40 ml .1 N HCl, with or without 10 g diet), Schaible and Bandemer (1942) concluded that solubility of manganese supplements in acid could not be used to predict availability because some sources, such as oxides, were more soluble when the acid also contained a sample of diet. Several researchers have reported low correlations between manganese availability for chicks and solubility in HCl, but solubility in neutral ammonium citrate was a more reliable predictor of manganese availability (Watson *et al.*, 1970, 1971; Black *et al.*, 1984; Wong-Valle *et al.*, 1989a). Solubility of inorganic manganese sources in neutral ammonium citrate was also a better predictor of bioavailability for sheep compared with water, .4% HCl, or 2% citric acid (Wong-Valle *et al.*, 1989b).

B. *In Vivo* Estimates of Bioavailability

1. Disappearance from Nylon Bags

Disappearance of manganese after a 48-hr incubation in nylon bags in the rumen of sheep was studied with two legumes and two grasses cut at 6 or 12 weeks of regrowth (Kabaija and Smith, 1988). Percentage disappearance of manganese increased with age of regrowth for legumes, *Gliricidia sepium* (Jacq.) Steud (4.2 *vs* 11.5%) and *Leucaena leucocephala* (Lam.) de Wit cultivar 'Peru' (1.9 *vs* 5.6%) and decreased with age of regrowth for grasses *Panicum maximum*, Schum. var. S112, Nchisi (29 *vs* 15%) and *Cynodon nlemfuensis* var. nlemfluensis IB8 (46 *vs* 25%). The manganese content (DM basis) of the respective forages at 6 and 12 weeks of regrowth was 60 *vs* 57, 66 *vs* 59, 81 *vs* 96, and 45 *vs* 38 ppm.

2. Absorption

Absorption of manganese in adult animals is on the order of 3 or 4%, but can be greater in younger animals. Consequently, measurements of absorption and retention of supplemental manganese sources are generally difficult to make. Apparent balance experiments in ruminants and nonruminants failed to provide values which could be used to calculate relative bioavailability values for supplemental sources.

3. Growth and Perosis Index

The earliest studies conducted on manganese bioavailability used deficient natural or purified diets that were often supplemented with high levels of calcium and phosphorus and that resulted in poor growth and perosis in young chicks. Wilgus *et al.* (1937) tested various feedstuffs for their manganese content and ability to prevent perosis in chicks. Feeding 10% standard wheat middlings (25 ppm manganese) resulted in a 63% incidence of perosis with a 23% severity index. Feeding 20% red dog flour also provided 25 ppm manganese, but resulted in a 54% incidence and 13% average severity index. Thus, the manganese in red dog flour seemed to be more available. Similarly, 20% wheat bran contributed 40 ppm manganese and resulted in a 48% incidence and 19% severity of perosis, while 20% standard wheat middlings (38 ppm manganese) produced only a 10% incidence and 2% severity index.

Schaible *et al.* (1938) conducted extensive studies measuring growth and incidence of perosis in chicks fed a natural diet containing 11 ppm manganese to which numerous sources and concentrations of inorganic manganese were added. Feeding the basal diet resulted in an 81% incidence of bone deformities at 5 weeks of age. There was no perosis recorded when manganese sulfate dihydrate ($MnSO_4 \cdot 2H_2O$), manganous chloride tetrahydrate ($MnCl_2 \cdot 4H_2O$), manganese carbonate ($MnCO_3$), potassium permanganate ($KMnO_4$), manganese dioxide (MnO_2), manganese sesquioxide (manganite; Mn_2O_3), manganese hematite, manganomanganic oxide (hausmannite; Mn_3O_4), pyrolusite (MnO_2), or psilomelane were added at 30 ppm but perosis was observed at a 20 ppm supplemental level. Rhodonite ($MnSiO_3$) and rhodochrosite ($MnCO_3$) did not prevent perosis when added at concentrations ranging from 20 to 450 ppm manganese. Growth was also poorer in chicks fed these two sources. Based on body weight of birds, it required 120 ppm manganese from rhodonite and 150 ppm from rhodochrosite to equal 20 ppm manganese from sulfate, chloride, carbonate, dioxide, or potassium permanganate.

Gallup and Norris (1939) conducted similar experiments with chicks fed a natural diet containing 10 ppm manganese for 6 weeks. Chicks fed the basal diet had an average body weight of 383 g and an 81.5% incidence of perosis. Birds fed 50 ppm manganese as $MnCl_2 \cdot 4H_2O$, $MnSO_4 \cdot 4H_2O$, $KMnO_4$, $MnCO_3$, and MnO_2 had body weights ranging from 547 to 591 g and an incidence of perosis ranging from 0 to 13% (Table I).

Van der Hoorn *et al.* (1938) compared growth and mortality in chicks fed a purified corn starch-casein diet supplemented with manganese sulfate or manganese dioxide for 12 weeks. Similar dietary additions of the element from the two sources were not used, consequently a relative value could not be calculated, but sulfate seemed to be more available than dioxide. Bandemer *et al.* (1940) conducted studies with 1-day-old chicks in which incidence of perosis resulting from feeding manganese from rhodochrosite samples ranging in particle size from 250 to 50 μm was compared with that resulting from addition of precipitated manganese carbonate. No perosis was observed in chicks fed 30 ppm manganese as precipitated manganese carbonate. Incidence of perosis ranged from 23 to 79% in chicks fed rhodochrosite and was not related linearly to particle size or levels of dietary addition ranging from 30 to 125 ppm.

Green manganese monoxide (MnO; 61% Mn) and a commercial manganese sulfate (28% Mn) were also studied by Dutch researchers (van Stratum *et al.*, 1964). One-day-old chicks were fed a low manganese diet for 10 days then assigned to treatments for a 6-weeks study. A natural diet (reported to contain 4 ppm manganese) was supplemented with 12.5, 25, 50, or 100 ppm from each source. All birds fed supplemented diets had greater body weights than birds fed the control diet, but there were no differences due to manganese source or level (Table I). There was still considerable perosis, even in chicks fed the greater concentrations of manganese, which seems to indicate that manganese supplementation is critical during the first 10 days of life. Both compounds were effective to some extent in decreasing the incidence and severity of perosis.

The first experiments in which it was stated clearly that there was pen replication of dietary treatments, as well as replicate experiments, were those of Watson *et al.* (1970, 1971). Reagent grade manganese sulfate monohydrate ($MnSO_4 \cdot H_2O$) was used as a standard and added to a soy-isolate purified diet (4 ppm manganese) at 0, 10, 20, and 30 ppm manganese. Two commercial FG manganous oxides were fed to provide 10 and 20 ppm manganese. The first oxide (52% Mn) contained manganosite (MnO) and hausmannite and the second (36% Mn) contained hausmannite and quartz. After 28 days, there was no difference among chicks fed the diets containing manganese. Leg deformity was assigned scores ranging from 0 = normal leg to 4 = swelling and marked slipping of the tendon. Based on leg scores, the mixture of MnO-Mn_3O_4 was more available than that of Mn_3O_4.

In another series of experiments, Watson *et al.* (1971) compared RG manganese sulfate and RG manganese carbonate with four FG manganese oxides and one FG manganese carbonate which was mostly rhodochrosite. The basal soy-isolate diet (5 ppm manganese) was supplemented with 10, 20, 30, 60, and 120 ppm manganese as sulfate and 10 ppm as other sources. Growth was similar among treatments but the perosis index was very poor for birds fed rhodochrosite, and also poorer for birds fed dioxide and the compound containing bixbyite. These experiments confirm the older studies that indicated that rhodochrosite provided less available manganese than other inorganic sources. The measurements of growth and perosis in early experiments were not sufficiently sensitive to estimate differences among the more available supplemental manganese sources. The concentration of dietary manganese necessary to promote growth was less than that necessary to minimize the incidence of perosis.

4. Tissue Concentrations

Watson *et al.* (1970) suggested that a useful bioassay for manganese may be developed using manganese sulfate as the standard and bone manganese concentration as the response criterion. Since the report of Black *et al.* (1984), tissue manganese concentrations, especially bone, have been used by numerous researchers to determine bioavailability of supplemental sources in chicks and sheep given plethoric dietary concentrations of the element (Table I). Generally, this method has not been useful for manganese in feedstuffs because concentration of the element is too low in most grains and forages to make sufficient contribution to the diet for differences in bioavailability to be measurable.

5. Manganese Radioisotopes

Few studies have been conducted with radiolabeled manganese to determine bioavailability of supplemental sources. The first such study was that of Hennig *et al.* (1966). A single oral dose of ^{54}Mn as the sulfate, chloride or dioxide was administered to chicks that had been fed diets containing the respective sources for 5 weeks. After 18 hr, activity of ^{54}Mn absorbed from manganese chloride was greater than that from the other sources. In research with rats, there was no difference in ^{54}Mn content of tibia, liver, kidney, or muscle of animals fed a single dose of either ^{54}MnCl$_2$ or ^{54}MnCO$_3$ (King *et al.*, 1979). Anke *et al.* (1968) reported with laying hens that 3.8% of ^{52}Mn injected into the crop as MnCl$_2$ was recovered from the body (excluding digestive tract and contents), while 3.0% of a dose as oxide was recovered. They reported that ^{52}Mn as MnCl$_2$ was absorbed and excreted more rapidly than that from oxide, and that ^{52}Mn as MnSO$_4$ was intermediate.

Extrinsic labeling with ^{54}Mn was used to determine bioavailability of manganese from milk products for rat pups at 2 weeks of age. A single oral dose (.5 ml) of labeled diet was administered by intubation and rats were killed 24 hr later. Based on the percentage of total dose retained, manganese bioavailability values were 81, 89, 77, and 65 for human milk, cow's milk, cow's milk formula, and soy formula, respectively. Lonnerdal *et al.* (1985) reported that distribution of an extrinsic ^{54}Mn label in human milk was 71% whey, 11%casein, and 18% lipid . The distribution in cow's milk was 32% whey, 67% casein, and 1% lipid. In the human whey fraction, most manganese was bound to lactoferrin, but in cow's whey most manganese was complexed to ligands with molecular weights less than 200.

III. FACTORS INFLUENCING BIOAVAILABILITY

A. Dietary Factors

1. Antibiotics

Several factors have been shown to influence the absorption and, thus, bioavailability of manganese. Henry *et al.* (1986a) reported a 10% increase in kidney manganese and 12.8% increase in bone manganese concentrations of chicks fed 12 ppm virginiamycin compared with birds not given antibiotics. In later experiments, virginiamycin at 10 ppm increased bone and kidney manganese concentrations from 12 to 49% and lincomycin at 4 ppm resulted in increases from 8 to 24% over that of birds fed the control diet (Henry *et al.*, 1987a).

2. Dietary Ingredients

Researchers at the University of Illinois have shown that addition of feedstuffs containing phytate and fiber to a purified casein diet for chicks decreased manganese absorption efficiency from 2.40 to 1.71% (Halpin *et al.*, 1986b). As little as 1% wheat bran, 2.5% fish meal, and 5% of a corn-soybean meal mixture added to a casein-dextrose diet supplemented with 1000 ppm manganese was capable of decreasing tissue manganese concentrations (Halpin and Baker, 1986b, 1987). Replacing rapeseed meal for half of the soybean meal in a chick starter diet decreased availability of added inorganic manganese by 30% (Luo, 1989). Substituting 14.5% feathermeal for soybean meal for chicks fed from 8 to 330 ppm manganese did not influence the incidence of perosis or tissue concentrations of manganese (Settle *et al.*, 1969). Tissue manganese concentrations were lower in swine fed diets in which cerelose was substituted for corn (Plumlee *et al.*, 1956). King *et al.* (1979), however, reported lower stable manganese concentrations in rats fed a purified casein-dextrose diet compared with those fed a corn-skim milk diet, but this was not observed in calves fed similar diets (King *et al.*, 1980b). When lactose was added to a similar purified diet, stable manganese concentrations tended to be greater in rats, although tissue concentration of ^{54}Mn 3 days after a single oral dose of ^{54}Mn was lower in rats fed lactose (King *et al.*, 1980a).

3. Minerals

Calcium and/or phosphorus have been shown to decrease manganese utilization in poultry (Wilgus *et al.*, 1936; Schaible and Bandemer, 1942) and dairy calves

(Hawkins *et al.*, 1955). Baker *et al.* (1986), Wedekind and Baker (1990b), and Scheideler (1991) reported no effect of high calcium on manganese utilization in chicks, but Smith and Kabaija (1985) reported that excess calcium from oyster shells decreased manganese utilization. Subsequent work confirmed that 1% excess calcium from oyster shells, but not from FG limestone, decreased manganese deposition in bone (Wedekind and Baker, 1990a,b). Also excess phosphorus, regardless of source, was found far more antagonistic to manganese utilization than excess calcium. In turnover studies (Wedekind *et al.*, 1991a) and isotope dilution experiments (Wedekind et al., 1991b), the antagonistic effect of excess phosphorus on manganese utilization was confirmed to exist at the gut level.

Thomson and Valberg (1972) reported that manganese uptake by the mucosal cells of duodenal loops from iron-deficient rats and transfer from the mucosa to the body was inhibited by cobalt and iron. In further research with rats on manganese interactions, iron supplementation at 140 ppm decreased absorption of ^{54}Mn compared with the basal diet containing 10 ppm iron (Johnson and Korynta, 1992). Work with chicks, however, showed no antagonism of manganese by excessive dietary intakes of either cobalt or iron (Halpin, 1985; Baker and Halpin, 1991). Bile, tibia, and kidney manganese concentrations were greater in chicks fed diets supplemented with 250 ppm cobalt than in birds fed a control diet (Brown and Southern, 1985). Addition of 5 ppm copper to a manganese-deficient diet for rats decreased manganese absorption and accelerated its turnover (Johnson and Korynta, 1992).

B. Animal Factors

Early work with poultry suggested that New Hampshire birds required more dietary manganese to prevent perosis than White Leghorns, but no indication of feed intake for the two breeds was provided (Gallup and Norris, 1939). Manganese absorption in rats increased during the last trimester of pregnancy, decreased shortly before parturition, and then increased again during lactation (Kirchgessner *et al.*, 1981). Black *et al.* (1985a) reported that liver manganese concentrations were similar in chicks killed at 1, 2, or 3 weeks, but that kidney, pancreas, plasma, and muscle concentrations decreased, while that of bone increased during the same time intervals. The decrease may have been due to dilution from increasing growth of the tissues. There is, however, some storage of excess manganese in bone which can serve as a reserve during periods of manganese deficit (Baker *et al.*, 1986).

IV. SUMMARY

Manganese bioavailability research has been conducted primarily with supplemental forms of the element which have potential use with domestic animals (Table II). Most of this research has been done with poultry for which there is a critical supplemental need for the element. A limited amount of research has been conducted with sheep. Earlier studies with poultry, in which growth or leg deformities were measured, were generally not sufficiently sensitive to detect differences in bioavailability among supplemental sources. One exception to this was rhodochrosite, an ore in which manganese exists as a natural manganese carbonate. The manganese in this ore is extremely low in bioavailability.

Much of the research since about 1980 to estimate manganese bioavailability of supplemental sources has measured tissue deposition of the element and frequently has involved dietary levels well in excess of the animals requirement. Manganese sulfate has almost always served as the standard in these studies. Based on current research, manganese chloride is equal in bioavailability and manganese methionine and manganese proteinate are utilized to a somewhat greater degree than is manganese sulfate. Manganese oxide, precipitated manganese carbonate, and manganese dioxide, in descending order, are less well utilized than is manganese sulfate for both poultry and sheep. Data with sheep are limited but results suggest that bioavailability of manganese sources is similar for both poultry and sheep.

Table I. Bioavailability of manganese sources for animals[a]

Source	RV	Standard	Response criterion	Meth cal	Type diet	Added level, ppm	Reference
Chickens							
Hausmannite (Mn_3O_4)	97	$MnSO_4 \cdot 2H_2O$	Growth	MR	N-11 ppm	20, 30	Schaible et al. (1938)
Manganese carbonate ($MnCO_3$)	101	$MnSO_4 \cdot 2H_2O$	Growth	MR	N-11 ppm	20, 30	Schaible et al. (1938)
$MnCO_3$ RG	94	$MnSO_4 \cdot 4H_2O$ RG	Growth	MR	N-10 ppm	50	Gallop and Norris (1939)
$MnCO_3$ RG (45% Mn)	93	$MnSO_4 \cdot H_2O$ RG	Bone Mn	MR	P-5 ppm	10	Watson et al. (1971)
$MnCO_3$ RG	98	$MnSO_4 \cdot H_2O$ RG	Pl [b]	MR	P-5 ppm	10	Watson et al. (1971)
$MnCO_3$ RG	77	$MnSO_4 \cdot H_2O$ RG	Bile Mn	SR	N-168 ppm	3000, 4000	Southern and Baker (1983)
$MnCO_3$ RG (47% Mn)	32	$MnSO_4 \cdot H_2O$	Bone Mn	SR	N-116ppm	1000, 2000, 4000	Black et al. (1984)
$MnCO_3$ RG	36	$MnSO_4 \cdot H_2O$	Liv Mn	SR	N-116ppm	1000, 2000, 4000	Black et al. (1984)
Manganese dioxide (MnO_2)	106	$MnSO_4 \cdot 2H_2O$	Growth	MR	N-11 ppm	20, 30	Schaible et al. (1938)
MnO_2 RG	95	$MnSO_4 \cdot 4H_2O$ RG	Growth	MR	N-10 ppm	50	Gallop and Norris (1939)
MnO_2 RG	29	$MnSO_4 \cdot H_2O$ RG	Bile Mn	SR	N-168 ppm	3000, 4000	Southern and Baker (1983)
MnO_2 RG (56.5% Mn)	34	MnO RG (77% Mn)	Bone Mn	SR	N-102 ppm	1000, 2000, 3000	Henry et al. (1987)
MnO_2 RG	46	MnO RG	Kid Mn	SR	N-102 ppm	1000, 2000, 3000	Henry et al. (1987)
MnO_2 FG (36% Mn)	37	MnO RG	Bone Mn	SR	N-102 ppm	1000, 2000, 3000	Henry et al. (1987)
MnO_2 FG	44	MnO RG	Kid Mn	SR	N-102 ppm	1000, 2000, 3000	Henry et al. (1987)

Table I. (continued)

Source	RV	Standard	Response criterion	Meth cal	Type diet	Added level, ppm	Reference
Manganese hematite	104	MnSO$_4$·2H$_2$O	Growth	MR	N-11 ppm	20, 30	Schaible et al. (1938)
Manganese-methionine	111	MnO	Bone Mn	MR	N	30, 60, 200	Scheideler (1991)
Manganese-methionine	101	MnO	Liv Mn	MR	N	30, 60, 200	Scheideler (1991)
Manganese-methionine (16% Mn)	130	MnO FG	Bone Mn	SR	P-1.4 ppm	13-1875	Fly et al. (1989)
Manganese-methionine	174	MnO FG	Bone Mn	SR	P + 10% N	13-175	Fly et al. (1989)
Manganese-methionine (16% Mn)	108	MnSO$_4$·H$_2$O	Bone Mn	SR	N-93 ppm	700, 1400, 2100	Henry et al. (1989)
Manganese-methionine	132	MnSO$_4$·H$_2$O	Kid Mn	SR	N-93 ppm	700, 1400, 2100	Henry et al. (1989)
Manganese monoxide RG (MnO) (76.7% Mn)	60	MnSO$_4$·H$_2$O	Bone Mn	SR	N-116 ppm	1000, 2000, 4000	Black et al. (1984)
MnO RG	77	MnSO$_4$·H$_2$O	Liv Mn	SR	N-116 ppm	1000, 2000, 4000	Black et al. (1984)
MnO RG	81	MnSO$_4$·H$_2$O	Bone Mn	SR	N-35 ppm	40, 80, 120	Henry et al. (1986)
MnO RG	46	MnSO$_4$·H$_2$O	Kid Mn	SR	N-35 ppm	40, 80, 120	Henry et al. (1986)
MnO RG	70	MnSO$_4$·H$_2$O	Liv Mn	SR	N-35 ppm	40, 80, 120	Henry et al. (1986)
MnO RG (73.0% Mn)	82	MnSO$_4$·H$_2$O	Bone Mn	SR	N-82 ppm	1000, 2000, 3000	Wong-Valle et al. (1989)
MnO RG	86	MnSO$_4$·H$_2$O	Kid Mn	SR	N-82 ppm	1000, 2000, 3000	Wong-Valle et al. (1989)
MnO RG (77.2% Mn)	96	MnSO$_4$·H$_2$O	Bone Mn	SR	N-93 ppm	700, 1400, 2100	Henry et al. (1989)
MnO RG	86	MnSO$_4$·H$_2$O	Kid Mn	SR	N-93 ppm	700, 1400, 2100	Henry et al. (1989)

248

Material	Value	Standard	Tissue	MR/SR	ppm	Levels	Reference
MnO FG (14.8% Mn)	82	$MnSO_4 \cdot H_2O$ RG	Bone Mn	MR	P-5 ppm	10	Watson et al. (1971)
MnO FG	73	$MnSO_4 \cdot H_2O$ RG	Pl[b]	MR	P-5 ppm	10	Watson et al. (1971)
MnO FG (61.0% Mn)	95	$MnSO_4 \cdot H_2O$ RG	Bone Mn	MR	P-5 ppm	10	Watson et al. (1971)
MnO FG	83	$MnSO_4 \cdot H_2O$ RG	Pl[b]	MR	P-5 ppm	10	Watson et al. (1971)
MnO FG (64.2% Mn)	93	$MnSO_4 \cdot H_2O$	Bone Mn	SR	N-82 ppm	1000, 2000, 3000	Wong-Valle et al. (1989)
MnO FG	68	$MnSO_4 \cdot H_2O$	Kid Mn	SR	N-82 ppm	1000, 2000, 3000	Wong-Valle et al. (1989)
MnO FG (45.6% Mn)	75	$MnSO_4 \cdot H_2O$	Bone Mn	SR	N-82 ppm	1000, 2000, 3000	Wong-Valle et al. (1989)
MnO FG	52	$MnSO_4 \cdot H_2O$	Kid Mn	SR	N-82 ppm	1000, 2000, 3000	Wong-Valle et al. (1989)
MnO FG (46% Mn)	83	$MnSO_4 \cdot H_2O$ RG	Bone Mn	SR	N-22 ppm	50, 100, 150, 200	Luo (1989)
MnO FG	83	$MnSO_4 \cdot H_2O$ RG	Toe Mn	SR	N-22 ppm	50, 100, 150, 200	Luo (1989)
Manganese oxide FG ($MnO + Mn_3O_4$)	103	$MnSO_4 \cdot H_2O$ RG	Bone Mn	MR	P-4 ppm	10, 20	Watson et al. (1970)
Manganese oxide FG ($MnO + Mn_3O_4$)	98	$MnSO_4 \cdot H_2O$ RG	Pl[b]	MR	P-4 ppm	10, 20	Watson et al. (1970)
Manganese oxide FG ($MnO + Mn_3O_4$)	70	$MnSO_4 \cdot H_2O$	Bone Mn	SR	N-82 ppm	1000, 2000, 3000	Wong-Valle et al. (1989)
Manganese oxide FG ($MnO + Mn_3O_4$)	53	$MnSO_4 \cdot H_2O$	Kid Mn	SR	N-82 ppm	1000, 2000, 3000	Wong-Valle et al. (1989)
Manganese oxide FG (Mn_2SiO_4) (58.0% Mn)	96	$MnSO_4 \cdot H_2O$ RG	Bone Mn	MR	P-5 ppm	10	Watson et al. (1971)

Table I. (continued)

Source	RV	Standard	Response criterion	Meth cal	Type diet	Added level, ppm	Reference
Manganese oxide FG ($MnO + Mn_2SiO_4$)	78	$MnSO_4 \cdot H_2O$ RG	PI[b]	MR	P-5 ppm	10	Watson et al. (1971)
Manganese oxide FG [$(Fe, Mn)_2O_3 + Mn_3O_4 + MnO + MnO_2$] (57.3% Mn)	86	$MnSO_4 \cdot H_2O$ RG	Bone Mn	MR	P-5 ppm	10	Watson et al. (1971)
Manganese oxide FG [$(Fe, Mn)_2O_3 + Mn_3O_4 + MnO + MnO_2$]	60	$MnSO_4 \cdot H_2O$ RG	PI[b]	MR	P-5 ppm	10	Watson et al. (1971)
Manganese-proteinate (10% Mn)	86	$MnSO_4 \cdot H_2O$	Bone Mn	MR	P-1.4 ppm	1000	Baker and Halpin (1987)
Manganese-proteinate	118	$MnSO_4 \cdot H_2O$	Bile Mn	MR	P-1.4 ppm	1000	Baker and Halpin (1987)
Manganese-proteinate	114	$MnSO_4 \cdot H_2O$	Bone Mn	MR	P + 10% wheat bran	1000	Baker and Halpin (1987)
Manganese-proteinate	122	$MnSO_4 \cdot H_2O$	Bile Mn	MR	P + 10% wheat bran	1000	Baker and Halpin (1987)
Manganite Mn_2O_3	93	$MnSO_4 \cdot 2H_2O$	Growth	MR	N-11 ppm	20, 30	Schaible et al. (1938)
Manganomanganic oxide FG (Mn_3O_4) (36.1% Mn)	101	$MnSO_4 \cdot H_2O$ RG	Bone Mn	MR	P-4 ppm	10, 20	Watson et al. (1970)
Mn_3O_4 FG	88	$MnSO_4 \cdot H_2O$ RG	PI[b]	MR	P-4 ppm	10, 20	Watson et al. (1970)
Manganous chloride ($MnCl_2 \cdot 4H_2O$)	101	$MnSO_4 \cdot 2H_2O$	Growth	MR	N-11 ppm	20, 30	Schaible et al. (1938)
$MnCl_2 \cdot 4H_2O$ RG	93	$MnSO_4 \cdot 4H_2O$ RG	Growth	MR	N-10 ppm	50	Gallop and Norris (1939)
$MnCl_2 \cdot 4H_2O$ RG	102	$MnSO_4 \cdot H_2O$ RG	Bile Mn	SR	N-168 ppm	3000, 4000	Southern and Baker (1983)

Potassium permanganate (KMnO$_4$)	109	MnSO$_4$·2H$_2$O	Growth	MR	N-11 ppm	20, 30	Schaible et al. (1938)
KMnO$_4$ RG	94	MnSO$_4$·4H$_2$O RG	Growth	MR	N-10 ppm	50	Gallop and Norris (1939)
Psilomelane	87	MnSO$_4$·2H$_2$O	Growth	MR	N-11 ppm	20, 30	Schaible et al. (1938)
Pyrolusite (MnO$_2$)	81	MnSO$_4$·2H$_2$O	Growth	MR	N-11 ppm	20, 30	Schaible et al. (1938)
Rhodochrosite (MnCO$_3$)	64	MnSO$_4$·2H$_2$O	Growth	MR	N-11 ppm	20, 30	Schaible et al. (1938)
Rhodochrosite FG (24% Mn)	80	MnSO$_4$·H$_2$O RG	Bone Mn	MR	P-5 ppm	10	Watson et al. (1971)
Rhodochrosite FG	39	MnSO$_4$·H$_2$O RG	Pl[b]	MR	P-5 ppm	10	Watson et al. (1971)
Rhodonite (MnSiO$_3$)	85	MnSO$_4$·2H$_2$O	Growth	MR	N-11 ppm	20, 30	Schaible et al. (1938)

Sheep

Manganese carbonate RG (MnCO$_3$)	93	MnO FG	Bone Mn	SR	N-31 ppm	500-8000	Black et al. (1985)
MnCO$_3$ RG	46	MnO FG	Kid Mn	SR	N-31 ppm	500-8000	Black et al. (1985)
MnCO$_3$ RG	23	MnSO$_4$·H$_2$O	Bone Mn	SR	N-38 ppm	1500, 3000	Wong-Valle et al. (1989)
MnCO$_3$ RG	20	MnSO$_4$·H$_2$O	Kid Mn	SR	N-38 ppm	1500, 3000	Wong-Valle et al. (1989)
MnCO$_3$ RG	40	MnSO$_4$·H$_2$O	Liv Mn	SR	N-38 ppm	1500, 3000	Wong-Valle et al. (1989)
Manganese dioxide RG (MnO$_2$)	39	MnSO$_4$·H$_2$O	Bone Mn	SR	N-38 ppm	1500, 3000	Wong-Valle et al. (1989)
MnO$_2$ RG	25	MnSO$_4$·H$_2$O	Kid Mn	SR	N-38 ppm	1500, 3000	Wong-Valle et al. (1989)
MnO$_2$ RG	35	MnSO$_4$·H$_2$O	Liv Mn	SR	N-38 ppm	1500, 3000	Wong-Valle et al. (1989)
Manganese-methionine (15.7% Mn)	157	MnSO$_4$·H$_2$O RG	Bone Mn	SR	N-34 ppm	900, 1800, 2700	Henry et al. (1992)
Manganese-methionine	102	MnSO$_4$·H$_2$O RG	Kid Mn	SR	N-34 ppm	900, 1800, 2700	Henry et al. (1992)

Table I. (continued)

Source	RV	Standard	Response criterion	Meth cal	Type diet	Added level, ppm	Reference
Manganese-methionine	132	$MnSO_4 \cdot H_2O$ RG	Bone Mn	SR	N-32 ppm	900 - 2700	Henry et al. (1992)
MnO RG (73.0% Mn)	57	$MnSO_4 \cdot H_2O$	Bone Mn	SR	N-38 ppm	1500, 3000	Wong Valle et al. (1989)
MnO RG	55	$MnSO_4 \cdot H_2O$	Kid Mn	SR	N-38 ppm	1500, 3000	Wong Valle et al. (1989)
MnO RG	61	$MnSO_4 \cdot H_2O$	Liv Mn	SR	N-38 ppm	1500, 3000	Wong Valle et al. (1989)
MnO FG (64.2% Mn)	70	$MnSO_4 \cdot H_2O$ RG	Bone Mn	SR	N-32 ppm	900 - 2700	Henry et al. (1992)
MnO FG	75	$MnSO_4 \cdot H_2O$ RG	Kid Mn	SR	N-32 ppm	900 - 2700	Henry et al. (1992)
MnO FG (58.1% Mn)	50	$MnSO_4 \cdot H_2O$ RG	Bone Mn	SR	N-32 ppm	900 - 2700	Henry et al. (1992)
MnO FG	59	$MnSO_4 \cdot H_2O$ RG	Kid Mn	SR	N-32 ppm	900 - 2700	Henry et al. (1992)
Rats							
$MnCO_3$	98	$^{54}MnCl_2$	^{54}Mn Upt	MR	N	SOD	King et al. (1979)
$MnCO_3$	107	$^{54}MnCl_2$	^{54}Mn Upt	MR	P <1 ppm	SOD	King et al. (1979)
Milk, cow's	89[c]	-	^{54}Mn Ret	-	-	SOD	Keen et al. (1986)
Milk, cow's, formula	77[c]	-	^{54}Mn Ret	-	-	SOD	Keen et al. (1986)
Milk, human	81[c]	-	^{54}Mn Ret	-	-	SOD	Keen et al. (1986)
Soy, formula	64[c]	-	^{54}Mn Ret	-	-	SOD	Keen et al. (1986)

[a] Abbreviations can be found in Appendix I. Chemical formula for a compound given only if provided by the author. RG indicates reagent grade, FG indicates feed grade.

[b] Authors provided a leg score of 0 = normal to 4 = swelling and marked slipping of tendon. Relative value calculated as: (Leg score test source -4)/ (Leg score standard source - 4) x 100.

[c] Value represents retention for treatment not relative value.

Table II. Relative bioavailability of supplemental manganese sources[a]

	Species	
Source	Poultry	Sheep
Manganese sulfate	100	100
Manganese carbonate, ppt.	55 (2)	30 (1)
Manganese dioxide	30 (3)	35 (1)
Manganese methionine	120 (1)	125 (2)
Manganese monoxide	75 (8)	60 (3)
Manganese proteinate	110 (2)	-
Manganous chloride	100 (1)	-

[a]Average values rounded to nearest "5" and expressed relative to response obtained with manganese sulfate. Number of studies or samples involved indicated within parentheses.

REFERENCES

Anke, M., H. Jeroch, M. Diettrich and G. Hoffmann. 1968. Incorporation and distribution of ^{52}Mn from different Mn salts in laying hens. *Nutr. Abstr. Rev.* **38**:148 [Abstract].

Baker, D. H. and K. M. Halpin. 1987. Efficacy of a manganese-protein chelate compound compared with that of manganese sulfate for chicks. *Poult. Sci.* **66**:1561.

Baker, D. H. and K. M. Halpin. 1991. Manganese and iron interrelationship in the chick. *Poult. Sci.* **70**:146.

Baker, D. H., K .M. Halpin, D. E. Laurin and L. L. Southern. 1986. Manganese for poultry: A review. *In* "Proceedings of theArkansas Nutrition Conference," pp. 1-6. University of Arkansas, Fayetteville.

Baker, D. H. and K. J. Wedekind. 1988. Manganese utilization in chicks as affected by excess calcium and phosphorus ingestion. *In* "Proceedings of the Maryland Nutrition Conference," pp. 29-34. University of Maryland, College Park, MD.

Bandemer, S. L., J. A. Davidson and P. J. Schaible. 1940. Availability of manganese in natural and precipitated manganese carbonate. *Poult. Sci.* **19**:116.

Black, J. R., C. B. Ammerman, P. R. Henry and R. D. Miles. 1984. Biological availability of manganese sources and effects of high dietary manganese on tissue mineral composition of broiler-type chicks. *Poult. Sci.* **63**:1999.

Black, J. R., C. B. Ammerman, P. R. Henry and R. D. Miles. 1985a. Effect of dietary manganese and age on tissue trace mineral composition of broiler-type chicks as a bioassay of manganese sources. *Poult. Sci.* **64**:688.

Black, J. R., C. B. Ammerman and P. R. Henry. 1985b. Effects of high dietary manganese as manganese oxide or manganese carbonate in sheep. *J. Anim. Sci.* **60**:861.

Brown, D. R. and L. L. Southern. 1985. Effect of *Eimeria acervulina* infection in chicks fed excess dietary cobalt and/or manganese. *J. Nutr.* **115**:347.

Combs, G. F., Jr. and S. B. Combs. 1986. " The Role of Selenium in Nutrition." Academic Press, New York.

Fly, A. D., O. A. Izquierdo, K. R. Lowry and D. H. Baker. 1989. Manganese bioavailability in a Mn-methionine chelate. *Nutr. Res.* **9**:901.

Gallup, W. D., and L. C. Norris. 1939. The amount of manganese required to prevent perosis in the chick. *Poult. Sci.* **18**:76.

Halpin, K. M. 1985. Factors affecting manganese homeostasis in the chick. Ph.D. Dissertation, University of Illinois, Urbana.

Halpin, K. M. and D. H. Baker. 1986a. Long-term effects of corn, soybean meal, wheat bran and fish meal on manganese utilization in the chick. *Poult. Sci.* **65**:1371.

Halpin, K. M. and D. H. Baker. 1986b. Manganese utilization in the chick: Effects of corn, soybean meal, fish meal, wheat bran and rice bran on tissue uptake of manganese. *Poult. Sci.* **65**:995.

Halpin, K. M. and D. H. Baker. 1987. Mechanism of the tissue manganese-lowering effect of corn, soybean meal, fish meal, wheat bran and rice bran. *Poult. Sci.* **66**:332.

Halpin, K. M., D. G. Chausow and D. H. Baker. 1986. Efficiency of manganese absorption in chicks fed corn-soy and casein diets. *J. Nutr.* **116**:1747.

Hawkins, G. E., Jr., G. H. Wise, G. Matrone, R. K. Waugh and W. L. Lott. 1955. Manganese in the nutrition of young dairy cattle fed different levels of calcium and phosphorus. *J. Dairy Sci.* **38**:536.

Hennig, A., M. Anke, H. Jeroch, H. Kaltwasser, W. Wiedner, G. Hoffman, M. Diettrich and H. Marcy. 1966. Utilization of manganese from different compounds and its distribution in the body of the chicken. *Archiv. Tierernaehr* **16**:545 [Biological Abstract 75618, 1967].

Henry, P. R., C. B. Ammerman and R. D. Miles. 1986a. Influence of virginiamycin and dietary manganese on performance, manganese utilization, and intestinal tract weight of broilers. *Poult. Sci.* **65**:321.

Henry, P. R., C. B. Ammerman and R. D. Miles. 1986b. Bioavailability of manganese sulfate and manganese monoxide in chicks as measured by tissue uptake of manganese from conventional dietary levels. *Poult. Sci.* **65**:983.

Henry, P. R., C. B. Ammerman, D. R. Campbell and R. D. Miles. 1987a. Effect of antibiotics on tissue trace mineral concentration and intestinal tract weight of broiler chicks. *Poult. Sci.* **66**:104.

Henry, P. R., C. B. Ammerman and R. D. Miles. 1987b. Bioavailability of manganese monoxide and manganese dioxide for broiler chicks. *Nutr. Rep. Int.* **36**:425.

Henry, P. R., C. B. Ammerman and R. D. Miles. 1989. Relative bioavailability of manganese in a manganese-methionine complex for broiler chicks. *Poult. Sci.* **68**:107.

Hurley, L. S. and C. L. Keen. 1987. Manganese. *In* "Trace Elements in Human and Animal Nutrition" (W. Mertz, Ed.), Vol. 1, p. 185. Academic Press, New York.

Johnson, P. E. and E. D. Korynta. 1992. Effects of copper, iron, and ascorbic acid on manganese availability to rats. *Proc. Soc. Exp. Biol. Med.* **199**:470.

Kabaija, E. and O. B. Smith. 1988. The effect of age of regrowth on content and release of manganese, iron, zinc and copper from four tropical forages incubated in sacco in rumen of sheep. *Anim. Feed Sci. Technol.* **20**:171.

Keen, C. L., J. G. Bell and B. Lonnerdal. 1986. The effect of age on manganese uptake and retention from milk and infant formulas in rats. *J. Nutr.* **116**:395.

Kemmerer, A. R., C. A. Elvehjem and E. B. Hart. 1931. Studies on the relation of manganese to the nutrition of the mouse. *J. Biol. Chem.* **92**:623.

King, B. D., J. W. Lassiter, M. W. Neathery, W. J. Miller and R. P. Gentry. 1979. Manganese retention in rats fed different diets and chemical forms of manganese. *J. Anim. Sci.* **49**:1235.

King, B. D., J. W. Lassiter, M. W. Neathery, W. J. Miller and R. P. Gentry. 1980a. Effect of lactose, copper and iron on manganese retention and tissue distribution in rats fed dextrose-casein diets. *J. Anim. Sci.* **50**:452.

King, B. D., J. W. Lassiter, M. W. Neathery, W. J. Miller and R. P. Gentry. 1980b. Effect of a purified or corn-skim milk diet on retention and tissue distribution of manganese-54 in calves. *J. Dairy Sci.* **3**:86.

Kirchegessner, M., F. J. Schwarz and D. A. Roth-Maier. 1981. Changes in the metabolism (retention, absorption, excretion) of copper, zinc, and manganese in gravidity and lactation. *In* "Trace Element Metabolism in Man and Animals-4" (J. McC. Howell, J. M. Gawthorne, and C. L. White, Eds.), p. 85. Australian Academy of Science, Canberra, Australia.

Lonnerdal, B., C. L. Keen and L. S. Hurley. 1985. Manganese binding proteins in human and cow's milk. *Am. J. Clin. Nutr.* **41**:550.

Luo, Xugang. 1989. Studies on the optimal manganese level and its bioavailability in a practical diet for broiler chicks. Ph.D. Dissertation. Chinese Acad. of Agric. Sci., Beijing, PRC.

Orent, E. R. and E. V. McCollum. 1931. Effects of deprivation of manganese in the rat. *J. Biol. Chem.* **92**:651.

Plumlee, M. P., D. M. Thrasher, W. M. Beeson, F. N. Andrews and H. E. Parker. 1956. The effects of a manganese deficiency upon the growth, development, and reproduction of swine. *J. Anim. Sci.* **15**:352.

Schaible, P. J. and S. L. Bandemer. 1942. The effect of mineral supplements on the availability of manganese. *Poult. Sci.* **21**:8.

Schaible, P. J., S. L. Bandemer and J. A. Davidson. 1938. The manganese content of feedstuffs and its relation to poultry nutrition. *Michigan Agric. Exp. Sta. Tech. Bull.* **159**.

Scheideler, S. E. 1991. Interaction of dietary calcium, manganese and manganese source (Mn oxide or Mn methionine chelate) on chick performance and manganese utilization. *Biol. Trace Element Res.* **29**:217.

Settle, E. A., F. R. Mraz, C. R. Douglas and J. K. Bletner. 1969. Effect of diet and manganese level on growth, perosis and [54]Mn uptake in chicks. *J. Nutr.* **97**:141.

Southern, L. L. and D. H. Baker. 1983a. *Eimeria acervulina* infection in chicks fed deficient or excess levels of manganese. *J. Nutr.* **113**:172.

Southern, L. L. and D. H. Baker. 1983b. Excess manganese ingestion in the chick. *Poult. Sci.* **62**:642.

Smith, O. B. and E. Kabaija. 1985. Effect of high dietary calcium and wide calcium-phosphorus ratios in broiler chicks. *Poult. Sci.* **64**:1713.

Thomson, A. B. R. and L. S. Valberg. 1972. Intestinal uptake of iron, cobalt, and manganese in the iron-deficient rat. *Am. J. Physiol.* **223**:1327.

Underwood, E. J. 1977. "Trace Elements in Human and Animal Nutrition," 4th ed. Academic Press, New York.

van der Hoorn, R., H. D. Branion and W. R. Graham, Jr. 1938. Studies in the nutrition of the chick. III. A maintenance factor present in wheat germ and the effect of the addition of a small amount of manganese dioxide to the diet. *Poult. Sci.* **17**:185.

Watson, L. T. 1968. Utilization of manganese from inorganic sources by ruminants. M.S. Thesis. University of Florida, Gainesville, FL.

Watson, L. T., C. B. Ammerman, S. M. Miller and R. H. Harms. 1970. Biological assay of inorganic manganese for chicks. *Poult. Sci.* **49**:1548.

Watson, L. T., C. B. Ammerman, S. M. Miller and R. H. Harms. 1971. Biological availability to chicks of manganese form different inorganic sources. *Poult. Sci.* **50**:1693.

Wedekind, K. J. and D. H. Baker. 1990a. Manganese utilization in chicks as affected by excess calcium and phosphorus ingestion. *Poult. Sci.* **69**:977.

Wedekind, K. J. and D. H. Baker. 1990b. Effect of varying calcium and phosphorus level on manganese utilization. *Poult. Sci.* **69**:1156.

Wilgus, H. S., Jr., L. C. Norris and G. F. Heuser. 1936. The role of certain inorganic elements in the cause and prevention of perosis. *Science* **84**:252.

Wilgus, H. S., Jr., L. C. Norris and G. F. Heuser. 1937. The role of manganese and certain other trace elements in the prevention of perosis. *J. Nutr.* **14**:155.

Wong-Valle, J., C. B. Ammerman, P. R. Henry, P. V. Rao and R. D. Miles. 1989a. Bioavailability of manganese from feed grade manganese oxides for broiler chicks. *Poult. Sci.* **68**:1368.

Wong-Valle, J., P. R. Henry, C. B. Ammerman and P. V. Rao. 1989b. Estimation of the relative bioavailability of manganese sources for sheep. *J. Anim. Sci.* **67**:2409.

12

PHOSPHORUS BIOAVAILABILITY

Joseph H. Soares, Jr.

Department of Animal Sciences
University of Maryland
College Park, Maryland

I. INTRODUCTION

About 80% of the body's phosphorus is in the skeleton. The remaining 20% is contained in nucleotides, such as ATP, nucleic acids, phospholipids, and a host of other phosphorylated compounds needed for metabolism. Most of the latter fraction is intracellular and does not readily cross cell membranes. Inorganic phosphate is also found in the cell and is important in acid-base balance. Phosphorus is a constituent of some lipid pools in the body and in this capacity plays several important roles, among which is its function in formation of the cell membrane bilayer. The phosphorus requirement of growing animals varies in proportion to the calcium requirement. There is evidence that an optimal dietary calcium to phosphorus ratio is approximately 2.2:1 (NRC, 1994). As an animal matures, the relative rate of bone growth slows such that the dietary phosphorus requirement declines. Practical diets require phosphorus supplementation in order to support optimal growth rate of animals. This is especially true for nonruminants when diets consist primarily of cereal grains which contain siginificant amounts of phosphorus in the phytin form.

A phosphorus deficiency will cause a reduction in bone mineralization and thereby impair calcium metabolism, which can lead to rickets. In the laying hen, phosphorus deficiency reduced the rate of egg production, probably through a reduction in feed intake (Bar and Hurwitz, 1984). Other factors, such as intake level, age of the animal, levels of dietary mineral antagonists, e.g., aluminum (Nelson *et al.*, 1968, Ammerman *et al.*, 1984), magnesium (Chester-Jones *et al.*, 1989) and intestinal pH (ruminants), all greatly influence phosphorus availability.

The variation in phosphorus availability from plant products and commercially used phosphorus supplements can be quite large. Since phosphorus is an expensive ingredient in the diet, and feedstuff phosphorus availability can be quite variable, knowledge of phosphorus bioavailability is critical to efficient animal production.

While it is quite common to supplement animal feeds with inorganic phosphates, such as dicalcium phosphate (anhydrous or hydrated), monocalcium phosphate, or defluorinated rock phosphate, in commercial feed manufacturing, it is important to note that these commercial products can contain other phosphate forms. Baker (1989) described the typical commercial products, dicalcium phosphate ($CaHPO_4$) and monocalcium phosphate [$Ca(H_2PO_4)_2·H_2O$] as containing mixtures of $CaHPO_4$, $Ca(H_2PO_4)_2·H_2O$, and $CaHPO_4·2H_2O$. Monocalcium phosphate generally contains 13% $CaHPO_4$, and 61% $Ca(H_2PO_4)_2·H_2O$, with the remainder small amounts of other phosphates and minerals. Commercial dicalcium phosphate generally contains about 14% $Ca(H_2PO_4)_2·H_2O$, 35% $CaHPO_4·2H_2O$, and 26% $CaHPO_4$. The data suggest at least eight different compounds contribute to the phosphorus content of commercial phosphates.

II. BIOAVAILABILITY STUDIES

A. Nonruminant Studies

Scheidler and Sell (1987) conducted research in which laying hens were fed varying concentrations of calcium, phosphorus, and phytate phosphorus in an attempt to determine the effect of phytase and calcium on phosphorus balance. Using a chromic oxide marker, the availability of dietary phosphorus could be calculated from the difference between fecal and dietary phosphorus, in much the same way as metabolizable energy is determined. Similarly, Hurwitz *et al.* (1978) determined the effect of calcium intake on phosphorus availability using this type of methodology, with the exception that ^{91}Y was used as the nonabsorbed marker in place of chromic oxide. Both studies demonstrated that high dietary calcium concentrations reduced the availability of phosphorus in the diet.

Cromwell (1992) described a slope ratio procedure using a low-phosphorus diet containing 65% dextrose and 30% soybean meal to evaluate phosphorus availability of feedstuffs fed to pigs. Diets were fed to pigs initially weighing 11 to 13 kg for a 5- to 6-week test period after which animals were terminated and third and fourth metacarpal and metatarsal bones were removed for breaking strength measurements. The results from a variety of feedstuffs (Table I) suggest that this procedure is a useful method for determining relative phosphorus bioavailability.

There have been several phosphorus standards used to measure phosphorus bioavailability. β-Tricalcium phosphate has been used as a standard in some studies

(Nelson and Peeler, 1961; Nelson and Walker, 1964), although others have used reagent grade dicalcium phosphate (Motzok, 1968; Potchanakorn and Potter, 1987), monocalcium phosphate (Damron and Harms, 1968; Yoshida and Hoshii, 1979; Apke *et al.*, 1987), monosodium or potassium phosphate (Waldroup *et al.*, 1965; Nelson *et al.*, 1968; Soares *et al.*, 1977; Corley *et al.*, 1980; Harrold *et al.*, 1983; Witt and Owens, 1983), or phosphoric acid (Pensack, 1974; Wozniak *et al.*, 1977). Determination of phosphorus availability is prone to the same problems experienced with other mineral elements. Since "availability" of phosphorus is a relative term and is dependent on the standard reference material used, it is entirely possible to obtain results that are greater than 100%. To minimize confusion and the generation of >100% results, investigators should strive to utilize the most efficiently utilized phosphate source possible for a standard. For example, reagent grade $CaHPO_4$, NaH_2PO_4, or KH_2PO_4 [preferably hydrated forms, since several reports have shown these to be most available (Supplee ,1962; Rucker *et al.*, 1968)] generally are most efficiently utilized and result in less variability in phosphorus availability from one source to another. Consequently, the availability of phosphorus from a number of commercial dicalcium phosphates has been determined to be greater than 100% when reagent grade monocalcium phosphate was used as a standard (Yoshida and Hoshii, 1979); from 89 to110% when compared to a typical commercial mono/dicalcium phosphate blend (Waibel *et al.*, 1984), and as low as 62% when reagent grade monosodium phosphate was the standard (Witt and Owens, 1983). The large variation in phosphorus availability determined for commercial dicalcium phosphates clearly suggests that relative phosphorus bioavailability varies markedly not only among commercial sources but also with reference standards used and experimental conditions.

Inorganic phosphorus sources were tested in a multilaboratory survey (Ellis *et al.*, 1945) where weanling rats were fed a semipurified basal diet limiting in calcium and phosphorus. These workers observed that when bone meal was used as the standard and growth and bone breaking strength were the criteria measured, six defluorinated phosphates ranged from 50 to 80% in available phosphorus. Calcium metaphosphate and β-pyrophosphate tested in this study were poorly available (Table I). Similar results were reported by Shrewsbury and Vestal (1945) using both growing swine and rats. In a series of comparative assays, Gobble *et al.* (1955) fed growing swine diets containing either dicalcium phosphate or soft rock phosphate. Their results suggested that phosphorus in soft rock phosphate was as available to growing swine as that in dicalcium phosphate. Plumlee *et al.* (1958), however, observed that weanling pigs were able to utilize only 72% of the phosphorus in soft rock phosphate compared with that in dicalcium phosphate. Harmon *et al.* (1970) confirmed these results. Phosphoric acid, bone meal, and monocalcium phosphate had phosphorus availability equal to dicalcium phosphate, while Curacao Island phosphate was of intermediate availability.

The phosphorus in defluorinated phosphate has been observed to be as available to the pig as dicalcium phosphate and monosodium phosphate but less available than bone char (Newman and Elliott, 1976; King, 1980; Clawson and Southern, 1985). Raw rock phosphate and triple superphosphate contain phosphorus that is generally less available than that in defluorinated phosphates (Table II).

B. Ruminant Studies

1. *In Vitro* Estimates of Bioavailability

Many studies have been conducted to determine the relative availability of different phosphorus sources for ruminants. Several investigators, including Hill *et al*. (1945) and Anderson *et a*l. (1956), have used cellulose digestion during *in vitro* ruminal fermentation cultures as a means of assessing phosphorus availability. In these studies, sodium metaphosphate, soft rock phosphate, sodium pyrophosphate, and Curacao Island phosphate proved to have significantly lower available phosphorus than dicalcium phosphate or bone meal. In contrast, Hall *et al.* (1961) found no differences in phosphorus availability among these sources and sodium or potassium orthophosphate. The latter results were also obtained in *in vivo* studies with sheep by Tillman and Brethour (1958b).

2. *In Vivo* Estimates of Bioavailability

Ammerman *et al.* (1957) fed wethers and steers a low phosphorus hay and concentrate diet in a series of absorption trials and showed that calcium metaphosphate (50%) and calcium pyrophosphate (0%) provided less available phosphorus than monocalcium phosphate monohydrate (100%). These authors also reported that Curacao Island phosphate was 90% the value of dicalcium phosphate, while soft rock phosphate and defluorinated phosphate had about 50% available phosphorus. Wise *et al.* (1961) reported similar results for soft rock phosphate, but Curacao Island phosphate and defluorinated phosphate were similar to the dicalcium phosphate control. Tillman and Brethour (1958a,b), Richardson *et al.* (1961), O'Donovan *et al.* (1965), and Webb *et al.* (1975) reported that phosphoric acid, defluorinated phosphate, Mexican rock phosphate, and sodium tripolyphosphate were as effective as dicalcium phosphate when fed to steers. Similarly, bone meal, ammonium phosphate, and superphosphate have been reported to have a phosphorus availability equal to dicalcium phosphate (Newlander *et al.*, 1936; Hodgson *et al.*, 1948; Long *et al.*, 1957; Johnson and McClure, 1961; Gutierrez *et al.*, 1983).

Comparisons of phosphorus availability in hays and grasses fed to ruminants have generally been reported as true or apparent absorption which may or may not be reported in comparison to a standard phosphorus source. Early studies by Turner *et al.* (1927) using lactating cows showed that phosphorus in chopped alfalfa and clover hays had apparent absorption values of 24 and 20%, respectively. Lofgreen and Kleiber (1953), on the other hand, reported that true phosphorus absorption in chopped alfalfa hay was 91% as determined by isotopic dilution in wether lambs. Although these studies are not directly comparable, they suggest an effect of age on phosphorus and/or calcium absorption. In contrast, Gutierrez *et al.* (1984) reported that calves tested in balance studies could only absorb (apparent) 26% of the phosphorus in a bermudagrass forage while Ellis and Tillman (1961) reported that growing wethers had a true phosphorus absorption of 26% from wheat bran.

III. FACTORS INFLUENCING BIOAVAILABILITY

A. Dietary Factors

1. Calcium

The ratio of calcium to phosphorus has a large influence on the availability of phosphorus from a feedstuff. The optimal dietary calcium concentration increased for each level of supplemental phosphorus according to studies by Damron and Harms (1968) and Fritz (1969). Motzok (1968) determined the bioavailability of phosphorus from a soft rock phosphate source when calcium to phosphorus ratios were optimal (between 2.2 and 2.5:1) and found that the bioavailability of phosphorus was 63 to 71%. Using ^{91}Y, a nonabsorbable marker, Hurwitz *et al.* (1978) demonstrated that apparent phosphorus absorption decreased progressively in young turkeys as the daily calcium intake exceeded 440 mg/bird. The inhibitory effect of excess calcium on phosphorus absorption was linear.

More recent reports (Starnes *et al.*, 1984; Kirk *et al.*, 1985; Kegley *et al.*, 1991) have indicated that calcium ionphores, such as monensin, lasalocid, and lysocellin, improved dietary phosphorus availability when added to ruminant diets.

2. Phytic Acid

A major consideration with respect to phosphorus availability is the proportion of phosphorus in plant products in the form of phytic acid. Phytic acid is myoinositol hexaphosphoric acid but it can also exist in the various partially phosphorylated forms. Phytic acid is synthesized by plants and phosphorus in this form is generally poorly utilized by monogastric animals. Plant seeds usually contain varying amounts of this compound in the aleuron/pericarp portions of cereals such as barley, rice, and wheat (Nelson et al., 1968; O'Dell et al., 1972). Corn grain has significant amounts of phytic acid in the germ. Some phytins are complexed very little with protein (e.g., corn germ, soybean meal), whereas others (e.g., sesame meal) are more insoluble protein-linked compounds heavily complexed with cations (deBoland et al., 1975; O'Dell and deBoland, 1976). The most common cations complexed to phytic acid are calcium, magnesium, and potassium, with lesser amounts of manganese, iron, and zinc (O'Dell et al. 1972; Ogawa et al. 1975; Morris and Ellis, 1976; Erdman, 1979). Although ionic calcium forms one of the weaker complexes with phytic acid, calcium phytates are among the most common insoluble phytate complexes in the digestive tract because calcium is present in most diets in the highest quantity among all the mineral elements. Phytic acid must be degraded by phytase to produce phosphoric acid and/or orthophosphate salts for animals to obtain phosphorus efficacy.

Naturally occurring phytases are known to occur in certain plants, fungi, yeasts and possibly other microbes. There is a question as to whether warm-blooded animals have any naturally occurring phytases that can effectively hydrolyze phytic acid (Nelson, 1980). It has been reported by Reid et al. (1947) and Nelson et al. (1976) that naturally occurring phytic acid is hydrolyzed in the rumen to produce available phosphate. Poultry and swine, however, are not able to utilize this complex (Nelson, 1980, 1989).

While there have been reports of intestinal phytases in chicks (Davies and Motzok, 1972) and rats (Pileggi et al., 1955; Roberts and Yudkin, 1960), Nelson (1980) has concluded after extensive review of the literature that monogastric animals cannot hydrolyze this compound. This is further supported by other studies (Waldroup et al., 1967; Nelson, 1976) that increasing age (chick vs laying hen) has no practical effect on phytate hydrolysis and phosphorus utilization. Swine, however, are reported to utilize up to 40% of the total phosphorus from some plant sources (Bayley et al., 1975; Besecker et al., 1967; Calvert et al., 1978; Cromwell, 1979). It is not clear whether this utilizable fraction contains phytate phosphorus. Some plant products contain phytase which enables partial hydrolysis of phytic acid to inositol and inorganic phosphate and thereby also releasing cations such as calcium (Ballam et al., 1985). Wheat bran is especially rich in this enzyme (Anderson, 1915; Boutwell, 1917). In recent years there has been a growing amount of data presented suggesting that phosphorus availability in feedstuffs of plant origin may vary considerably. Studies by Bayley and Thompson (1969), Tonroy et al. (1973), Calvert et al. (1978), Cromwell (1980, 1992), and others have shown low phosphorus availability in pelleted corn, corn grain, grain sorghum, and hominy feed ranging from about 9 to 25%. Krieger et al. (1941), Taylor (1965), Pointillart et al.

(1984, 1987), and Pointillart (1991) showed distinct differences in phytate phosphorus utilization among cereal grains. Wheat, rye, and triticale phytate complexes are more labile because phytases are present in these grains. Corn, oats, and most other cereal grains are significantly poorer sources of available phosphorus to nonruminants, partly because of the lack of plant phytases in these grains.

Nelson (1976) and Simons et al. (1990) have shown that additions of a crude microbial phytase increased phosphorus availability (up to 92% hydrolysis of phytate molecules) from plant sources fed to monogastric animals. Other recent studies using broilers and pigs (Simons et al., 1990; Cromwell et al., 1993; Edwards, 1993; Lei et al., 1994; Mroz et al., 1994), rats (Shah et al., 1990) and trout (Ketola et al., 1993) indicated that dietary addition of phytase increased the utilization of phytate phosphorus by monogastric animals. This increase in the availability of phytate phosphorus has resulted in significantly increased weight gain and bone mineralization (Pointillart, 1991). The use of phytase in diets for monogastric animals has three distinct advantages: (1) the incorporation of phytase will reduce the amount of nonphytate phosphorus (including that supplied by animal protein) needed and, as a result, will reduce feed costs; (2) the phytate complex binds other elements, such as zinc, calcium, and magnesium, and therefore, when phytase is added, other essential minerals are released as well; and (3) improved utilization of dietary phosphorus will decrease the environmental burden of the element.

Ketaren et al. (1993a,b) assessed phosphorus bioavailability for pigs and rats. They observed that bone variables, such as bone bending moment, were a more reliable criteria to measure phosphorus bioavailability than bone ash. Furthermore, phosphorus bioavailability determined with rats appeared to overestimate that for pigs. Soybean phosphorus bioavailability (as determined by apparent absorption) was optimal when 1000 units of aspergillis phytase were added per kilogram of diet. Bioavailabity of soybean meal varied depending on the bone characteristic measured but was always improved by phytase addition.

While phytate phosphorus is poorly utilized by nonruminants, the majority of data published studying utilization of phytate phosphorus by ruminants suggested complete hydrolysis of the molecule in the rumen by microorganisms (Reid et al., 1947; Raun et al., 1956; Tillman and Brethour, 1958c; Barth and Hansard, 1962; Clark et al., 1986). These reports indicated that phytate phosphorus was equal to, or only slightly less available than, inorganic phosphorus for ruminants.

It was suggested by NRC (1988) ,based upon research from Cromwell's laboratory (Cromwell et al., 1993), that phosphorus in corn was 12% available to swine and that in soybean meal was 25% available. Thus, a value of 15% is generally assumed for the bioavailability of phosphorus in corn-soybean meal diets for swine. It was concluded that poultry (NRC, 1994) can usually absorb 30 to 40% of total plant phosphorus. The remaining phosphorus in the plant is present as phytate and is poorly utilized by poultry.

IV. SUMMARY

Phosphorus bioavailability has been studied more extensively than most other elements since it is a much more costly item in commercial diet formulations. It appeared that bone ash percentage or bone breaking measurements were the most appropriate dependent variables for assays. The range of bioavailability is great and the following is a brief summary of relative phosphorus bioavailability in feedstuffs when compared with highly available inorganic phosphate such as hydrated dicalcium phosphate or monosodium phosphate. The phosphorus in many inorganic sources and in meat and fish meals is highly available to monogastric animals. In general, and when compared to several highly available standard phosphate sources, sources and feedstuffs with greater than 95% phosphorus bioavailability include ammonium polyphosphate, dicalcium phosphate, fish meal, meat meal, meat and bone meal, monocalcium phosphate, potassium phosphate monobasic, monosodium phosphate, phosphoric acid, poultry by-product meal, tricalcium phosphate, and urea phosphate. Somewhat less available (85 to 90%) but still considered to be highly available are bone meal, blood meal, Curacao Island phosphate, defluorinated phosphate, and dried poultry waste. It should be noted that defluorinated phosphates have significantly greater phosphorus bioavailability today than in the past due to improved processing methods. Low phosphorus bioavailability for nonruminant animals has been reported for alfalfa meal, cereal grains, and most plant-source oilseed meals. Essentially all the phosphorus in metaphosphates and pyrophosphates is unavailable to nonruminant animals. Ruminants, however, appear to be able to utilize these sources to a greater degree. Microbial phytase added to diets for poultry, pigs and fish appears to increase phytate phosphorus bioavailability by as much as 50%. Recent evidence also shows that adding 5 to 10 µg of dihydroxycholecalciferol to a vitamin D-adequate diet increased phytate phosphorus bioavailability by 50%.

Table I. Bioavailability of phosphorus sources for animals[a]

Source	RV	Standard	Response criterion	Meth cal	Type diet	Added level, %	Reference
Chickens							
Alfalfa meal	77	Monosodium phosphate	Bone ash	SR	N	.15-4	Huang and Allee (1981)
Ammonium polyphosphate	118	Tricalcium phosphate	Bone ash	SC	N	.1-3	Jensen and Edwards (1980)
Barley	50	Monosodium phosphate, hyd	Bone ash	SC	SP	.27-44	Hayes et al. (1979)
Barley	35	Potassium phosphate, MB	Bone ash	SR	P	NG	Harrold et al. (1979)
Bone ash	89	β-Tricalcium phosphate	Bone ash	SC	SP	.25-35	Gillis et al. (1954)
Bone char	84	β-Tricalcium phosphate	Bone ash	SC	SP	.25-35	Gillis et al. (1954)
Bone meal, steamed	94	Potassium phosphate, MB	Bone ash	MR	SP	.40-80	Gillis et al. (1948)
Bone meal, steamed	93	β-Tricalcium phosphate	Bone ash	SC	SP	.25-35	Gillis et al. (1954)
Calcium phosphate, vitreous	45	β-Tricalcium phosphate	Bone ash	SC	SP	.40-80	Gillis et al. (1954)
Calcium-aluminum-iron phosphate	15	Monobasic phosphate	BBS	SR	N	.14-35	Huyghebaert et al. (1980)
Corn	33	Monosodium phosphate	Bone ash	SR	N	.15-4	Huang and Allee (1981)

Table I. (continued)

Source	RV	Standard	Response criterion	Meth cal	Type diet	Added level, %	Reference
Corn	12	Monosodium phosphate, hyd	Bone ash	SC	SP	.27-.44	Hayes et al. (1979)
Cottonseed meal	42	Monosodium phosphate	Bone ash	SR	N	.15-.4	Huang and Allee (1981)
Curacao Island phosphate	87	Tricalcium phosphate	Bone ash	SC	SP	.25-.35	Gillis et al. (1984)
Curacao Island phosphate	100	Dicalcium phosphate	Egg qual	MR	N	.50-.80	Damron et al. (1974)
Defluorinated phosphate FG	79	Tricalcium phosphate	Bone ash	MR	N	NG	Bird et al. (1945)
Defluorinated phosphate FG	83	Potassium phosphate, MB	Bone ash	MR	SP	.40-.80	Gillis et al. (1948)
Defluorinated phosphate FG	92	β-Tricalcium phosphate	Bone ash	SC	SP	.25-.35	Gillis et al. (1954)
Defluorinated phosphate FG	95	Dicalcium phosphate RG	Bone ash	SR	SP	.45-.58	Hurwitz (1964)
Defluorinated phosphate FG	84	Monosodium phosphate, hyd	Bone ash	SC	N	.15-.25	Dilworth and Day (1964)
Defluorinated phosphate FG	86	Monosodium phosphate	Bone ash	SC	N	NG	Day et al. (1973)
Defluorinated phosphate FG	69	Phosphoric acid	Bone ash	SC	SP	.2	Pensack (1974)
Defluorinated phosphate FG	96	Potassium phosphate, MB	Bone ash & growth	SC	N	.51-.71	Soares et al. (1977)

Defluorinated phosphate FG	111	Tricalcium phosphate	Bone ash	SC	N	.1-.3	Jensen and Edwards (1980)
Defluorinated phosphate FG	96	Disodium phosphate	BBS	SR	N	.14-.35	Huyghebaert et al. (1980)
Defluorinated phosphate FG	91	Dicalcium phosphate, dihyd	Bone ash	SR	N	.05-.15	Garlich and Mian (1986)
Defluorinated phosphate FG (.05-2.0 mm)	94	Monosodium phosphate, monohyd	Bone ash & BBS	SR	N	.05-.40	Burnell et al. (1990)
Defluorinated super-phosphate	30	Tricalcium phosphate	Bone ash	MR	N	NG	Bird et al. (1945)
Dicalcium phosphate RG	94	Potassium phosphate, MB	Bone ash	MR	SP	.40-.80	Gillis et al. (1948)
Dicalcium phosphate FG	95	β-Tricalcium phosphate	Bone ash	SC	SP	.25-.35	Gillis et al. (1954)
Dicalcium phosphate RG	98	β-Tricalcium phosphate	Bone ash	SC	SP	.25-.35	Gillis et al. (1954)
Dicalcium phosphate, hyd (USP)	99	Monocalcium phosphate, hyd	Bone ash	MR	N	.20-.35	Gillis et al. (1962)
Dicalcium phosphate, anhydrous RG	95	Monocalcium phosphate, hyd	Bone ash	MR	P	.20-.35	Gillis et al. (1962)
Dicalcium phosphate FG	100	Monosodium phosphate, hyd	Bone ash & growth	SC	SP	.05-.15	Waldroup et al. (1965)
Dicalcium phosphate	85	Monosodium phosphate	Bone ash	SC	N	NG	Day et al. (1973)
Dicalcium phosphate FG	81	Phosphoric acid	Bone ash	SC	SP	.2	Pensack (1974)
Dicalcium phosphate, anhydrous RG	86	Disodium phosphate	BBS	SR	N	.14-.35	Huyghebaert et al. (1980)

267

Table I. (continued)

Source	RV	Standard	Response criterion	Meth cal	Type diet	Added level, %	Reference
Dicalcium phosphate, hyd	96	Disodium phosphate	BBS	SR	N	.14-.35	Huyghebaert et al. (1980)
Dicalcium phosphate	123	Tricalcium phosphate	Bone ash	SC	N	.1-.3	Jensen and Edwards (1980)
Dicalcium phosphate	95	Monosodium phosphate	Bone ash	SR	N	.15-.40	Huang and Allee (1981)
Dicalcium phosphate	87	Potassium phosphate, MB	BBS	SR	P	.05-.10	Chung and Baker (1990)
Fish meal	88[b]	-	Ret	-	SP	NG	Huque and Jensen (1985)
Fish meal	102	Monosodium phosphate, hyd	Bone ash	SC	SP	.05-.15	Waldroup et al. (1965)
Fish meal, Menhaden	100	Dicalcium phosphate	Bone ash	SC	SP	.1-.7	Spandorf and Leong (1965)
Fused rock phosphate	88	Potassium phosphate, MB	Bone ash	MR	SP	.40-.80	Gillis et al. (1948)
Meat and bone meal	90	Disodium phosphate	BBS	SR	N	.14-.35	Huyghebaert et al. (1965)
Meat and bone meal	102	Monosodium phosphate, hyd	Bone ash	SC	SP	.05-.15	Waldroup et al. (1965)
Meat and bone meal	99	Monosodium phosphate	Bone ash	SR	N	.15-.40	Huang and Allee (1981)
Metaphosphate, calcium	0	Potassium phosphate, MB	Bone ash	MR	SP	.40-.80	Gillis et al. (1948)
Metaphosphate, calcium	30	Potassium phosphate, MB	Bone ash	MR	SP	.40-.80	Gillis et al. (1948)

Metaphosphate, calcium, vitreous	68	Potassium phosphate, MB	Bone ash	MR	SP	.40-.80	Gillis et al. (1948)
Metaphosphate, calcium, vitreous	45	β-Tricalcium phosphate	Bone ash	SC	SP	.25-.35	Gillis et al. (1954)
Metaphosphate, calcium	0	β-Tricalcium phosphate	Bone ash	SC	SP	.25-.35	Gillis et al. (1954)
Metaphosphate, potassium	0	Potassium phosphate, MB	Bone ash	MR	SP	.40-.80	Gillis et al. (1948)
Metaphosphate, potassium	0	β-Tricalcium phosphate	Bone ash	SC	SP	.25-.35	Gillis et al. (1954)
Metaphosphate, sodium	0	β-Tricalcium phosphate	Bone ash	SC	SP	.25-.35	Gillis et al. (1954)
Metaphosphate, sodium, vitreous	69	Potassium phosphate, MB	Bone ash	MR	SP	.40-.80	Gillis et al. (1948)
Monocalcium phosphate monohyd	99	Potassium phosphate, MB	Bone ash	MR	SP	.25-.35	Gillis et al. (1948)
Monosodium phosphate	101	Tricalcium phosphate	Bone ash	SC	SP	.25-.35	Gillis et al. (1954)
Monosodium phosphate	96	Disodium phosphate	BBS	SR	N	.14-.35	Huyghebaert et al. (1980)
Oats	37	Monosodium phosphate	Bone ash	SR	N	.15-.40	Huang and Allee (1981)
Oat bran	60	Potassium phosphate, MB	Bone ash	SR	SP	150-428 mg/day	Hahn et al. (1990)
Oat flour	42	Potassium phosphate, MB	Bone ash	SR	SP	150-428 mg/day	Hahn et al. (1990)
Phosphate slag	54	β-Tricalcium phosphate	Bone ash	MR	N	NG	Bird et al. (1945)

Table I. (continued)

Source	RV	Standard	Response criterion	Meth cal	Type diet	Added level, %	Reference
Phosphoric acid	128	Dicalcium phosphate FG	Bone ash & growth	SC	N	.028-.111	Summers et al. (1959)
Phytate, calcium	0	Potassium phosphate, MB	Bone ash	MR	SP	.40-.80	Gillis et al. (1948)
Phytin	60	Monosodium phosphate	Ret	-	N	NG	Temperton and Cassidy (1964)
Phytin	60	Dicalcium phosphate	Bone ash & growth	SC	N	.05-.15	Waldroup et al. (1964)
Phytin, cereal	0	Inorganic phosphate	Bone ash	MR	N	.46-.86	McGinnis et al. (1944)
Phytin, corn	0	Disodium phosphate	Bone ash	SC	SP	.66-.83	Lowe et al. (1939)
Phytin, oat	20[b]	Potassium phosphate, MB	Ret	-	SP	NG	Ashton et al. (1960)
Potassium phosphate, MB	109	β-Tricalcium phosphate	Bone ash	SC	SP	.25-.35	Gillis et al. (1954)
Poultry by-product	101	Monosodium phosphate, hyd RG	Bone ash & growth	SC	SP	.05-.15	Waldroup et al. (1965)
Poultry waste, dried	90	Dicalcium phosphate, dihyd	Bone ash	SR	N	.2-.6	Steinsberger et al. (1987)
Pyrophosphate, calcium	1	β-Tricalcium phosphate	Bone ash	MR	N	NG	Bird et al. (1945)
Pyrophosphate, calcium	0	Potassium phosphate, MB	Bone ash	MR	SP	.40-.80	Gillis et al. (1948)

Pyrophosphate, calcium	0	Potassium phosphate, MB	Bone ash	MR	SP	.40-.80	Gillis et al. (1948)
Pyrophosphate, calcium β	0	Potassium phosphate, MB	Bone ash	MR	SP	.40-.80	Gillis et al. (1948)
Pyrophosphates, calcium β	0	β-Tricalcium phosphate	Bone ash	SC	SP	.25-.35	Gillis et al. (1954)
Pyrophosphate, sodium, decahyd	57	Tricalcium phosphate	Bone ash	SC	SP	.25-.35	Gillis et al. (1954)
RNA, yeast	67	Potassium phosphate, MB	Bone ash	SR	P	.1-.72	Burns and Baker (1976)
Rock phosphate, calcined	86	Potassium phosphate, MB	Bone ash	MR	SP	.40-.80	Gillis et al. (1948)
Single cell protein	98	Potassium phosphate, MB	Bone ash	SR	P	.1-.72	Burns and Baker (1976)
Soft rock phosphate	25	β-Tricalcium phosphate	Bone ash	SC	N	.25-.35	Gillis et al. (1954)
Soft rock phosphate	47	Dicalcium phosphate FG	Bone ash & growth	SC	N	.028-.111	Summers et al. (1959)
Soft rock phosphate	38	Monosodium phosphate, hyd	Bone ash	SC	N	.15-.25	Dilworth and Day (1964)
Soft rock phosphate	76	Dicalcium phosphate RG	Bone ash	SR	SP	.45-.48	Hurwitz (1964)
Sorghum	36	Monosodium phosphate	Bone ash	SR	N	.15-.4	Huang and Allee (1981)
Soybeans	50	Dicalcium phosphate, dihyd	Bone ash	SC	N	.28-.51	Nelson et al. (1968)
Soybean meal (44%)	40	Monosodium phosphate	Bone ash	SR	N	.15-.40	Huang and Allee (1981)

Table I. (continued)

Source	RV	Standard	Response criterion	Meth cal	Type diet	Added level, %	Reference
Sunflower meal	23	Potassium phosphate, MB	Bone ash	SC	P	.07-.48	Harrold et al. (1983)
Tricalcium phosphate, RG	90	Monocalcium phosphate, hyd	Bone ash	MR	P	.20-.35	Gillis et al. (1962)
Tricalcium phosphate	92	Dicalcium phosphate	Bone ash	SR	SP	.45-.58	Hurwitz (1964)
Tricalcium phosphate, β	95	Potassium phosphate, MB	Bone ash	MR	SP	.40-.80	Gillis et al. (1948)
Tricalcium phosphate, β	80	Monocalcium phosphate, hyd	Bone ash	MR	P	.20-.35	Gillis et al. (1962)
Tricalcium phosphate, β	93	Monosodium phosphate, hyd	Bone ash	SC	N	.15-.25	Dilworth and Day (1964)
Urea phosphate	100	Dicalcium phosphate	Egg prod	SC	N	.24-.40	Kiiskinen (1983)
Venezuelan rock phosphate	67	Dicalcium & monocalcium phosphate	Bone ash	SR	N	.24-.36	Osorio and Jensen (1986)
Wheat	38	Monosodium phosphate	Bone ash	SR	N	.15-.40	Huang and Allee (1981)
Wheat, hard	43	Monosodium phosphate, hyd	Bone ash	SC	SP	.15-.25	Dilworth and Day (1964)
Wheat, soft	58	Monosodium phosphate, hyd	Bone ash	SC	SP	.27-.44	Hayes et al. (1979)
Wheat bran	23	Potassium phosphate, MB	Bone ash	SR	P	451-885 mg	Corley et al. (1980)

Turkeys

Ammonium polyphosphate	95	Monosodium phosphate	Bone ash & growth	SC	N	.14-.36	Sullivan (1967)
Corn	80	Monosodium phosphate	Bone ash & growth	SC	N	.38-.80	Andrews et al. (1972)
Cottonseed meal	80	Monosodium phosphate	Bone ash & growth	SC	N	.38-.80	Andrews et al. (1972)
Curacao Island phosphate	55	Monocalcium phosphate	Bone ash	SC	N	.09-.27	Potter (1988)
Defluorinated phosphate	93	Monosodium phosphate, monohyd	Bone ash	SC	N	.20-.35	Sullivan (1966)
Defluorinated phosphate	89	Monosodium phosphate	Bone ash & growth	SC	N	.14-.36	Sullivan (1967)
Defluorinated phosphate	70	Monocalcium phosphate, monohyd	Bone ash	SR	N	.44-.65	Waibel et al. (1984)
Defluorinated phosphate	70	Dicalcium phosphate, dihyd	Bone ash	SC	N	.09-.45	Potchanakorn and Potter (1987)
Defluorinated phosphate	79	Monocalcium phosphate	Bone ash	SC	N	.09-.27	Potter (1988)
Diammonium phosphate	97	Monosodium phosphate, monohyd	Bone ash	SC	N	.15-.36	Struwe et al. (1976)
Dicalcium phosphate, anhyd RG	80	Monocalcium phosphate, hyd	Bone ash	MR	P	.20-.35	Gillis et al. (1962)
Dicalcium phosphate	96	Monosodium phosphate, monohyd	Bone ash	SC	N	.20-.35	Sullivan (1966)

273

Table I. (continued)

Source	RV	Standard	Response criterion	Meth cal	Type diet	Added level, %	Reference
Dicalcium phosphate FG	80	Dicalcium phosphate, dihyd	Bone ash	SR	N	NG	Griffith et al. (1966)
Dicalcium phosphate FG	97	Monosodium phosphate	Bone ash & growth	SC	N	.14-.36	Sullivan (1967)
Dicalcium phosphate	88	Monocalcium phosphate monohyd	Bone ash	SR	N	.44-.65	Waibel et al. (1984)
Dicalcium phosphate, anhyd	71	Dicalcium phosphate, monohyd	Bone ash	SR	N	NG	Grimbergen et al. (1985)
Dicalcium phosphate FG	81	Dicalcium phosphate, dihyd	Bone ash	SC	N	.09-.45	Potchanakorn and Potter (1987)
Dicalcium phosphate	100	Monocalcium phosphate	Bone ash	SC	N	.09-.27	Potter (1988)
Phosphate/soda FG	100	Monosodium phosphate, monohyd	Bone ash	SC	N	.20-.35	Sullivan (1966)
Monocalcium phosphate FG	93	Dicalcium phosphate, dihyd	Bone ash	SC	N	.09-.45	Potchanakorn and Potter (1987)
Monocalcium phosphate, hyd	100	Monosodium phosphate, monohyd	Bone ash	SC	N	.20-.35	Sullivan (1966)
Mono/dicalcium phosphate	94	Monocalcium phosphate, monohyd	Bone ash	SR	N	.44-.65	Waibel et al. (1984)

Ingredient	Value	Phosphorus source	Standard		Basis	Range	Reference
Poultry litter ash	80	Dicalcium phosphate, dihyd	Bone ash	SR	N	.44-.65	Apke et al. (1984)
Raw rock phosphate	91	Monosodium phosphate, monohyd	Bone ash	SC	N	.20-.35	Sullivan (1966)
Superphosphate	95	Monosodium phosphate, monohyd	Bone ash	SC	N	.15-.36	Struwe et al. (1976)
Tricalcium phosphate	100	Monosodium phosphate, monohyd	Bone ash	SC	N	.20-.35	Sullivan (1966)

Swine

Ingredient	Value	Phosphorus source	Standard		Basis	Range	Reference
Alfalfa meal	42	Monosodium phosphate	Bone ash	SR	N	.15-.4	Huang and Allee (1981)
Barley	28[b]	-	App abs	-	N	.3-.5	Calvert et al. (1978)
Barley	30	Monosodium phosphate, hyd	Bone ash & BBS	SR	N	.30-.45	Cromwell (1992)
Blood meal	92	Monosodium phosphate, hyd	BBS	SR	SP	.05-.2	Burnell et al. (1989c)
Bone char	48[b]	-	App abs	-	N	.36-.56	King (1980)
Bone meal, steamed	82	Monosodium phosphate, hyd	Bone ash & BBS	SR	N	.30-.45	Cromwell (1992)
Canola meal	21	Monosodium phosphate, hyd	Bone ash & BBS	SR	N	.30-.45	Cromwell (1992)
Chloroapatite	45[b]	-	App abs	-	N	[c]	Ammerman et al. (1963)
Corn	15[b]	-	App abs	-	N	.30-.65	Pierce et al. (1977)
Corn	12[b]	-	App abs	-	N	.3-.5	Calvert et al. (1978)

Table I. (continued)

Source	RV	Standard	Response criterion	Meth cal	Type diet	Added level, %	Reference
Corn	29[b]	-	App abs	-	N	.33-.36	Pointillart et al. (1984)
Corn	48[b]	-	App abs	-	N	NG	Pointillart et al. (1987)
Corn	29	Monosodium phosphate	Bone ash	SR	N	.15-.4	Huang and Allee (1981)
Corn	14	Monosodium phosphate, hyd	Bone ash & BBS	SR	N	.30-.45	Cromwell (1992)
Corn, high moisture	44	Potassium phosphate, dibasic	Alk phos	SC	SP	.26-.44	Boyd et al. (1983)
Corn, high moisture	41	Potassium phosphate, dibasic	BBS	SC	SP	.26-.44	Boyd et al. (1983)
Corn, high moisture	53	Monosodium phosphate, hyd	Bone ash & BBS	SR	N	.30-.45	Cromwell (1992)
Corn, pelleted	12	Monosodium phosphate, hyd	Bone ash & BBS	SR	N	.30-.45	Cromwell (1992)
Corn gluten feed	59	Monosodium phosphate, hyd	BBS	SR	SP	.1-.2	Burnell et al. (1989b)
Cottonseed meal	1	Monosodium phosphate, hyd	Bone ash & BBS	SR	N	.30-.45	Cromwell (1992)
Cottonseed meal	42	Monosodium phosphate	Bone ash	SR	N	.15-.4	Huang and Allee (1981)
Curacao Island phosphate	48[b]	-	App abs	-	N	.31-.52	Harmon et al. (1974)
Curacao Island phosphate	93	Dicalcium phosphate	Bone ash	SC	N	.275-.300	Plumlee et al. (1958)
Defluorinated phosphate	41[b]	-	App abs	-	N	c	Ammerman et al. (1963)

Defluorinated phosphate	87	Monosodium phosphate, hyd	Bone ash & BBS	SR	N	.30-.45	Cromwell (1992)
Defluorinated phosphate	73[b]	-	True abs	-	SP	.61-.75	Partridge (1981)
Defluorinated phosphate	100	Dicalcium phosphate	Growth & Bone ash	MR	N	.30-.61	Hagemeier et al. (1981)
Dicalcium phosphate	35[b]	-	App abs	-	N	[c]	Ammerman et al. (1963)
Dicalcium phosphate	62[b]	-	App abs	-	SP	.3-.5	Tonroy (1973)
Dicalcium phosphate	48[b]	-	App abs	-	N	.31-.52	Harmon et al. (1974)
Dicalcium phosphate	71[b]	-	App abs	-	N	.31-.52	Harmon et al. (1974)
Dicalcium phosphate	65[b]	-	App abs	-	N	.3-.5	Calvert et al. (1978)
Dicalcium phosphate	32[b]	-	App abs	-	N	.36-.56	King (1980)
Dicalcium phosphate	70[b]	-	Trua abs	-	SP	.61-.75	Partridge (1981)
Dicalcium phosphate	95	Monosodium phosphate	Bone ash	SR	N	.15-.4	Huang and Allee (1981)
Dicalcium phosphate, anhyd.	89	Dicalcium phosphate, hyd	Bone ash	SR	N	NG	Grimbergen et al. (1985)
Dicalcium phosphate	107	Monosodium phosphate, hyd	Bone ash & BBS	SR	N	.30-.45	Cromwell (1992)
Distiller's grain	71	Monosodium phosphate, hyd	BBS	SR	SP	.05-.2	Burnell et al. (1989c)
Distiller's grains and solubles	77	Monosodium phosphate, hyd	Bone ash & BBS	SR	N	.30-.45	Cromwell (1992)
Fish meal	100	Monosodium phosphate, hyd	Bone ash & BBS	SR	N	.30-.45	Cromwell (1992)
Hominy feed	14	Monosodium phosphate, hyd	Bone ash & BBS	SR	N	.30-.45	Cromwell (1992)

Table I. (continued)

Source	RV	Standard	Response criterion	Meth cal	Type diet	Added level, %	Reference
Hominy feed	14	Monosodium phosphate hyd	BBS	SR	SP	.1-2	Burnell et al. (1989b)
Iron aluminum rock phosphate	7[b]	-	App abs	-	N	[c]	Ammerman et al. (1963)
Meat and bone meal	102	Monosodium phosphate	Bone ash	SR	N	.15-.4	Huang and Allee (1981)
Meat and bone meal	64	Monosodium phosphate	BBS	SR	N	.30-.45	Burnell et al. (1989a)
Monocalcium phosphate	101	Dicalcium phosphate	Bone ash	SC	N	.275-.30	Plumlee et al. (1958)
Monocalcium phosphate	121	Dicalcium phosphate, hyd	Bone ash	SR	N	NG	Grimbergen et al. (1985)
Oats	36	Monosodium phosphate	Bone ash	SR	N	.15-.4	Huang and Allee (1981)
Oats	22	Monosodium phosphate, hyd	Bone ash & BBS	SR	N	.30-.45	Cromwell (1992)
Palm kernal cake	11	Monosodium phosphate, hyd	Bone ash & BBS	SR	N	.30-.45	Cromwell (1992)
Peanut meal	12	Monosodium phosphate, hyd	Bone ash & BBS	SR	N	.30-.45	Cromwell (1992)
Phosphoric acid	100	Dicalcium phosphate	Bone ash	SC	N	.275-.30	Plumlee et al. (1958)
Rice bran	25	Monosodium phosphate, hyd	Bone ash & BBS	SR	N	.30-.45	Cromwell (1992)

Feedstuff		Form	Method		Availability column	Value	Reference
Rock phosphate (Christmas Island)	31[b]	-	App abs	-	N	.36-.56	King (1980)
Soft rock phosphate	72	Dicalcium phosphate	Bone ash	SC	N	.275-.30	Plumlee et al. (1958)
Soft rock phosphate	28[b]	-	App abs	-	N	c	Ammerman et al. (1963)
Soft rock phosphate	57[b]	-	App abs	-	N	.31-.52	Harmon et al. (1974)
Sorghum	25	Monosodium phosphate	Bone ash	SR	N	.15-.4	Huang and Allee (1981)
Sorghum	20	Monosodium phosphate, hyd	Bone ash & BBS	SR	N	.30-.45	Cromwell (1992)
Sorghum	3[b]	-	App abs	-	SP	.3-.5	Tonroy et al. (1973)
Sorghum, high moisture	43	Monosodium phosphate, hyd	Bone ash & BBS	SR	N	.30-.45	Cromwell (1992)
Soybean hulls	78	Monosodium phosphate, hyd	Bone ash & BBS	SR	N	.30-.45	Cromwell (1992)
Soybean meal (44%)	27[b]	-	App abs	-	SP	.3-.5	Tonroy et al. (1973)
Soybean meal (44%)	36	Monosodium phosphate	Bone ash	SR	N	.15-.4	Huang and Allee (1981)
Soybean meal, dehulled	23	Monosodium phosphate, hyd	Bone ash &BBS	SR	N	.30-.45	Cromwell (1992
Soybean meal (44%)	31	Monosodium phosphate, hyd	Bone ash & BBS	SR	N	.30-.45	Cromwell (1992)
Sunflower meal	3	Monosodium phosphate, hyd	Bone ash & BBS	SR	N	.30-.45	Cromwell (1992)
Triticale	65[b]	-	App abs	-	N	NG	Pointillart et al. (1987)
Triticale	46	Monosodium phosphate, hyd	BBS	SR	SP	.1-.2	Burnell et al. (1989b)

Table I. (continued)

Source	RV	Standard	Response criterion	Meth cal	Type diet	Added level, %	Reference
Triticale	46	Monosodium phosphate, hyd	Bone ash & BBS	SR	N	.30-.45	Cromwell (1992)
Wheat	51	Monosodium phosphate	Bone ash	SR	N	.15-.4	Huang and Allee (1981)
Wheat	46[b]	-	App abs	-	N	.33-.36	Pointhillart et al. (1984)
Wheat	49	Monosodium phosphate, hyd	Bone ash & BBS	SR	N	.30-.45	Cromwell (1992)
Wheat bran	29	Monosodium phosphate, hyd	Bone ash & BBS	SR	N	.30-.45	Cromwell (1992)
Wheat middlings	41	Monosodium phosphate, hyd	Bone ash & BBS	SR	N	.30-.45	Cromwell (1992)
Wheat offal	77	Dicalcium phosphate FG	App abs	-	N	.4-.5%	Frape et al. (1979)
Whey, dried	76	Monosodium phosphate, hyd	BBS	SR	SP	.05-.2	Burnell et al. (1989c)
In Vitro							
Bone meal, steamed	28	Sodium & potassium phosphates	Cell dig	MR	-	10-40 µg/ml medium	Anderson et al. (1956)
Curacao Island phosphate	12	Sodium & potassium phosphates	Cell dig	MR	-	10-40 µg/ml medium	Anderson et al. (1956)
Dicalcium phosphate	93	Sodium & potassium phosphates	Cell dig	MR	-	10-40 µg/ml medium	Anderson et al. (1956)

Metaphosphate, calcium	78	Monocalcium phosphate	Cell dig	MR	-	1.5-4.5 mg/tube	Chicco et al. (1965)
Metaphosphate, sodium	98	Monocalcium phosphate	Cell dig	MR	-	1.5-4.5 mg/tube	Chicco et al. (1965)
Pyrophosphate, calcium	0	Monocalcium phosphate	Cell dig	MR	-	1.5-4.5 mg/tube	Chicco et al. (1965)
Pyrophosphate, sodium	100	Monocalcium phosphate	Cell dig	MR	-	1.5-4.5 mg/tube	Chicco et al. (1965)
Soft rock phosphate	2	Sodium & potassium phosphates	Cell dig	MR	-	10-40 µg/ml medium	Anderson et al. (1956)

Cattle

Bermudagrass	24[b]	-	App abs	-	N	.25-.26	Gutierrez et al. (1984)
Bone meal	30[b]	-	Ret	-	SP	.09	Ammerman et al. (1957)
Clover, hay	44[b]	-	App abs	-	N	.15-.75	Turner et al. (1927)
Curacao Island phosphate	25[b]	-	Ret	-	SP	.09	Ammerman et al. (1957)
Defluorinated phosphate	29[b]	-	Ret	-	SP	.09	Ammerman et al. (1957)
Defluorinated phosphate	61[b]	-	App abs	-	N	[c]	Arrington et al. (1963)
Defluorinated phosphate	85	-	App abs	-	N	.09-.12	O'Donovan et al. (1965)
Defluorinated phosphate	100	Dicalcium phosphate FG	Bone ash & growth	MR	N	.06-.24	Miller et al. (1987)
Dicalcium phosphate FG	33[b]	-	Ret	-	SP	.09	Ammerman et al. (1957)
Dicalcium phosphate FG	31[b]	-	Ret	-	SP	.09	Ammerman et al. (1957)
Dicalcium phosphate	75[b]	-	True abs	-	SP	.13	Tillman and Brethour (1958a)
Dicalcium phosphate FG	70[b]	-	App abs	-	N	[c]	Arrington et al. (1963)

Table I. (continued)

Source	RV	Standard	Response criterion	Meth cal	Type diet	Added level, %	Reference
Dicalcium phosphate RG	86[b]	-	App abs	-	N	.09-.12	O'Donovan et al. (1965)
Dicalcium phosphate FG	85[b]	-	App abs	-	N	.09-.12	O'Donovan et al. (1965)
Dicalcium phosphate RG	44[b]	-	App abs	-	N	.25-.26	Gutierrez et al. (1984)
Phosphorus acid	76[b]	-	True abs	-	SP	.13	Tillman and Brethour (1958a)
Soft rock phosphate	17	Dicalcium phosphate	Growth	TP	N	.05	Long et al. (1956)
Soft rock phosphate	28[b]	-	Ret	-	SP	.09	Ammerman et al. (1957)
Soft rock phosphate	54[b]	-	App abs	-	N	c	Arrington et al. (1963)
Urea ammonium polyphosphate	100	Dicalcium phosphate	Bone ash	MR	SP	.24-.31	Teh et al. (1982)
Sheep							
Alfalfa, chaff	56[b]	-	True abs	-	N	.56-.62	Grace (1981)
Alfalfa, hay	94[b]	-	True abs	-	N	-	Lofgreen and Kleiber (1954)
Alfalfa, hay	91[b]	-	True abs	-	N	-	Lofgreen and Kleiber (1953)
Bone meal	46[b]	-	True abs	-	N	-	Lofgreen (1960)
Broiler litter	55[b]	-	App abs	-	N	.15-.31	Cooke and Fontenot (1990)
Bromegrass, smooth	21[b]	-	App abs	-	N	.22-.31	Powell et al. (1978)
Calcium phytate	63[b]	-	App abs	-	SP	.22	Tillman and Brethour (1958c)
Calcium phytate	90	Monocalcium phosphate	True abs	MR	SP	.22	Tillman and Brethour (1958c)
Calcium phytate	33[b]	-	True abs	-	N	-	Lofgreen (1960)

Item							Reference
Clover, white	22[b]	-	App abs	-	N	.56-.62	Grace et al. (1974)
Corn silage	75[b]	-	True abs	-	N	-	Dayrell and Ivan (1989)
Curacao Island phosphate	90[b]	-	True abs	-	SP	.12	Ammerman et al. (1957)
Defluorinated phosphate	54[b]	-	True abs	-	SP	.12	Ammerman et al. (1957)
Dicalcium phosphate	100[b]	-	True abs	-	SP	.12	Ammerman et al. (1957)
Dicalcium phosphate FG	50[b]	-	True abs	-	N	-	Lofgreen (1960)
Dicalcium phosphate	67[b]	-	True abs	-	N	-	Dayrell and Ivan (1989)
Dicalcium phosphate	30[b]	-	App abs	-	N	.15-.31	Cooke and Fontenot (1990)
Fescue, tall	0[b]	-	App abs	-	N	.22-.31	Powell et al. (1978)
Metaphosphate, calcium [Ca(PO$_4$)$_2$]	34[b]	-	True abs	-	SP	.10	Ammerman et al. (1957)
Metaphosphate, calcium	33[b]	-	App abs	-	N	c	Chicco et al. (1965)
Metaphosphate, sodium vitreous	87[b]	-	True abs	-	SP	-	Tillman and Brethour (1958a)
Metaphosphate, sodium	46[b]	-	App abs	-	N	c	Chicco et al. (1965)
Milk, sheep's	99[b]	-	App abs	-	N	NG	Dillion and Scott (1979)
Monocalcium phosphate, hyd	63[b]	-	True abs	-	SP	.10	Ammerman et al. (1957)
Monocalcium phosphate	70[b]	-	App abs	-	SP	.22	Tillman and Brethour (1958c)
Monocalcium phosphate	47[b]	-	App abs	-	N	c	Chicco et al. (1965)
Monosodium phosphate	89[b]	-	True abs	-	SP	-	Tillman and Brethour (1958a)
Orchardgrass	15[b]	-	App abs	-	N	.15-.31	Powell et al. (1978)
Poultry manure	55[b]	-	App abs	-	N	6.81 g/day	Ben-Ghedalia et al. (1982)

Table I. (continued)

Source	RV	Standard	Response criterion	Meth cal	Type diet	Added level, %	Reference
Pyrophosphate, calcium ($Ca_2P_2O_7$)	0^b	-	True abs	-	SP	.10	Ammerman et al. (1957)
Pyrophosphate, calcium	26^b	-	App abs	-	N	c	Chicco et al. (1965)
Pyrophosphate, sodium	90^b	-	True abs	-	SP	-	Tillman and Brethour (1958a)
Pyrophosphate, sodium	39^b	-	App abs	-	N	c	Chicco et al. (1965)
Rock phosphate	48^b	-	True abs	-	N	-	Dayrell and Ivan (1989)
Ryegrass, perennial	21^b	-	App abs	-	N	.56-.62	Grace et al. (1974)
Ryegrass, perennial	15^b	-	App abs	-	N	.15-.31	Powell et al. (1978)
Ryegrass, perennial	62^b	-	True abs	-	N	.56-.62	Grace (1981)
Ryegrass, short rotation	26^b	-	App abs	-	N	.56-.62	Grace et al. (1974)
Soft rock phosphate	50^b	-	True abs	-	SP	.12	Ammerman et al. (1957)
Soft rock phosphate	14^b	-	True abs	-	N	NG	Lofgreen (1960)
Soybean meal	43^b	-	App abs	-	N	.15-.31	Cooke and Fontenot (1990)
Swine waste	64^b	-	App abs	-	N	.15-.31	Cooke and Fontenot (1990)
Wheat bran	25^b	-	True abs	-	N	-	Ellis and Tillman (1961)
Horses							
Soybean meal	56^b	-	App abs	-	N	4.5 g/day	Ben-Ghedalia et al. (1982)
Bone meal	100	Bonemeal & tricalcium phosphate	Bone ash	MR	SP	.03-.39	Ellis et al. (1945)

284

Calcium phosphate	49	Bone meal & tricalcium phosphate	Bone ash	MR	SP	.03-.39	Ellis *et al.* (1945)
Defluorinated phosphate	61	Bone meal & tricalcium phosphate	Bone ash	MR	SP	.03-.39	Ellis *et al.* (1945)
Phosphate slag	70	Bone meal & tricalcium phosphate	Bone ash	MR	SP	.03-.39	Ellis *et al.* (1945)
Pyrophosphate, γ-calcium	33	Bone meal & tricalcium phosphate	Bone ash	MR	SP	.03-.39	Ellis *et al.* (1945)
Pyrophosphate, β-calcium	30	Bone meal & tricalcium phosphate	Bone ash	MR	SP	.03-.39	Ellis *et al.* (1945)
Tricalcium phosphate	100	Bone meal & tricalcium phosphate	Bone ash	MR	SP	.03-.39	Ellis *et al.* (1945)

[a]Abbreviations can be found in Appendix 1. Chemical formula for a compound given only if provided by the author; RG indicates reagent grade, FG indicates feed grade.
[b]Percentage absorption or retention, not relative value.
[c]Phosphate containing ^{32}P administered as single oral dose.

Table II. Relative bioavailability of supplemental phosphorus sources[a]

Source	Poultry	Swine
Sodium or potassium phosphate	100	100
Ammonium polyphosphate	95 (1)	-
Bone meal	95 (1)	80 (1)
Defluorinated phosphate	90 (8)	85 (1)
Diammonium phosphate	95 (1)	-
Dicalcium phosphate	95 (8)	100 (2)
Monocalcium phosphate	100 (1)	-
Soft rock phosphate	40 (1)	-

[a]Average values rounded to nearest "5" and expressed relative to response with either sodium or potassium phosphate. Number of studies or samples involved indicated within parentheses. Sources are identified according to AAFCO (1994). Dicalcium phosphate identified as such without indication of degree of hydration or presence of monocalcium phosphate.

REFERENCES

Ammerman, C. B., L. R. Arrington, J. T. McCall, J. P. Feaster, G. E. Combs and G. K. Davis. 1963. Inorganic phosphorus utilization by swine as measured by an isotope technique. *J. Anim. Sci.* **22**:890.

Ammerman, C. B., R. M. Forbes, U. S. Garrigus, A. L. Neumann, H. W. Norton and E. E. Hatfield. 1957. Ruminant utilization of inorganic phosphates. *J. Anim. Sci.* **16**:796.

Ammerman, C. B., R. Valdivia, I. V. Rosa, P. R. Henry, J. P. Feaster and W. G. Blue. 1984. Effect of sand or soil as a dietary component on phosphorus utilization by sheep. *J. Anim. Sci.* **59**:1092.

Anderson, R., E. Cheng and W. Burroughs. 1956. A laboratory technique for measuring phosphorus availability of feed supplements fed to ruminants. *J. Anim. Sci.* **15**:489.

Anderson, R. J. 1915. The hydrolysis of phytin by the enzyme phytase contained in wheat bran. *J. Biol. Chem.* **20**:475.

Andrews, T. L., B. L. Damron and R. H. Harms. 1972. Utilization of various sources of plant phosphorus by the turkey poult. *Nutr. Rep. Int.* **6**:251.

Apke, M. P., P. E. Waibel, K. Larntz, A. L. Metz, S. L. Noll and M. M. Walser. 1987. Phosphorus availability bioassay using bone ash and bone densitometry as response criteria. *Poult. Sci.* **66**:713.

Apke, M. P., P. E. Waibel and R. V. Morey. 1984. Bioavailability of phosphorus in poultry litter biomass ash residues for turkeys. *Poult. Sci.* **63**:2100.

Arrington, L. R., J. C. Outler, C. B. Ammerman and G. K. Davis. 1963. Absorption, retention and tissue deposition of labeled inorganic phosphates by cattle. *J. Anim. Sci.* **22**:940.

Ashton, W. M., C. Evans and P. C. Williams. 1960. Phosphorus compounds of oats. II. The utilization of phytate phosphorus by growing chicks. *J. Sci. Food Agric.* **11**:722.

Association of American Feed Control Officials (AAFCO). 1994. Official publication. AAFCO, Atlanta, GA.

Baker, D. H. 1989. Phosphorus supplements for poultry. *Multistate Poult. Exten. Res. Newsletter.* University Illinois 1(5):5.

Ballam, G. C., T. S. Nelson and L. K. Kirby. 1985. Effect of different dietary levels of calcium and phosphorus on phytate hydrolysis by chicks. *Nutr. Rep. Int.* **32**:909.

Bar, A. and S. Hurwitz. 1984. Egg shell quality, medullary bone ash, intestinal calcium and phosphorus absorption and calcium-binding protein in phosphorus-deficient hens. *Poult. Sci.* **63**:1975.

Barth, J. and S. L. Hansard. 1962. Comparative availability of phytin and inorganic phosphorus to rumen microorganisms, *in vitro. Proc. Soc. Exp. Biol. Med.* **109**:448.

Bayley, H. S. and R. G. Thomson. 1969. Phosphorus requirements of growing pigs and effect of steam pelleting on phosphorus availability. *J. Anim. Sci.* **28**:484.

Bayley, H. S., J. Pos and R. G. Thomson. 1975. Influence of steam pelleting and dietary level on utilization of phosphorus by the pig. *J. Anim. Sci.* **40**:859.

Ben-Ghedalia, D., H. Tagari, A. Geva and S. Zamwel. 1982. Availability of macroelements from a concentrate diet supplemented with soybean meal or poultry manure fed to sheep. *J. Dairy Sci.* **65**:1760.

Besecker, R. J., Jr., M. P. Plumlee, R. A. Pickett and J. H. Conrad. 1967. Phosphorus from barley grain for growing swine. *J. Anim. Sci.* **26**:1477 [Abstract].

Bird, H. R., J. P. Mattingly, H. W. Titus, J. C. Hammond. W. L. Kellogg, T. B. Clark, C. E. Weakley, Jr. and A. H. van Landingham. 1945. Nutritive evaluation of defluorinated phosphates and other phosphorus supplements. *J. Assoc. Off. Agric. Chem.* **28**:118.

Boutwell, P. W. 1917. The phytic acid of the wheat kernel and some of its salts. *J. Am. Chem. Soc.* **39**:491.

Boyd, R. D., D. Hall and J. F. Wu. 1983. Plasma alkaline phosphatase as a criterion for determining biological availability of phosphorus for swine. *J. Anim. Sci.* **57**:396.

Burnell, T. W., G. L. Cromwell and T. S. Stahly. 1990. Effects of particle size on the biological availability of calcium and phosphorus in defluorinated phosphate for chicks. *Poult. Sci.* **69**:1110.

Burnell, T. W., G. L. Cromwell and T. S. Stahly. 1989a. Bioavailability of phosphorus in meat and bone meal for pigs. *J. Anim. Sci.* **67**(Suppl. 2):38 [Abstract].

Burnell, T. W., G. L. Cromwell, and T. S. Stahly. 1989b. Bioavailability of phosphorus in triticale, hominy feed and corn gluten feed for pigs. *J. Anim. Sci.* **67**(Suppl. 2):126 [Abstract].

Burnell, T. W., G. L. Cromwell and T. S. Stahly. 1989c. Bioavailability of phosphorus in dried whey, blood meal, and distillers grains for pigs. *J. Anim. Sci.* **67**(Suppl. 1):262 [Abstract].

Burns, J. M., and D. H. Baker. 1976. Assessment of the quantity of biologically available phosphorus in yeast RNA and single-cell protein. *Poult. Sci.* **55**:2447.

Calvert, C. C., R. J. Besecker, M. P. Plumlee, T. R. Cline and D. M. Forsyth. 1978. Apparent digestibility of phosphorus in barley and corn for growing swine. *J. Anim. Sci.* **47**:420.

Chester-Jones, H., J. P. Fontenot, H. P. Veit and K. E. Webb, Jr. 1989. Physiological effects of feeding high levels of magnesium to sheep. *J. Anim. Sci.* **67**:1070.

Chicco, C. F., C. B. Ammerman, J. E. Moore, P. A. van Walleghem, L. R. Arrington and R. L. Shirley. 1965. Utilization of inorganic ortho-, meta-, and pyrophosphates by lambs and by cellulolytic rumen micro-organisms *in vitro*. *J. Anim. Sci.* **24**:355.

Chung, T. K. and D. H. Baker. 1990. Phosphorus utilization in chicks fed hydrated sodium calcium aluminosilicate. *J. Anim. Sci.* **68**:1992.

Clark, W. D., J. E. Wohlt, R. L. Gilbreath and P. K. Zajac. 1986. Phytate phosphorus intake and disappearance in the gastrointestinal tract of high producing dairy cows. *J. Dairy Sci.* **69**:3151.

Clawson, A. J. and L. L. Southern. 1985. Effect of level and source of phosphorus on performance of growing-finishing swine. *Nutr. Rep. Int.* **31**:429.

Cooke, J. A. and J. P. Fontenot. 1990. Utilization of phosphorus and certain other minerals from swine waste and broiler litter. *J. Anim. Sci.* **68**:2852.

Corley, J. R ., D. H. Baker and R. A. Easter. 1980. Biological availability of phosphorus in rice bran and wheat bran as affected by pelleting. *J. Anim. Sci.* **50**:286.

Cromwell, G. L. 1979. Availability of phosphorus in feedstuffs for swine. *Proc. Dist. Feed Res. Council* **34**:40.

Cromwell, G. L. 1980. Biological availability of phosphorus for pigs. *Feedstuffs* **52**(9):38.

Cromwell, G. L. 1992. The biological availability of phosphorus in feedstuffs for pigs. *Pig News Inform.* **13**:75.

Cromwell, G. L., T. S. Stahly, R. D. Coffey, H. J. Monegue and J. H. Randolph. 1993. Efficacy of phytase in improving the bioavailibility of phosphorus in soybean meal and corn-soybean meal diets for pigs. *J. Anim. Sci.* **71**:1831.

Damron, B. L. and R. H. Harms. 1968. A comparison of phosphorus assay techniques with chicks. 3. Development of calcium standard curve for soft phosphate, defluorinated phosphate, and calcium phosphate. *Poult. Sci.* **47**:1878.

Damron, B. L., T. L. Andrews and R. H. Harms. 1974. Effect of diet composition upon the performance of laying hens receiving Curacao Island phosphate. *Poult. Sci.* **53**:99.

Davies, M. I. and I. Motzok. 1972. Properties of chick intestinal phytase. *Poult. Sci.* **51**:494.

Day, E. J., J. McNaughton and B. C. Dilworth. 1973. Chemical versus chick bioassay for phosphorus availability of feed grade sources. *Poult. Sci.* **52**:393.

Dayrell, M. de S. and M. Ivan. 1989. True absorption of phorphorus in sheep fed corn silage and corn silage supplemented with dicalcium or rock phosphate. *Can. J. Anim. Sci.* **69**:181.

deBoland, A. R., G. B. Garner and B. L. O'Dell. 1975. Identification and properties of "phytate" in cereal grains and oilseed products. *J. Agric. Food Chem.* **23**:1186.

Dillon, J. and D. Scott. 1979. Digesta flow and mineral absorption in lambs before and after weaning. *J. Agric. Sci. Camb.* **92**:229.

Dilworth. B. C. and E. J. Day. 1964. Phosphorus availability studies with feed grade phosphates. *Poult. Sci.* **43**:1039.

Edwards, H. 1993. Dietary 1,25 dihydroxycholecalciferol supplementation increases natural phytate phosphorus utilization in chickens. *J. Nutr.* **123**:567.

Ellis, N. R., C. A. Cabell, W. P. Elmslie, G. S. Frape, P. H. Phillips and D. E. Williams. 1945. Nutritive evaluation of defluorinated phosphates and other phosphorus supplements. III. Utilization experiments with rats. *J. Assoc. Off. Agric. Chem.* **28**:129.

Ellis, L. C. and A. D. Tillman. 1961. Utilization of phytin phosphorus in wheat bran by sheep. *J. Anim. Sci.* **20**:606.

Erdman, J. W., Jr. 1979. Oilseed phytates: Nutritional implications. *J. Am. Oil Chem. Soc.* **56**:736.

Frape, D. L., B. J. Wayman and M. G. Tuck. 1979. The utilization of phosphorus and nitrogen in wheat offal by growing pigs. *J. Agric. Sci. Camb.* **93**:133.

Fritz, J. C. 1969. Availability of mineral nutrients. *In* "Proceedings of the Maryland Nutrition Conference," p. 1.

Garlich, J. D. and M. Mian. 1986. Slope ratio assay for available phosphorus from defluorinated phosphates. *Poult. Sci.* **65**(Suppl. 1):168 [Abstract].

Gillis, M. B., H. M. Edwards, Jr. and R. J. Young. 1962. Studies on the availability of calcium orthophosphates to chickens and turkeys. *J. Nutr.* **78**:155.

Gillis, M. B., L. C. Norris and G. F. Heuser. 1948. The utilization by the chick of phosphorus from different sources. *J. Nutr.* **35**:195.

Gillis, M. B., L. C. Norris and G. F. Heuser. 1954. Studies on the biological value of inorganic phosphates. *J. Nutr.* **54**:115.

Gobble, J. L., R. C. Miller, G. W. Sherritt and H. W. Dunne. 1955. Soft phosphate with colloidal clay as a source of phosphorus for growing and fattening pigs. *Pennsylvania Agric. Exp. Sta. Bull.* **609**.

Grace, N. D. 1981. Phosphorus kinetics in the sheep. *Br. J. Nutr.* **45**:367.

Grace, N. D., M. J. Ulyatt and J. C. McCrae. 1974. Quantitative digestion of fresh herbage by sheep. III. The movement of Mg, Ca, P, K, and Na in the digestive tract. *J. Agric. Sci. Camb.* **82**:321.

Griffith, M., R. J. Young and M. L. Scott. 1966. Influence of soybean on growth and phosphorus availability in turkey poults. *Poult. Sci.* **45**:189.

Grimbergen, A. H. M., J. P. Cornelissen and H. P. Stappers. 1985. The relative availability of phosphorus in inorganic feed phosphates for young turkeys and pigs. *Anim. Feed Sci. Technol.* **13**:131.

Gutierrez, O., C. M. Geetken and A. Diaz. 1983. A note on the phosphorus balance of calves fed natural superphosphate supplemented diets. *Cuban J. Agric. Sci.* **17**:51.

Gutierrez, O., C. M. Geetken and A. Diaz. 1984. Apparent digestibility and retention of Ca and P in calves fed forage diets alone or supplemented with dicalcium phosphate. *Cuban J. Agric. Sci.* **18**:157.

Hagemeier, D. L., E. R. Peo, Jr., T. D. Crenshaw, A. J. Lewis and B. D. Moser. 1981. The bioavailability of phosphorus from defluorinated rock phosphate for growing-finishing swine. *Nutr. Rep. Int.* **23**:189.

Hahn, J. D., T. K. Chung and D. H. Baker. 1990. Nutritive value of oat flour and oat bran. *J. Anim. Sci.* **68**:4253.

Hall, O. G., H. D. Baxter and C. S. Hobbs. 1961. Effect of phosphorus in different chemical forms on *in vitro* cellulose digestion by rumen microorganisms. *J. Anim. Sci.* **20**:817.

Harmon, B. G., C. T. Liu, S. G. Cornelius, J. E. Pettigrew, D. H. Baker and A. H. Jensen. 1974. Efficacy of different phosphorus supplements for sows during gestation and lactation. *J. Anim. Sci.* **39**:1117.

Harmon, B. G., J. Simon, D. E. Becker, A. H. Jensen and D. H. Baker. 1970. Effect of source and level of dietary phosphorus on structure and composition of turbinate and long bones. *J. Anim. Sci.* **30**:742.

Harrold, R. L., W. D. Slanger, C. N. Haugse and R. L. Johnson. 1979. Availability of barley phosphorus: A modified chick bioassay. *J. Anim. Sci.* **49**(Suppl. 1):97 [Abstract].

Harrold, R. L., W. D. Slanger, C. N. Haugse and R. L. Johnson. 1983. Phosphorus bioavailability in the chick: Effects of protein source and calcium level. *J. Anim. Sci.* **57**:1173.

Hayes, S. H., G. L. Cromwell, T. S. Stahly and T. H. Johnson. 1979. Availability of phosphorus in corn, wheat and barley for the chick. *J. Anim. Sci.* **49**:992.

Hill, W. L., D. S. Reynolds, S. B. Hendricks and K. D. Jacob. 1945. Nutritive evaluation of defluorinated phosphates and other phosphorus supplements. *J. Assoc. Off. Agric. Chem.* **28**:105.

Hintz, H. F., A. J. Williams, J. Rogoff and H. F. Schryver. 1973. Availability of phosphorus in wheat bran when fed to ponies. *J. Anim. Sci.* **36**:522.

Hodgson, C. W., R. F. Johnson, A. C. Wiese and C. W. Hickman. 1948. A comparison of steamed bonemeal and defluorinated superphosphate as phosphorus supplements for fattening steers. *J. Anim. Sci.* **7**:273.

Huang, K. C. and G. L. Allee. 1981. Bioavailability of phosphorus in selected feedstuffs for young chicks and pigs. *J. Anim. Sci.* **53**(Suppl. 1):248 [Abstract].

Huque, Q. M. E. and J. F. Jensen. 1985. Biological availability of selenium and phosphorus in fish meal as affected by condition of fish and type of meal. *Br. Poult. Sci.* **26**:289.

Hurwitz, S., D. Dubrov, U. Eisner, G. Riserfeld and A. Bar. 1978. Phosphate absorption and excretion in the young turkey as influenced by calcium intake. *J. Nutr.* **108**:1329.

Hurwitz, S. 1964. Estimation of net phosphorus utilization by the "slope" method. *J. Nutr.* **84**:83.

Huyghebaert. G., G. de Groote and L. Keppens. 1980. The relative biological availability of phosphorus in feed phosphates for broilers. *Ann. Zootech.* **29**:245.

Jensen, L. S. and H. M. Edwards, Jr. 1980. Availability of phosphorus from ammonium polyphosphate for growing chickens. *Poult. Sci.* **59**:1280.

Kegley, E. B., R. W. Harvey and J. W. Spears. 1991. Effects of lysocellin and calcium level on mineral metabolism, performance and ruminal and plasma characteristics of beef steers. *J. Anim. Sci.* **69**:782.

Ketaren, P. P., E. S. Batterham, E. B. Dettmann and D. J. Farrell. 1993a. Phosphorus studies in pigs. 2. Assessing phosphorus availability for pigs and rats. *Br. J. Nutr.* **70**:269.

Ketaren, P. P., E. S. Batterham, E. B. Dettmann and D. J. Farrell. 1993b. Phosphorus studies in pigs. 3. Effect of phytase supplementation on the digestibility and availability of phosphorus in soya-bean meal for grower pigs. *Br. J. Nutr.* **70**:289.

Ketola, G. H. and B. F. Harland. 1993. Influence of phosphorus in rainbow trout diets on phosphorus discharges in effluent water. *Trans. Am. Fisheries Soc.* **122**:1120.

Kiiskinen, T. 1983. Urea phosphate as a source of supplemental phosphorus for poultry. *Ann. Agric. Fenniae.* **22**:86.

King. R. H. 1980. Various sources of supplemental phosphorus for grower /finisher pig diets based on plant protein. *Aust. J. Exp. Agric. Anim. Husb.* **20**:433.

Kirk, D. J., L. W. Green, G. T. Schelling and F. M. Byers. 1985. Effects of monensin on Mg, Ca, P, and Zn metabolism and tissue concentrations in lambs. *J. Anim. Sci.* **60**:1485.

Krieger, C. H., R. Bunkfeldt, C. R. Thompson and H. Steenbock. 1941. Cereals and Rickets. XIII. Phytic acid, yeast nucleic acid, soybean phosphatides and inorganic salts as sources of phosphorus for bone calcification. *J. Nutr.* **21**:213.

Lei, X. G., P. K. Ku, E. R. Miller, M. T. Yokoyama and D. E. Ullrey. 1994. Calcium level affects the efficacy of supplemental microbial phytase in corn-soybean meal diets of weanling pigs. *J. Anim. Sci.* **72**:139.

Lofgreen, G. P. 1960. The availability of the phosphorus in dicalcium phosphate, bonemeal, soft phosphate and calcium phytate for mature wethers. *J. Nutr.* **70**:58.

Lofgreen, G. P. and M. Kleiber. 1953. The availability of the phosphorus in alfalfa hay. *J. Anim. Sci.* **12**:366.

Lofgreen, G. P. and M. Kleiber. 1954. Further studies on the availability of phosphorus in alfalfa hay. *J. Anim. Sci.* **13**:258.

Long, T. A., A. D. Tillman, A. B. Nelson, W. D. Gallup and B. Davis. 1957. Availability of phosphorus in mineral supplements for beef cattle. *J. Anim. Sci.* **16**:444.

Long, T. A., A. D. Tillman, A. B. Nelson, B. Davis and W. D. Gallup. 1956. Dicalcium phosphate and soft phosphate with colloidal clay as sources of phosphorus for beef heifers. *J. Anim. Sci.* **15**:1112.

Lowe, J. T., H. Steenbock and C. H. Krieger. 1939. Cereals and rickets. IX. The availability of phytin-P to the chick. *Poult. Sci.* **18**:40.

McGinnis, J., L. C. Norris and G. F. Heuser. 1944. Poor utilization of phosphorus in cereals and legumes by chicks for bone development. *Poult. Sci.* **23**:157.

Miller, W. J., M. W. Neathery, R. P. Gentry, D. M. Blackmon, C. T. Crowe, G. O. Ware and A. S. Fielding. 1987. Bioavailability of phosphorus from defluorinated and dicalcium phosphates and phosphorus requirement of calves. *J. Dairy Sci.* **70**:1885.

Morris, E. R. and R. Ellis. 1976. Isolation of monoferric phytate from wheat bran and its biological value as an iron source to the rat. *J. Nutr.* **106**:753.

Motzok, I. 1968. Studies on phosphorus assay techniques. I. The assay of soft phosphorus with chicks. *Poult. Sci.* **47**:967.

Mroz, Z., A. W. Jongbloed and P. A. Kemme. 1994. Apparent digestibility and retention of nutrients bound to phytate complexes as influenced by microbial phytase and feeding regimen in pigs. J. Anim. Sci. 72:126.

National Research Council (NRC). 1988. " Nutrient Requirements of Swine," 9th ed. Nat. Acad. Press, Washington, DC.,

National Research Council (NRC). 1994. "Nutrient Requirements of Poulty," 9th ed. Nat. Acad. Press, Washington, DC.

Nelson, T. S. 1976. The hydrolysis of phytate phosphorus by chicks and laying hens. *Poult. Sci.* **55**:2262.

Nelson, T. S. 1980. Phosphorus availability in plant origin feedstuffs for poultry and swine. *In* "Proceedings of the 3rd Annual International Mineral Conference," p.59.

Nelson, T. S. 1989. Phosphorus requirements. II. Availability of phosphorus in plant origin feed ingredients to poultry. *In* "Feed Phosphates in Monogastric Nutrition," Proceedings of the Texas Gulf Nutrition Symposium, Raleigh, NC.

Nelson, T. S., L. B. Daniels, J. R. Hall and L. G. Shields. 1976. Hydrolysis of natural phytate phosphorus in the digestive tract of calves. *J. Anim. Sci.* **42**:1509.

Nelson, T. S. and H. T. Peeler. 1961. The availability of phosphorus from single and combined phosphates to chicks. Poult. Sci. 40:1321.

Nelson, T. S., T. R. Shieh, R. J. Wodzinski and J. H. Ware. 1968. The availability of phytate phosphorus in soybean meal before and after treatment with a mold phytase. *Poult. Sci.* **47**:1842.

Nelson, T. S. and A. C. Walker. 1964. The biological evaluation of phosphorus compounds - A summary. *Poult. Sci.* **43**:94.

Newlander, J. A., H. B. Ellenberger and C. H. Jones. 1936. Calcium and phosphorus requirements of dairy cows. III. Relative values of dicalcium phosphate and bone meal as mineral supplements. *Vermont Agric. Exp. Sta. Bull.* **406**.

Newman, C. W. and D. O. Elliott. 1976. Source and level of phosphorus for growing-finishing swine. *J. Anim. Sci.* **42**:92.

O'Dell, B. L., A. R. deBoland and S. R. Koirtyohann. 1972. Distribution of phytate and nutritionally important elements among the morphological components of cereal grains. *J. Agric. Food Chem.* **20**:718.

O'Dell, B. L. and A. R. deBoland. 1976. Complexation of phytate with proteins and cations in corn germ and oilseed meals. *J. Agric. Food Chem.* **24**:804.

O'Donovan, J. P., M. P. Plumlee, W. H. Smith and W. M. Beeson. 1965. Availability of phosphorus in dicalcium phosphates and defluorinated phosphate for steers. *J. Anim. Sci.* **24**:981.

Ogawa, M., K. Tanaka and Z. Kasai. 1975. Isolation of high phytin containing particles from rice grains using an aqueous polymer two phase system. *Agric. Biol. Chem.* **39**:695.

Osorio, J. G. and L. S. Jensen. 1986. Biological availability of phosphorus from a Venezuelan rock phosphate for broiler chicks. *Nutr. Rep. Int.* **33**:545.

Partridge, I. G. 1981. Comparison of defluorinated rock phosphate and dicalcium phosphate in diets containing either skim milk powder or soya bean meal as the main protein supplement, for early-weaned pigs. *Anim. Prod.* **32**:67.

Pensack, J. M. 1974. Biological availability of commercial feed phosphates. *Poult. Sci.* **53**:143.

Pierce, A. B., C. E. Doige, J. M. Bell and D. B. Owen. 1977. Availability of phytate phosphorus to the growing pigs receiving isonitrogenous diets based on wheat or corn. *Can J. Anim. Sci.* **57**:573.

Pileggi, V. J., H. F. DeLuca and H. Steenbock. 1955. The role of vitamin D and intestinal phytase in the prevention of rickets in rats on cereal diets. *Arch. Biochem. Biophys.* **58**:194.

Plumlee, M. P., C. E. Jordan, M. H. Kennington and W. M. Beeson. 1958. Availability of the phosphorus from various phosphate materials for swine. *J. Anim. Sci.* **17**:73.

Pointillart, A. 1991. Enhancement of phosphorus utilization in growing pigs fed phytate-rich diets by using rye bran. *J. Anim. Sci.* **69**:1109.

Pointillart, A., N. Fontaine and M. Thomasset. 1984. Phytate phosphorus utilization and intestinal phosphatases in pigs fed low phosphorus: Wheat or corn diets. *Nutr. Rep. Int.* **29**:473.

Pointillart, A., A. Fourdin and N. Fontaine. 1987. Importance of cereal phytase activity for phytate phosphorus utilization by growing pigs fed diets containing triticale or corn. *J. Nutr.* **117**:907.

Potchanakorn, M. and L. M. Potter. 1987. Biological values of phosphorus from various sources for young turkeys. *Poult. Sci.* **66**:505.

Potter, L. M. 1988. Bioavailability of phosphorus from various phosphates based on body weight and toe ash measurements. *Poult. Sci.* **67**:96.

Powell, K., R. L. Reid and J. A. Balasko. 1978. Performance of lambs on perennial ryegrass, smooth bromegrass, orchardgrass and tall fescue pastures. II. Mineral utilization, *in vitro* digestibility and chemical composition of herbage. *J. Anim. Sci.* **46**:1503.

Raun A., E. Cheng and W. Burroughs. 1956. Phytate phosphorus hydrolysis and availability to rumen microorganisms. *J. Agric. Food Chem.* **4**:869.

Reid, R. L., M. C. Franklin and E. G. Hallsworth. 1947. The utilization of phytate phosphorus by sheep. *Aust. Vet. J.* **23**:136.

Richardson, D., F. H. Baker, E. F. Smith and R. F. Cox. 1961. Phosphoric acid as a phosphorus source for beef cattle. *J. Anim. Sci.* **20**:522.

Roberts, A. H. and J. Yudkin. 1960. Dietary phytate as a possible cause of magnesium deficiency. *Nature* **185**:823.

Rucker, R. B., H. E. Parker and J. C. Rogler. 1968. Utilization of calcium and phosphorus from hydrous and anhydrous dicalcium phosphates. *J. Nutr.* **96**:513.

Scheidler, S. E. and J. L. Sell. 1987. Utilization of phytate phosphorus in laying hens as influenced by dietary phosphorus and calcium. *Nutr. Rep. Int.* **35**:1073.

Shah, B. G., S. Malcolm, B. Belonje, K. D. Trick, R. Brassard and R. Mongeau. 1990. Effect of dietary cereal brans on the metabolism of calcium, phosphorus and magnesium in a long term rat study. *Nutr. Res.* **10**:1015.

Shrewsbury, C. L. and C. M. Vestal. 1945. A comparison of different phosphate supplements for hogs and rats. *J. Anim. Sci.* **4**:403.

Simons, P. C. M., H. A .J. Versteegh, A. W. Jongbloed, P. A. Kemme, P. Slump, K. D. Bos, M. G. E. Wolters, R. F. Beudeker and G. J. Verschoor. 1990. Improvement of phosphorus availability by microbial phytase in broilers and pigs. *Br. J. Nutr.* **64**:525.

Soares, J. H., Jr., M. R. Swerdel and E. H. Bossard. 1977. Phosphorus availability. 1. The effect of chick age and vitamin D metabolites on the availability of phosphorus in defluorinated phosphate. *Poult. Sci.* **57**:1305.

Spandorf, A. H. and K. C. Leong. 1965. Biological bioavailability of calcium and phosphorus in menhaden fish meals. *Poult. Sci.* **44**:1107.

Starnes, S. R., J. W. Spears, M. A. Froeschel and W. J. Croom, Jr. 1984. Influence of monensin and lasalocid on mineral metabolism and ruminal urease activity in steers. *J. Nutr.* **114**:518.

Steinsberger, S. C., J. F. Ort and J. C. Shih. 1987. Composition and phosphorus bioavailability of a solid by-product from anaerobically digested waste from caged layer hens. *Poult. Sci.* **66**:634.

Struwe, F. J., T. W. Sullivan, and H. J. Kuhl, Jr. 1976. Evaluation of phosphated egg-shell and fertilizer phosphates in turkey starter diets. *Poult. Sci.* **55**:1691.

Sullivan, T. W. 1966. A triple response method for determining biological value of phosphorus sources with young turkeys. *Poult. Sci.* **45**:1236.

Sullivan, T. W. 1967. Relative biological value of ammonium polyphosphate and two high phosphate supplements. *Poult. Sci.* **45**:1324.

Summers, J. D., S. J. Slinger, W. F. Pepper, I. Motzok and G. C. Ashton. 1959. Availability of phosphorus in soft phosphate and phosphoric acid and the effect of acidulation of soft phosphate. *Poult. Sci.* **38**:1168.

Supplee, W. C. 1962. Anhydrous dicalcium phosphate as a source of phosphorus in poult diets. *Poult. Sci.* **41**:1984.

Taylor, T. G. 1965. The availability of the calcium and phosphorus of plant materials for animals. *Proc. Nutr. Soc.* **24**:105.

Teh Thian Hor, R. W. Hemken and L. S. Bull. 1982. Evaluation of urea ammonium polyphosphate as a phosphorus source for dairy calves. *J. Anim. Sci.* **55**:174.

Temperton, H. and J. Cassidy. 1964. Phosphorus requirements of poultry. I. The utilization of phytin phosphorus by the chick as indicated by balance experiments. *Br. Poult. Sci.* **5**:75.

Tillman, A. D. and J. R. Brethour. 1958a. Dicalcium phosphate and phosphoric acid as phosphorus sources for beef cattle. *J. Anim. Sci.* **17**:100.

Tillman, A. D. and J. R. Brethour. 1958b. Ruminant utilization of sodium meta-, ortho-, and pyrophosphates. *J. Anim. Sci.* **17**:792.

Tillman, A. D. and J. R. Brethour. 1958c. Utilization of phytin phosphorus by sheep. *J. Anim. Sci.* **17**:104.

Tonroy, B., M. P. Plumlee, J. H. Conrad and T. R. Cline. 1973. Apparent digestibility of the phosphorus in sorghum grain and soybean meal for growing swine. *J. Anim. Sci.* **36**:669.

Turner, W. A., T. S. Harding, and A. M. Hartman. 1927. The relative assimilation by dairy cows of clover and alfalfa hays and of rations of different calcium and phosphorus content. *J. Agric. Res.* **35**:625.

Waibel, P. E., N. A. Nahorniak, H. E. Dzuik, M. M. Walser and W. G. Olson. 1984. Bioavailability of phosphorus in commercial phosphate supplements for turkeys. *Poult. Sci.* **63**:730.

Waldroup, P. W., C. B. Ammerman and R. H. Harms. 1964. The availability of phytic acid phosphorus for chicks. 3. Effect of calcium and vitamin D_3 levels on the utilization of calcium phytate. *Poult. Sci.* **43**:426.

Waldroup, P. W., C. B. Ammerman and R. H. Harms. 1965. The utilization of phosphorus from animal protein sources for chicks. *Poult. Sci.* **44**:1302.

Waldroup, P. W., C. F. Simpson, B. L. Damron and R. H. Harms. 1967. The effectiveness of plant and inorganic phosphorus in supporting egg production in hens and hatchability and bone development in chick embryos. *Poult. Sci.* **46**:659.

Webb, K. E. Jr., J. P. Fontenot and M. B. Wise. 1975. Utilization of phosphorus from different supplements for growing-finishing beef steers. *J. Anim. Sci.* **40**:760.

Wise M. B., R. A. Wentworth and S. E. Smith. 1961. Availability of the phosphorus in various sources for calves. *J. Anim. Sci.* **20**:329.

Witt, K. E. and F. N. Owens. 1983. Phosphorus: Ruminal availability and effects on digestion. *J. Anim. Sci.* **56**:930.

Wozniak, L. A., J. M. Pensack, V. Stryeski and R. D. Wilbur. 1977. Biological availability of feed grade phosphates using a corn-soybean meal basal diet. *Poult. Sci.* **56**:366.

Yoshida, M. and H. Hoshii. 1979. Monobasic calcium phosphate as a standard for bioassay of phosphorus availability. *Jpn. Poult. Sci.* **16**:271.

13

POTASSIUM BIOAVAILABILITY

Elwyn R. Miller

Department of Animal Science
Michigan State University
East Lansing, Michigan

I. INTRODUCTION

Potassium is a dietary essential for all animals and is the third most abundant mineral element in the animal body. It is readily absorbed mainly from the upper small intestine and is excreted from the body primarily through the urine. The functions of potassium in the body include osmotic pressure regulation, maintenance of water balance and acid-base balance, nerve impulse conduction, muscle contraction and enzymatic reactions. Potassium is found predominantly within body cells with a small but important amount of the element occurring extracellularly. Obvious deficiencies of potassium are seldom encountered in domestic animals and, in normal circumstances, dietary deficiencies of the element are not observed in humans.

Forages, especially those that are young and growing rapidly, frequently contain potassium at concentrations well in excess of the ruminant animal's requirement. The element is readily leached from dry plant tissue, however, and mature forages that have been subjected to weathering may not contain adaquate amounts. Grains tend to be lower in potassium than forages but typical grain-soybean meal diets will usually meet the potassium requirements for both swine and poultry.

Reviews by Peeler (1972) and Miller (1980) concluded that potassium from potassium chloride (KCl), potassium carbonate (K_2CO_3), potassium sulfate (K_2SO_4), potassium acetate ($KC_2H_3O_2$), potassium bicarbonate ($KHCO_3$), dibasic potassium phosphate (K_2HPO_4) and potassium citrate monohydrate ($K_3C_6H_5O_7 \cdot H_2O$) was highly biologically available to animals and that potassium present in natural feedstuffs was probably well utilized.

BIOAVAILABILITY OF NUTRIENTS FOR ANIMALS:
AMINO ACIDS, MINERALS, AND VITAMINS
Copyright © 1995 by Academic Press, Inc.

295

II. BIOAVAILABILITY STUDIES

A. Ruminants

Disappearance of potassium from fresh, lyophilized, and ground samples of Kentucky 31 tall fescue, Kenhy fescue, and red clover-tall fescue pasture when suspended in dacron bags in the bovine rumen was 90, 94, and 92%, respectively, after 3 hr of incubation (van Eys and Reid, 1987). These values increased to 98, 99, and 98%, respectively, after 48 hr of incubation. Disappearance was decreased slightly with plant maturity. Emanuele and Staples (1990) and Emanuele *et al.* (1991) observed very rapid and complete release of potassium from ground samples of six forage species from dacron bags that were suspended in the rumen of the adult bovine.

Apparent absorption was used by Paquay *et al.* (1969) to determine the utilization of potassium from forages and forage-concentrate combinations in 41 different diets by dairy cows. The apparent absorption of potassium from alfalfa silage, clover silage, and cabbage silage varied from 87 to 94%. Potassium absorption from a mixed pea and oat silage was lower and the addition of concentrates including barley generally decreased potassium absorption. Perdomo *et al.* (1977) found apparent absorption of potassium to be 80 to 90% when four tropical forages, Pangola digitgrass (*Digitaria decumbens* Stent), guineagrass (*Panicum maximum* Jaq.), stargrass (*Cynodon plectostachyum* Pilger), and sheepgrass *(Brachiaria decumbens* Stapf)*, were fed fresh to sheep. The forages were harvested at 28, 42, and 56 days of regrowth and potassium absorption was not influenced greatly by maturity. Apparent absorption by sheep of potassium from combinations of two grass hays (orchardgrass, perennial ryegrass) and two legume hays (alfalfa and red clover) was approximately 82% with little effect of grass-legume proportion (Reid *et al.*, 1987).

B. Nonruminants

Combs *et al.* (1985) fed young pigs .06 and .12% potassium as the acetate or bicarbonate forms in a bioassay procedure and examined growth and a number of urinary and hematological measurements for linear response. Plasma potassium concentration was the only hematological measure that showed a significant linear response to dietary concentrations of the element. Urinary concentration and daily urinary excretion of potassium showed highly significant linear responses to dietary potassium. Based on these results, a potassium bioavailability assay using urinary potassium as the primary response variable and plasma potassium concentration as the secondary response variable seemed most promising. Patience *et al.* (1987) also found a linear relation between dietary potassium intake and retention of the element in short-term balance trials with young pigs. Using slope ratios of potassium retention in young pigs, Combs and Miller (1985) determined relative biological availabilities for potassium of 103% for potassium carbonate, 107% for potassium bicarbonate, 93% for corn, and 97% for soybean meal compared to a value of 100% for that in potassium acetate (Table I). Based on urinary potassium from a single oral dose to human subjects, Koenig *et al.* (1991) reported that potassium citrate, potassium chloride, and potassium-magnesium citrate were equal in bioavailability of potassium.

In a study with rats, Schricker (1985) obtained an apparent absorption of 98% for potassium from potassium bicarbonate, 97% from Dynamate® (Pitman-Moore, Mundelein, IL) ($K_2SO_4 \cdot 2MgSO_4$), and 98% from potassium chloride. Supplemental dietary concentrations of .1 or .4% potassium did not influence its apparent absorption when expressed as a percentage. Potassium retention was 73% of intake when .1% potassium from potassium bicarbonate was added to the diet but fell to 16% due to urinary excretion when .4% potassium from the same source was added. Potassium retention values were 67 and 18%, respectively, for rats fed diets suppplemented with either .1 or .4% potassium from Dynamate and 74 and 22%, respectively, for rats fed diets supplemented with either .1 or .4% potassium from potassium chloride. With dietary potassium additions of .4 or 1.2% from potassium citrate monohydrate, apparent absorption of the element was 98% for both concentrations and retentions were 37 and 8%, respectively. Thus, apparent absorption of potassium did not seem to be influenced by dietary source or concentration of the element. Endogenous potassium excretion was minimal, and concentrations of potassium in plasma, tibia, heart, and kidney tissues did not differ significantly. Hence, regulation of this electrolyte is closely controlled even with wide variations in dietary intake. Based on the results of this study, the use of apparent absorption appeared to be a useful technique for determining bioavailability of potassium from different sources.

Supplee and Combs (1959) and Supplee (1965) observed similar dietary potassium requirements for turkey poults when either potassium citrate monohydrate or dibasic potassium phosphate provided the element in a purified diet. Potassium chloride was 85% as effective as potassium acetate in requirement studies with the weanling guinea pig (Grace and O'Dell, 1968).

III. FACTORS INFLUENCING BIOAVAILABILITY

O'Dell and Savage (1966) found that chicks increased weight gain with supplemental potassium when arginine was limiting in the diet. Leibholz *et al.* (1966) observed that supplemental dietary potassium increased weight gains in pigs when dietary lysine was limiting. Scott and Austic (1978) found that chicks fed a high lysine diet gained weight faster when the diet was supplemented with potassium, primarily as a consequence of increased feed intake and, to a lesser extent, from alleviation of metabolic manifestations of the lysine-arginine antagonism. Whether some sources of potassium may be more effective than others in alleviating the lysine-arginine antagonism in poultry is yet to be determined.

IV. SUMMARY

Research that has measured the utilization of potassium by animals from feeds and supplements is limited. It appears, however, that potassium present in organic and inorganic salts of the element is of high bioavailability. The bioavailability of potassium from forage and concentrates that have been evaluated is more variable but, in general, the element appears to be well utilized. The average apparent absorption of potassium in eight forages tested in either cattle or sheep was about 85%. Because potassium is excreted from the animal body primarily in the urine, urinary excretion and apparent absorption are effective criteria for the estimation of bioavailability.

Table 1. Bioavailability of potassium sources for animals[a]

Source	RV	Standard	Response criterion	Meth cal	Type diet	Added level, %	Reference
Swine							
Corn	93	$KC_2H_3O_2$	App ret	SR	P	.12	Combs and Miller (1985)
Potassium bicarbonate ($KHCO_3$)	107	$KC_2H_3O_2$	App ret	SR	P	.12	Combs and Miller (1985)
Potassium carbonate (K_2CO_3)	103	$KC_2H_3O_2$	App ret	SR	P	.12	Combs and Miller (1985)
Soybean meal	97	$KC_2H_3O_2$	App ret	SR	P	.06, .12	Combs and Miller (1985)
Cattle							
Alfalfa silage	87[b]	--	App abs	--	N	163 g/day	Paquay et al. (1969)
Alfalfa silage	92	--	App abs	--	N	149 g/day	Paquay et al. (1969)
Cabbage silage	94	--	App abs	--	N	128 g/day	Paquay et al. (1969)
Clover silage	89	--	App abs	--	N	160 g/day	Paquay et al. (1969)
Pea and oat silage	67	--	App abs	--	N	151 g/day	Paquay et al. (1969)
Sheep							
Guineagrass[c]	89[b]	--	App abs	--	N	2.71	Perdomo et al. (1977)
Pangola digitgrass[c]	81	--	App abs	--	N	1.46	Perdomo et al. (1977)
Sheepgrass (Brachiaria decumbens Stapf)[c]	86	--	App abs	--	N	2.74	Perdomo et al. (1977)
Stargrass[c]	90	--	App abs	--	N	2.74	Perdomo et al. (1977)

Table I. (continued)

Source	RV	Standard	Response criterion	Meth cal	Type diet	Added level, %	Reference
Rats							
Potassium bicarbonate	98[b]	--	App abs	--	P	.1, .4	Schricker (1985)
Potassium citrate	98[b]	--	App abs	--	P	.4, 1.2	Schricker (1985)
Potassium chloride	98[b]	--	App abs	--	P	.1, .4	Schricker (1985)
Potassium magnesium sulfate[d], ($K_2SO_4 \cdot 2MgSO_4$)	97[b]	--	App abs	--	P	.1, .4	Schricker (1985)

[a]Abbreviations are found in Appendix I. Chemical formula for a compound given only if provided by the author.
[b]Values represent apparent absorption of potassium as percentage of total potassium intake.
[c]Forage fed fresh after 28-day regrowth.
[d]Dynamate, Pitman-Moore (Mundelein, IL).

REFERENCES

Combs, N. R., E. R. Miller and P. K. Ku. 1985. Development of an assay to determine the bioavailability of potassium in feedstuffs for the young pig. *J. Anim. Sci.* **60**:709.

Combs, N. R. and E. R. Miller. 1985. Determination of potassium availability in K_2CO_3, $KHCO_3$, corn and soybean meal for the young pig. *J. Anim. Sci.* **60**:715.

Emanuele, S. M. and C. R. Staples. 1990. Ruminal release of minerals from six forage species. *J. Anim. Sci.* **68**:2052.

Emanuele, S. M., C. R. Staples and C. J. Wilcox. 1991. Extent and site of mineral release from six forage species incubated in mobile dacron bags. *J. Anim. Sci.* **69**:801.

Grace, N. D. and B. L. O'Dell. 1968. Potassium requirement of the weanling guinea pig. *J. Nutr.* **94**:166.

Koenig, K., P. Padalino, G. Alexandrides and C. Y. C. Pak. 1991. Bioavailability of potassium and magnesium, and citraturic response from potassium magnesium citrate. *J. Urology* **145**:330.

Leibholz, J. M., J. T. McCall, V. W. Hays and V. C. Speer. 1966. Potassium, protein and basic amino acid relationships in swine. *J. Anim. Sci.* **25**:37.

Miller, E. R. 1980. Bioavailability of minerals. *In* "Proceedings of the 41st Minnesota Nutrition Conference," p. 144 Bloomington, MN.

O'Dell, B. L. and J. E. Savage. 1966. Arginine-lysine antagonism in the chick and its relationship to dietary cations. *J. Nutr.* **90**:364.

Paquay, R., F. Lomba, A. Lousse and V. Bienfet. 1969. Statistical research on the fate of dietary mineral elements in dry lactating cows. V. Potassium. *J. Agric. Sci. Camb.* **73**:445.

Patience, J. F., R. E. Austic and R. D. Boyd. 1987. Effect of dietary supplements of sodium or potassium bicarbonate on short-term macromineral balance in swine. *J. Anim. Sci.* **64**:1079.

Peeler, H.T. 1972. Biological availability of nutrients in feeds: Availability of major mineral ions. *J. Anim. Sci.* **35**:695.

Perdomo, J. T., R. L. Shirley and C. F. Chicco. 1977. Availability of nutrient minerals in four tropical forages fed freshly chopped to sheep. *J. Anim. Sci.* **45**:1114.

Reid, R. L., W. C. Templeton, Jr., T. S. Ranney and W. V. Thayne. 1987. Digestibility, intake and mineral utilization of combinations of grasses and legumes by lambs. *J. Anim. Sci.* **64**:1725.

Schricker, B. R. 1985. Effect of dietary potassium sources on apparent absorption and retention of potassium, magnesium and sodium. *Nutr. Rep. Int.* **31**:615.

Scott, R. L. and R. E. Austic. 1978. Influence of dietary potassium on lysine metabolism in the chick. *J. Nutr.* **108**:137.

Supplee, W. C. and G. F. Combs. 1959. Studies of the potassium requirement of turkey poults fed purified diets. *Poult. Sci.* **38**:833.

Supplee, W. C. 1965. Observations on the requirement of young turkeys for dietary potassium. *Poult. Sci.* **44**:1142.

van Eys, J. E. and R. L. Reid. 1987. Ruminal solubility of nitrogen and minerals from fescue and fescue-red clover herbage. *J. Anim. Sci.* **65**:1101.

14

SELENIUM BIOAVAILABILITY

Pamela R. Henry
Clarence B. Ammerman

Department of Animal Science
University of Florida
Gainesville, Florida

I. INTRODUCTION

Early interest in selenium resulted from its role as a toxic element. Signs of selenium toxicosis in horses were recorded in the travel journals of Marco Polo and by a U.S. Army surgeon at Fort Randall, Nebraska Territory in 1857 (Madison, 1860). Selenium was finally reported to be an essential element in the prevention of liver necrosis in rats (Schwarz and Foltz, 1957) and exudative diathesis in chicks (Patterson et al., 1957). Eggert et al. (1957) found that selenium prevented hepatosis diatetica in swine, and white muscle disease in young ruminants was also alleviated with selenium supplementation (Muth et al., 1958; Hogue, 1958).

Selenium was identified by Rotruck et al. (1973) as an integral part of the enzyme glutathione peroxidase (GSH-Px), which destroys lipid peroxides and functions by protecting cell membranes against peroxidative damage. The element's role as a component of the transport protein, liver selenoprotein-P was reported by Burk and Gregory (1982). A monomeric selenium-containing phospholipid hydroperoxide glutathione peroxidase was discovered by Ursisi et al. (1985) and was proposed by Sunde et al. (1993) to be the primary selenium-containing antioxidant enzyme. Most recently, selenium was identified as a component of 5'-iodothyronine deiodinase which converts tetra- to triiodothyronine and functions in nonshivering thermoregulation (Behne et al., 1992).

Selenium deficiency is a serious problem in livestock worldwide. Severe deficiencies can be found in Finland, New Zealand, China, the United States, and Japan, but areas of selenium toxicity can also be found in China, the United States, and other areas of the world. Because of selenium's long history of toxicity, supplementation of the element for domestic livestock with inorganic sources was not approved in the United States until the late 1970s. Selenium was noted to be essential for humans when its role in prevention of Keshan disease, a cardiomyopathy, was reported by Chinese scientists (NRC, 1989). At the present time, bioavailability of various selenium sources is somewhat of a moot point because only sodium selenite and sodium selenate can be used legally as supplemental sources in the United States (AAFCO, 1994).

II. BIOAVAILABILITY STUDIES

Selenomethionine is preferentially incorporated into protein, particularly muscle, *in lieu* of methionine (Beilstein and Whanger, 1986a,b). In animals injected with [^{75}Se]-selenite, most of the ^{75}Se was recovered as [^{75}Se]-selenocysteine, while in those injected with selenomethionine, it was found in that form and was only slowly converted to selenocysteine, the active component of GSH-Px. Selenite is more readily metabolized to the immediate precursors of selenocysteine than are the orally consumed organic forms, including selenocysteine (Sunde and Hoekstra, 1980). Based on immediate utilization for a biological function, selenite is the reference standard most commonly used for evaluation of bioavailability (Gabrielsen and Opstvedt, 1980a,b; Douglass *et al.*, 1981; Alexander *et al.*, 1983; Chansler *et al.*, 1986). The relative activity of pure selenium compounds for biological functions depends, in part, on the criterion of assessment.

A. Selenium Radioisotopes

Essentially all selenium absorption studies have been done *in vivo* with the aid of a radioisotopic tracer. Whole-body retention of ^{75}Se-labeled selenite, selenate, and selenomethionine, as well as both extrinsically and intrinsically labeled soy protein, has been used in the rat to estimate true absorption (Thomson and Stewart, 1973; Mason and Weaver, 1986). The absorption of selenite ranged from 86 to 92% and that of selenomethionine from 89 to 95%. Absorption of selenate and soy protein selenium also ranged from 86 to 95% (Mason and Weaver, 1986). The absorption of selenocystine by rats was 81 compared to 86% for selenomethionine, while the urinary excretion of absorbed Se during the first week after administration of the two compounds was 13.9 and 5.8%, respectively (Thomson *et al.*, 1975b).

Whole body retention of [^{75}Se]-selenomethionine was greater than [^{75}Se]-selenite (Thomson and Stewart, 1973; Mason and Weaver, 1986); liver, testes, and kidney retained more of an oral dose than did lung or blood (Mason and Weaver, 1986).

B. Prevention of Selenium Deficiency Disorders

Selenium deprivation results in several pathological syndromes depending, in part, on the species involved and on vitamin E status. These include liver necrosis in rats, exudative diathesis and pancreatic fibrosis in chicks, white muscle disease in calves and lambs, and eventual death in all species. Schwarz and Foltz (1958) first used the prevention of liver necrosis to compare the bioavailability of various selenium compounds. Combs and Combs (1986) compiled a table of bioavailability values relative to sodium selenite which summarized the extensive experiments of Schwarz and co-workers. Evaluations were made with 291 inorganic and organic selenium sources to determine their efficacy in preventing liver necrosis in vitamin E-deficient rats. Only results from inorganic sources and amino acid complexes are found in Table I (Schwarz and Foltz, 1958).

Schwarz and Fredga (1969) studied aliphatic monoseleno- and diseleno-dicarboxylic acids and found that asymmetric monoseleno-dicarboxylic acids with the general structure R_1-Se-R_2 had bioavailability values less than 30% of sodium selenite. Bioavailability of symmetric monoseleno-dicarboxylic acids (HOOC-$(CH_2)_n$-Se-$(CH_2)_n$-COOH) was less than 20% except for those with an odd number of carbon atoms, starting with 5, which averaged 50 to 80% for 5 and 7 carbon atoms and 130 to 170% for 9 and 11 carbon atoms. In contrast, the symmetric diseleno-dicarboxylic acids (HOOC-$(CH_2)_n$-Se-Se-$(CH_2)_n$-COOH) with 2 to 5 or 9 to 11 carbon atoms were available (96 to 122 and 79 to 110%, respectively), but those with 6 to 8 carbon atoms were relatively inactive (34 to 69%). In branched-chain acids, attaching the selenium atom at carbon position four or five resulted in greater availability than attaching it at carbon two or three. Branching by a single methyl group resulted in a moderate decrease in activity (46 to 100%), while introducing two methyl groups to give a quartenary carbon in the chain greatly depressed activity (<5%). The symmetric diseleno-dicarboxylic acid amides (H_2N-CO-$(CH_2)_n$-Se-Se-$(CH_2)_n$-CO-NH_2) had activity values similar to that of corresponding free monoseleno-dicarboxylic acids.

Generally, odd-numbered carbon chains attached to the selenium atom resulted in greater activity, while even-numbered chains have lower activity in aliphatic seleno-carboxylic acids of the structure CH_3-$(CH_2)_m$-Se-$(CH_2)_n$-COOH (Schwarz and Fredga, 1972a) especially when the selenium atom was located near the center of the molecule. Alkyl residues of three or four carbons strongly depressed activity. The corresponding acid amides were more potent than free acids for compounds with one selenium atom.

Compounds with odd-numbered carbon chains were also more potent than even-numbered chains for the 2,4-dinitrophenylseleno-carboxylic acids. Activity was

170% or greater for odd-numbered chains of more than four carbons for the benzylseleno-*n*-carboxylic acids (Schwarz and Fredga, 1972b).

The symmetrical straigt chain dialkyl monoselenides with the general formula $CH_3-(CH_2)_n-Se-(CH_2)_n-CH_3$ have low activity with 2 to 4 carbon atoms and with 5 or more, those with odd-numbered chains are more active than the even-numbered (Schwarz *et al.*, 1974). The diselenides with similar structure are slightly active with 2, 3, or more than 13 carbon units, and for those with 5 to 12 carbons, those with an odd number are more potent.

Regarding the diselenides of alcohols and amines (Schwarz and Fredga, 1974), like carboxylic acids, a methyl group adjacent to the selenium atom depressed activity, while those with a quarternary carbon atom had no activity. The diselenides of aliphatic and heterocyclic amines also had low activity. However, monoseleno-ketones with the ketone oxygen in the β or γ position to the selenium atom had good activity.

Liver necrosis in rats and exudative diathesis in chicks have been used to compare sodium selenite to the selenium of alfalfa grown under different agronomic conditions with that of sodium selenite (Mathias *et al.*, 1965). Since vitamin E interacts with selenium in the prevention of these disorders, it is necessary to keep the vitamin E level low and constant in such assays. Cantor *et al.* (1975a) fed chicks graded levels of selenium and used the prevention of exudative diathesis as an index of selenium bioavailability. They used a basal diet low in both selenium and vitamin E and extracted the feedstuffs with hexane to remove vitamin E. Feedstuffs of both plant and animal origin were compared to selenite at levels of 20, 40, and 60 ppb. When compared to the standard response curve, selenium of plant-derived feedstuffs was highly available, ranging from 60 to 90%; that of animal origin was less than 25% available. On average, selenomethionine was 38% as potent in this assay as selenite but the variation was wide. Osman and Latshaw (1976) also found selenomethionine less effective than selenite or selenocystine in the prevention of exudative diathesis.

For the prevention of exudative diathesis in chicks, quadrivalent selenium is most active; hexavalent selenium is about 70% as potent. While selenomethionine is the predominant form of selenium in natural products, its activity in preventing exudative diathesis is approximately 38% of that of selenite; similar relationships were found for the restoration of GSH-Px activity (Cantor *et al.*, 1975a). While this general difference has been found by others (Osman and Latshaw, 1976; Gabrielson and Opstvedt, 1980b), some investigators (Omaye and Tappel, 1974) have observed little or no difference in the activity of the two compounds for support of GSH-Px activity.

Prevention of pancreatic fibrosis has been used to measure the efficacy of various selenium sources (Cantor *et al.*, 1975b). This syndrome has the advantage that it is specific for Se, vitamin E being essentially inactive. Using a crystalline amino acid diet that contained 12 ppb selenium and 15 IU/kg of vitamin E, it was found that addition of selenomethionine or wheat protected against pancreatic damage at 20 ppb selenium, while 80 ppb was required for selenium in the form of selenite or tuna. It appears that protection against pancreatic fibrosis, as an index, gives a distinctly different comparison of selenium sources than does exudative diathesis. For the prevention of pancreatic fibrosis in chicks, the selenium in selenomethionine proved to be considerably more active than that in selenite.

C. Glutathione Peroxidase Activity

Rotruck et al. (1973) first showed that a major biochemical role of selenium is as a component of GSH-Px. Soon Omaye and Tappel (1974) found a semilogarithmic relationship between GSH-Px activity in several chick tissues and the amount of dietary selenium. Since this is the most important biochemical function of selenium in vertebrates, GSH-Px activity is considered one of the best indices of selenium status and utilization. It has the advantage that it is not affected directly by vitamin E and can be measured quantitatively.

Gabrielson and Opstvedt (1980a) used slope ratios of the plasma GSH-Px activity in chicks to compare bioavailablity of selenium in fish meal to that of sodium selenite (Table I). The method was found to provide statistically valid data over a range of 20 to 100 ppb added selenium. Fish meal selenium had low bioavailability, less than 50%, while that of selenomethionine was 78% that of selenite (100%). The bioavailability of selenium in raw and processed tuna, as well as that in wheat flour and bread, has been determined by a similar method using the rat (Alexander et al., 1983). A standard curve assay based on restoration of erythrocyte GSH-Px activity was used to evaluate selenium bioavailability in tuna, kidney, and wheat (Douglass et al., 1981). Rats were depleted for 4 weeks, then fed 100, 200, or 300 ppb selenium as selenite to establish the reponse curve, while test sources were supplied at 200 ppb. In both studies, tuna selenium was less available than that of wheat. A variation of the slope ratio assay based on GSH-Px activity in the growing rat involved measurement of activity in the milk of lactating dams and in the pups' red blood cells (Smith and Picciano, 1987). In contrast to most GSH-Px-based assays, both yeast selenium and selenomethionine were appreciably more active than selenite selenium.

D. Tissue Selenium Concentrations

Tissue concentrations of selenium after dietary repletion have been used for quantitative evaluation of bioavailability (Table I). Although the estimates obtained agree qualitatively with those based on GSH-Px activity, they tend to give greater values relative to sodium selenite. This probably arises from the fact that most selenium in natural products occurs as selenomethionine (Beilstein and Whanger, 1986a). Furthermore, selenomethionine selenium was retained to a greater extent in tissues of lambs (Ehlig *et al.*, 1967), rats (Cary *et al.*, 1973; Mason and Weaver, 1986), and chicks (Miller *et al.*, 1972). Tissue selenium concentrations following plethoric dosing with inorganic sources have also been used to estimate bioavailability of the element for chicks (Echevarria *et al.*, 1988) and lambs (Henry *et al.*, 1988). In studies conducted with plethoric dietary concentrations, elemental selenium appeared to have 50 to 97% the bioavailability of sodium selenite, while this source was generally unavailable when selenium-deficient diets were fed and GSH-Px or exudative diathesis was the response criterion.

E. Slow Release Ruminal Boluses

Several forms of slow release ruminal boluses are used in various locations worldwide for selenium supplementation of grazing livestock. Compressed pellets containing sodium selenite, barium selenate, and calcium selenate were more effective in raising selenium status of sheep than elemental selenium (Kuchel and Buckley, 1969; Langlands *et al.*, 1990a). Sustained release (Hidiroglou *et al.*, 1985; Koh and Judson, 1987; Lawson *et al.*, 1990; 1991; Donald *et al.*, 1993) and soluble glass boluses (Carlos *et al.*, 1985; Care *et al.*, 1985; Judson *et al.*, 1985; Petterson *et al.*, 1985; Buckley *et al.*, 1987; Hidiroglou *et al.*, 1987; Koh and Judson, 1987; Langlands *et al.*, 1990b) have been shown to increase blood and liver concentrations of selenium and GSH-Px in cattle and sheep.

III. FACTORS INFLUENCING BIOAVAILABILITY

In contrast to the cationic elements, selenium bioavailability is not affected appreciably by chelation, but it is affected by interaction with other elements.

A. Metal-Ion Interactions

Metabolic interactions occur between selenium and iron, copper, zinc, cadmium, mercury, silver, arsenic, and others, but the concentrations required exceed those commonly found in feedstuffs by as much as 1000-fold (Hill, 1976). The exudative diathesis induced in chicks by silver ions was alleviated by selenium supplementation (Peterson and Jensen, 1975). Both exudative diathesis and muscular dystrophy induced by high copper (800 to 1600 ppm) and zinc (2000 to 4000 ppm) were prevented by addition of .5 ppm selenium (Jensen, 1975). Rahim *et al.* (1986) found no effect on whole-body retention or tissue distribution of [^{75}Se]-selenite fed or injected in rats also supplemented with copper (1-200 ppm), iron (20-500 ppm), cadmium (.02-5 ppm), molybdenum (.3-50 ppm), and manganese (.2-200 ppm). At 200 ppm, copper reduced GSH-Px activity in blood, liver, kidney, and testis.

B. Other Dietary Components

The bioavailability of selenium in natural products differs widely, ranging from high (100% compared to selenite) in Brazil nuts to low (<15%) in mushrooms (Chansler *et al.*, 1986). Wheat and its by-products have high selenium availability, while tuna and fish meals have low bioavailability (Douglass *et al.*, 1981; Alexander *et al.*, 1983; Gabrielson and Opstvedt, 1980b). The basis of these differences is not clear. In general, selenomethionine is less available than selenite and it is the chief selenium component of most feedstuffs. Other selenium compounds, such as selenocystathionine, as well as selenium inhibitors, may be present. No evidence of an inhibitor was found in the mushrooms that had low bioavailability (Chansler *et al.*, 1986).

The nature and quantity of dietary protein plays a role in selenium absorption and utilization. Supplemental methionine increased the biopotency of selenomethionine when methionine was limiting, but it was without effect on selenite (Sunde *et al.*, 1981b; Waschulewski and Sunde, 1988). Zhou and Combs (1984) fed chicks two levels of protein, 16.9 and 22.5%, supplemented with selenite and selenomethionine. The low protein diet resulted in a lower incidence of exudative diathesis, and thus, of greater apparent bioavailability from both sources. Dietary restriction with the same daily intake of selenium also reduced exudative diathesis.

Antioxidants decrease the incidence of exudative diathesis and increase the activity of plasma GSH-Px. Ethoxyquin also appeared to increase selenium utilization without affecting vitamin E function (Combs and Scott, 1974). Absorbic acid enhanced potency of selenite and selenate, apparently increasing both absorption and utilization (Combs and Pesti, 1976). It is not clear how antioxidants increased selenium utilization, but certainly selenium was reduced before incorporation into selenocysteine. The antioxidants, being reducing agents, may have promoted that process.

IV. SUMMARY

Bioavailability estimates for selenium sources vary based on the criterion used in the assessment (Table II).   The greatest discrepancy occurs between sources containing selenium as selenite compared to selenomethionine, due to a difference in the manner in which they are metabolized to selenocysteine for incorporation into GSH-Px. In addition, selenomethionine can be incorporated directly into body proteins and stored as such, thereby inflating bioavailability estimates based on body retention. In general, selenium in animal products is 60 to 90% as bioavailable as sodium selenite, while the selenium in plant products averages 25% or less. Elemental selenium is unavailable when selenium-deficient diets are fed and GSH-Px or exudative diathesis is the response criterion.   In studies utilizing plethoric dosing, however, elemental selenium is 50 to 95% as available as sodium selenite. Sodium selenite and sodium selenate are the only supplemental selenium sources currently approved for use in the United States and both are highly available forms. Several kinds of slow release boluses have been used for supplementation of ruminants.

Table I. Bioavailability of selenium sources for animals[a]

Source	RV	Standard	Response criterion	Meth cal	Type diet	Added level, ppm	Reference
Chickens							
Alfalfa	75	Sodium selenite	ED	-	P	.05	Mathias et al. (1965)
Alfalfa meal	83	Sodium selenite	Egg yolk Se	TP	N-.08 ppm	.1	Martello and Latshaw (1982)
Alfalfa meal (.21 ppm Se)	210	Sodium selenite	ED[b]	-	P-.02-.04 ppm	.02, .04, .06, .08	Cantor et al. (1975a)
Barley (.16 ppm)	113	Sodium selenite	ED[b]	-	P-.01 ppm	.01 - .08	Seier and Bragg (1973)
Beef, cooked	35	Sodium selenite	WB GSH-Px	TP	SP	.03	Laws et al. (1986)
Beef, cooked	94	Sodium selenite	Egg yolk Se	TP	N-.045 ppm	.1	Laws et al. (1986)
Beef, raw	55	Sodium selenite	WB GSH-Px	TP	SP	.03	Laws et al. (1986)
Beef, raw	67	Sodium selenite	Egg yolk Se	TP	N-.045 ppm	.1	Laws et al. (1986)
Brewers grains (.7 ppm Se)	80	Sodium selenite	ED[b]	-	P-.02-.04 ppm	.02, .04, .06, .08	Cantor et al. (1975a)
Brewers yeast (1.5 ppm Se)	89	Sodium selenite	ED[b]	-	P-.02-.04 ppm	.02, .04, .06, .08	Cantor et al. (1975a)
Calcium selenite (3CaSeO₃·4H₂O) (41.4% Se)	95	Na₂SeO₃ RG	Liv Se	SR	N-.18 ppm	3, 6, 9	Echevarria et al. (1988)
3CaSeO₃·4H₂O	113	Na₂SeO₃ RG	Kid Se	SR	N-.18 ppm	3, 6, 9	Echevarria et al. (1988)

Table I. (continued)

Source	RV	Standard	Response criterion	Meth cal	Type diet	Added level, ppm	Reference
Chicken, raw	82	Sodium selenite	Egg yolk Se	TP	N-.045 ppm	.1	Laws et al. (1986)
Corn (1.0 ppm Se)	86	Sodium selenite	ED[b]	-	P-.02-.04 ppm	.02, .04, .06, .08	Cantor et al. (1975a)
Corn (.30 ppm Se)	46	Na_2SeO_3	ED[b]	SR	P	.03, .06, .09	Combs et al. (1980)
Corn gluten meal	26	$NaHSeO_3$	WB GSH-Px	SR	SP-.04 ppm	.02, .04, .06, .08, .10, .12	Gabrielsen and Opstvedt (1980b)
Cottonseed meal (.96 ppm Se)	86	Sodium selenite	ED[b]	-	P-.02-.04 ppm	.02, .04, .06, .08	Cantor et al. (1975a)
Distiller's dried grains + solubles (.32 ppm Se)	65	Sodium selenite	ED[b]	-	P-.02-.04 ppm	.02, .04, .06, .08	Cantor et al. (1975a)
Fish, lyophilized	38	Sodium selenite	WB GSH-Px	TP	SP	.03	Laws et al. (1986)
Fish, dried	38	Sodium selenite	WB GSH-Px	TP	SP	.03	Laws et al., 1986
Fish meal	41	$NaHSeO_3$	WB GSH-Px	SR	SP-.04 ppm	.02, .04, .06, .08, .10, .12	Gabrielsen and Opstvedt (1980a)
Fish meal	60	$NaHSeO_3$	WB GSH-Px	SR	SP-.04 ppm	.02, .04, .06, .08, .10, .12	Gabrielsen and Opstvedt (1980a)
Fish meal	36	$NaHSeO_3$	WB GSH-Px	SR	SP-.04 ppm	.02, .04, .06, .08, .10, .12	Gabrielsen and Opstvedt (1980a)
Fish meal	32	$NaHSeO_3$	WB GSH-Px	SR	SP-.04 ppm	.02, .04, .06, .08, .10, .12	Gabrielsen and Opstvedt (1980a)
Fish meal, capelin	48	$NaHSeO_3$	WB GSH-Px	SR	SP-.04 ppm	.02, .04, .06, .08, .10, .12	Gabrielsen and Opstvedt (1980b)

Ingredient	No.	Source	Criterion		Supplementation	Se levels	Reference
Fish meal, mackerel	34	NaHSeO$_3$	WB GSH-Px	SR	SP-.04 ppm	.02, .04, .06, .08, .10, .12	Gabrielsen and Opstvedt (1980b)
Fish meal, pressed cake, sprat & small herring	59	NaHSeO$_3$	Pla GSH-Px	SR	SP-.04 ppm	.04, .08, .12	Huque and Jensen (1985)
Fish meal, sprat & whiting (2.0 ppm Se)	77	NaHSeO$_3$	Pla GSH-Px	SR	SP-.04 ppm	.04, .08, .12	Huque and Jensen (1985)
Fish meal, partly decomposed whiting & herring (2.54 ppm Se)	51	NaHSeO$_3$	Pla GSH-Px	SR	SP-.04 ppm	.04, .08, .12	Huque and Jensen (1985)
Fish meal	93	Sodium selenite	Whole body Se	TP	P	.05, .10	Miller et al. (1972)
Fish meal	45	Sodium selenite	Egg yolk Se	TP	N-.08 ppm	.1	Martello and Latshaw (1982)
Fish meal, menhaden (2.6 ppm Se)	16	Sodium selenite	ED[b]	-	P-.02-.04 ppm	.02, .04, .06, .08	Cantor et al. (1975a)
Fish meal, herring (3.6 ppm Se)	25	Sodium selenite	ED[b]	-	P-.02-.04 ppm	.02, .04, .06, .08	Cantor et al. (1975a)
Fish meal, menhaden, (2.33 ppm Se)	48	Na$_2$SeO$_3$	ED	-	SP-.03 ppm	.03	Whitacre and Latshaw (1982)
Fish meal, menhaden, lyophilized (2.04 ppm Se)	140	Na$_2$SeO$_3$	ED	-	SP-.03 ppm	.03	Whitacre and Latshaw (1982)
Fish meal	70	Sodium selenite	Egg yolk Se	TP	N-.045 ppm	.1	Laws et al. (1986)
Fish solubles	67	Sodium selenite	Whole Body Se	TP	P	.05, .10	Miller et al. (1972)
Fish solubles (2.1 ppm Se)	9	Sodium selenite	ED[b]	-	P-.02-.04 ppm	.02, .04, .06, .08	Cantor et al. (1975a)

Table I. (continued)

Source	RV	Standard	Response criterion	Meth cal	Type diet	Added level, ppm	Reference
Meat and bone meal (.69 ppm Se)	15	Sodium selenite	ED[b]	-	P-.02-.04 ppm	.02, .04, .06, .08	Cantor et al. (1975a)
Milk, cow, high Se (.28 ppm)	132	Sodium selenite	ED	MR	P	.028	Mathias et al. (1967)
Oats	76	Sodium selenite	Egg yolk Se	TP	N-.045 ppm	.1	Laws et al. (1986)
Poultry by-product meal	50	Na_2SeO_3	ED	-	P	.02, .04	Scott and Cantor (1971)
Poultry by-product meal (1.7 ppm Se)	18	Sodium selenite	ED[b]	-	P-.02-.04 ppm	.02, .04, .06, .08	Cantor et al. (1975a)
Se, elemental (99.9% Se)	97	Na_2SeO_3 RG	Liv Se	SR	N-.18 ppm	3, 6, 9	Echevarria et al. (1988)
Se, elemental (99.9% Se)	55	Na_2SeO_3 RG	Kid Se	SR	N-.18 ppm	3, 6, 9	Echevarria et al. (1988)
Se, elemental	7	Sodium selenite	ED[b]	-	P-.02-.04 ppm	.02, .04, .06, .08	Cantor et al. (1975a)
Selenocystine	122	Sodium selenite	Yolk Se	TP	N-.07 ppm	.1	Latshaw and Osman (1975)
Selenocystine	89	Sodium selenite	App abs	TP	N-.07 ppm	.1	Latshaw and Osman (1975)
Seleno-DL-cystine	110	Sodium selenite	Panc fib	-	P	.02, .04	Cantor et al. (1975b)
Seleno-DL-cystine	74	Sodium selenite	ED[b]	-	P-.02-.04 ppm	.02, .04, .06, .08	Cantor et al. (1975a)
Seleno-DL-cystine	98	Na_2SeO_3	Liv Se	TP	SP-.03 ppm	.06	Osman and Latshaw (1976)
Seleno-DL-cystine	110	Na_2SeO_3	Kid Se	TP	SP-.03 ppm	.06	Osman and Latshaw (1976)
Selenodicysteine	100	Na_2SeO_3	ED	MR	P	.2	Jenkins et al. (1970)
Selenodicysteine	100	Sodium selenite	Pla GSH-Px	SR	N-.03-.04 ppm	.05, .1, .15	Cantor et al. (1983)

				SR			
Selenodicysteine	91	Sodium selenite	Liv Se	SR	N-.03-.04 ppm	.05, .1, .15	Cantor et al. (1983)
Seleno-DL-ethionine	44	Sodium selenite	ED[b]	-	P-.02 - .04 ppm	.02, .04, .06, .08	Cantor et al. (1975a)
Selenomethionine	119	Sodium selenite	Pla GSH-Px	MR	P-.02 ppm	.1	Omaye and Tappel (1974)
Selenomethionine	73	Sodium selenite	RBC GSH-Px	MR	P-.02 ppm	.1	Omaye and Tappel (1974)
Selenomethionine	125	Sodium selenite	Liv GSH-Px	MR	P-.02 ppm	.1	Omaye and Tappel (1974)
Selenomethionine	72	Sodium selenite	Yolk Se	TP	N-.07 ppm	.1	Latshaw and Osman (1975)
Selenomethionine	115	Sodium selenite	App abs	TP	N-.07 ppm	.1	Latshaw and Osman (1975)
Selenomethionine	169	Sodium selenite	Egg prod	TP	N-.027 ppm	.1	Cantor and Scott (1974)
Selenomethionine	97	Sodium selenite	Hat eggs	TP	N-.027 ppm	.1	Cantor and Scott (1974)
Selenomethionine	103	Sodium selenite	Egg Se	TP	N-.027 ppm	.1	Cantor and Scott (1974)
Selenomethionine	118	Sodium selenite	Liv Se	TP	N-.08 ppm	.1	Abdel-Ati et al. (1984)
Selenomethionine	107	Sodium selenite	Kid Se	TP	N-.08 ppm	.1	Abdel-Ati et al. (1984)
Selenomethionine	46	Sodium selenite	Pla GSH-Px	TP	P	SOD-5 μg	Bunk and Combs (1980)
Selenomethionine	117	Sodium selenite	Liv GSH-Px	TP	P	SOD-5 μg	Bunk and Combs (1980)
Selenomethionine	53	Sodium selenite	WB GSH-Px	TP	SP	.03	Laws et al. (1986)
Selenomethionine	105	Sodium selenite	^{75}Se upt	MR	N	Intraluminal SOD	Mykkanen and Humaloja (1984)

Table I. (continued)

Source	RV	Standard	Response criterion	Meth cal	Type diet	Added level, ppm	Reference
Selenomethionine	108	Sodium selenite	^{75}Se upt	MR	N	Intraluminal SOD	Mykkanen and Mutanen (1986)
Selenomethionine	133	Sodium selenite	Whole body Se	TP	P	.05, .10	Miller et al. (1972)
Selenomethionine	95	Sodium selenite	Egg yolk Se	TP	N-.08 ppm	.1	Martello and Latshaw (1982)
Selenomethionine	78	$NaHSeO_3$	WB GSH-Px	SR	SP-.04 ppm	.02, .04, .06, .08, .10, .12	Gabrielsen and Opstvedt (1980b)
Selenomethionine	88	Sodium selenite	Egg yolk Se	TP	N-.045 ppm	.1	Laws et al. (1986)
Seleno-L-methionine	124	Na_2SeO_3	Se^{75} upt	MR	P	SOD	Humaloja and Mykkanen (1986)
Seleno-DL-methionine	60	Na_2SeO_3	Pla GSH-Px	TP	P <.02 ppm	.03, .06, .09	Zhou and Combs (1984)
Seleno-DL-methionine	53	Sodium selenite	Pla GSH-Px	SR	P	.02, .04, .06	Noguchi et al. (1973)
Seleno-DL-methionine	213	Sodium selenite	Panc fib	-	P	.02, .04	Cantor et al. (1975b)
Seleno-DL-methionine	37	Sodium selenite	ED^b	-	P-.02 - .04 ppm	.02, .04, .06, .08	Cantor et al. (1975a)
Seleno-DL-methionine	84	Na_2SeO_3	Liv Se	TP	SP-.03 ppm	.06	Osman and Latshaw (1976)
Seleno-DL-methionine	87	Na_2SeO_3	Kid Se	TP	SP-.03 ppm	.06	Osman and Latshaw (1976)
6 - Selenopurine	20	Sodium selenite	ED^b	-	P-.02 - .04 ppm	.02, .04, .06, .08	Cantor et al. (1975a)

Selenoyeast (131 ppm)	100	Na₂SeO₃	ED	-	NG-.02 ppm	SOD-1.4 µg/100g BW	Combs et al. (1984)
Selenoyeast (131 ppm)	61	Na₂SeO₃	Plasma GSH-Px	-	NG-.02 ppm	SOD-1.4 µg/100g BW	Combs et al. (1984)
Na₂SeO₄ (41.8% Se)	117	Na₂SeO₃ RG	Liv Se	SR	N-.18 ppm	3, 6, 9	Echevarria et al. (1988)
Na₂SeO₄	123	Na₂SeO₃ RG	Kid Se	SR	N-.18 ppm	3, 6, 9	Echevarria et al. (1988)
Sodium selenate	74	Sodium selenite	ED[b]	-	P-.02 - .04 ppm	.02, .04, .06, .08	Cantor et al. (1975a)
Sodium selenate	104	Sodium selenite	75Se upt	MR	N	Intraluminal SOD	Mykkanen and Mutanen (1986)
Sodium selenide	42	Sodium selenite	ED[b]	-	P-.02 - .04 ppm	.02, .04, .06, .08	Cantor et al. (1975a)
Na₂SeO₃ + fumed amorphous carrier (29.3% Se)	92	Na₂SeO₃ RG	Liv Se	SR	N-.18 ppm	3, 6, 9	Echevarria et al. (1988)
Na₂SeO₃ + fumed amorphous carrier	104	Na₂SeO₃ RG	Kid Se	SR	N-.18 ppm	3, 6, 9	Echevarria et al. (1988)
Soybean meal (.44 ppm Se)	60	Sodium selenite	ED[b]	-	P-.02 - .04 ppm	.02, .04, .06, .08	Cantor et al. (1975a)
Soybean meal	73	Sodium selenite	Egg yolk Se	TP	N-.08 ppm	.1	Martello and Latshaw (1982)
Soybean meal	18	NaHSeO₃	WB GSH-Px	SR	SP-.04 ppm	.02, .04, .06, .08, .10, .12	Gabrielsen and Opstvedt (1980b)
Swine kidney	53	Sodium selenite	Egg yolk Se	TP	N-.08 ppm	.1	Martello and Latshaw (1982)
Tuna	48	Sodium selenite	Egg yolk Se	TP	N-.045 ppm	.1	Laws et al. (1986)
Tuna meal	40	Na₂SeO₃	ED	-	P	.02, .04	Scott and Cantor (1971)

Table I. (continued)

Source	RV	Standard	Response criterion	Meth cal	Type diet	Added level, ppm	Reference
Tuna meal (5 ppm Se)	22	Sodium selenite	ED[b]	-	P-.02 - .04 ppm	.02, .04, .06, .08	Cantor et al. (1975a)
Wheat (.58 ppm)	65	Sodium selenite	ED[b]	TP	P-.01 ppm	.01 - .08	Seier and Bragg (1973)
Wheat (.20 - .29 ppm)	96	Sodium selenite	ED[b]	TP	P-.01 ppm	.01 - .08	Seier and Bragg (1973)
Wheat (.09 ppm)	161	Sodium selenite	ED[b]	TP	P-.01 ppm	.01 - .08	Seier and Bragg (1973)
Wheat	100	Na_2SeO_3	ED	-	P	.02, .04	Scott and Cantor (1971)
Wheat (2.0 ppm)	71	Sodium selenite	ED[b]	TP	P-.02 - .04 ppm	.02, .04, .06, .08	Cantor et al. (1975a)
Wheat flakes	48	Sodium selenite	Egg yolk Se	TP	N-.045 ppm	.1	Laws et al. (1986)
Yeast	106	Sodium selenite	Egg yolk Se	TP	N-.045 ppm	.1	Laws et al. (1986)

Turkeys

Source	RV	Standard	Response criterion	Meth cal	Type diet	Added level, ppm	Reference
Fish meal, menhaden (2.95 ppm Se)	36	Na_2SeO_3	Pla Se	TP	SP-.05 ppm	.1	Cantor and Tarino (1982)
Fish meal, menhaden (2.95 ppm Se)	46	Na_2SeO_3	Pla GSH-Px	TP	SP-.05 ppm	.1	Cantor and Tarino (1982)
Seleno-DL-cystine	118	Na_2SeO_3	Pla Se	TP	SP-.05 ppm	.2	Cantor and Tarino (1982)
Seleno-DL-cystine	123	Na_2SeO_3	WB Se	TP	SP-.05 ppm	.2	Cantor and Tarino (1982)
Seleno-DL-cystine	147	Na_2SeO_3	Pla GSH-Px	TP	SP-.05 ppm	.2	Cantor and Tarino (1982)
Seleno-DL-ethionine	93	Na_2SeO_3	Pla Se	TP	SP-.05 ppm	.2	Cantor and Tarino (1982)
Seleno-DL-ethionine	121	Na_2SeO_3	WB Se	TP	SP-.05 ppm	.2	Cantor and Tarino (1982)

Seleno-DL-ethionine	70	Na_2SeO_3	Pla GSH-Px	TP	SP-.05 ppm	.2	Cantor and Tarino (1982)
Seleno-DL-methionine	127	Na_2SeO_3	Pla Se	TP	SP-.05 ppm	.2	Cantor and Tarino (1982)
Seleno-DL-methionine	159	Na_2SeO_3	WB Se	TP	SP-.05 ppm	.2	Cantor and Tarino (1982)
Seleno-DL-methionine	78	Na_2SeO_3	Pla GSH-Px	TP	SP-.05 ppm	.2	Cantor and Tarino (1982)
Seleno-DL-methionine	124	Na_2SeO_3	Pla Se	TP	SP-.05 ppm	.04, .08, .12	Cantor et al. (1982)
Seleno-DL-methionine	97	Na_2SeO_3	Pla GSH-Px	TP	SP-.05 ppm	.04, .08, .12	Cantor et al. (1982)
Seleno-DL-methionine	101	Na_2SeO_3	Liv Se	TP	SP-.05 ppm	.04, .08, .12	Cantor et al. (1982)
Sodium selenate Na_2SeO_4	141	Na_2SeO_3	Pla Se	TP	SP-.05 ppm	.2	Cantor and Tarino (1982)
Na_2SeO_4	126	Na_2SeO_3	WB Se	TP	SP-.05 ppm	.2	Cantor and Tarino (1982)
Na_2SeO_4	220	Na_2SeO_3	Pla GSH-Px	TP	SP-.05 ppm	.2	Cantor and Tarino (1982)

Swine

Brewers grains (.7 ppm Se)	80	Sodium selenite	Liv Se	TP	N	.1	Mahan and Moxon (1978)
Brewers grains (.7 ppm Se)	79	Sodium selenite	Kid Se	TP	N	.1	Mahan and Moxon (1978)
Brewers grains	119	Sodium selenite	Liv Se	MR	N	.1, .4	Mahan and Moxon (1978)
Brewers grains	106	Sodium selenite	Kid Se	MR	N	.1, .4	Mahan and Moxon (1978)
Calcium selenite RG (47.4% Se)	102	Sodium selenite	Ser GSH-Px	MR	N	.3, 5.0, 15.0	Mahan and Magee (1991)
Calcium selenite RG	100	Sodium selenite	Liv & kid Se	MR	N	.3, 5.0, 15.0	Mahan and Magee (1991)
Clover, white (Melilotus alba) (70 ppm Se)	66	Na_2SeO_3	WB Se	TP	N-.06 ppm	3.5, 7.0	Mandisodza et al. (1979)

319

Table I. (continued)

Source	RV	Standard	Response criterion	Meth cal	Type diet	Added level, ppm	Reference
Clover, white	115	Na$_2$SeO$_3$	Liv Se	TP	N-.06 ppm	3.5, 7.0	Mandisodza et al. (1979)
Clover, white	167	Na$_2$SeO$_3$	Kid Se	TP	N-.06 ppm	3.5, 7.0	Mandisodza et al. (1979)
Corn (25 ppm Se)	89	Sodium selenite	App abs	MR	N-.04 ppm	.2	Groce et al. (1973)
Corn (25 ppm Se)	59	Sodium selenite	Ser Se	MR	N-.04 ppm	.2	Groce et al. (1973)
Distillers grains + solubles (.33 ppm Se)	70	Sodium selenite	Liv Se	TP	N	.1	Mahan and Moxon (1978)
Distillers grains + solubles	68	Sodium selenite	Kid Se	TP	N	.1	Mahan and Moxon (1978)
Fish meal, menhaden (2.6 ppm Se)	53	Sodium selenite	Liv Se	TP	N	.1	Mahan and Moxon (1978)
Fish meal, menhaden	57	Sodium selenite	Kid Se	TP	N	.1	Mahan and Moxon (1978)
Fish meal, menhaden	86	Sodium selenite	Liv Se	MR	N	.1, .4	Mahan and Moxon (1978)
Fish meal, menhaden	96	Sodium selenite	Kid Se	MR	N	.1, .4	Mahan and Moxon (1978)
Selenomethionine	102	Sodium selenite	App abs	MR	SP	.11	Parsons et al. (1985)
Selenomethionine (.12 mg/day)	153	Sodium selenite (.18 mg/d)	Liv Se	MR	SP	-	Parsons et al. (1985)
Selenomethionine	141	Sodium selenite	GSH-Px	MR	SP	-	Parsons et al. (1985)
Selenomethionine	100	Sodium selenite	Pla GSH-Px	MR	N	.3	Sankari (1985)

Cattle

Alfalfa cubes (.05 ppm Se)	32[c]	-	App abs	-	N	.43-.53 mg/day	Harrison and Conrad (1984)
Barley	68[d]	-	Int lab	-	N	SOD	Symonds et al. (1981)
Cobalt selenite	103	Sodium selenite	RBC GSH-Px	MR	N-.02 ppm	.5-1.2 mg/day	Pehrson et al. (1989)
Linseed meal (1.2 ppm Se)	131	Sodium selenite	Liv Se	MR	N	.1	Byers and Moxon (1980)
Linseed meal	128	Sodium selenite	Liv Se	MR	N	1.0 mg/day total	Ammerman et al. (1980)
Linseed meal	123	Sodium selenite	Pla Se	MR	N	1.0 mg/day total	Ammerman et al. (1980)
Orchardgrass cubes (.07 ppm Se)	28[c]	-	App abs	-	N	.6-.7 mg/day	Harrison and Conrad (1984)
Selenium-baker's yeast	288	Sodium selenite	RBC GSH-Px	MR	N	.5-1.2 mg/day	Pehrson et al. (1989)
Selenomethionine	246	Sodium selenite	RBC GSH-Px	MR	N	.5-1.2 mg/day	Pehrson et al. (1989)
Timothy, hay, Se-fert 25g/ha (.6 ppm Se)	116	Sodium selenite	WB Se	MR	N-1.25mg/day	3.0 mg/day	Overnes et al. (1986)
Timothy, hay, Se-fert 25g/ha	103	Sodium selenite	WB GSH-Px	MR	N-1.25 mg/day	3.0 mg/day	Overnes et al. (1986)
Timothy, hay, Se-fert 25g/ha	114	Sodium selenite	Liv Se	MR	N-1.25 mg/day	3.0 mg/day	Overnes et al. (1986)

Sheep

Barium selenate	183	Se, elemental	WB Se	TP	N-.03-.05 ppm	Single ruminal pellet	Kuchel and Buckley (1969)
Barium selenate	52	Se, elemental	Liv Se	TP	N-.03-.05 ppm	Single ruminal pellet	Kuchel and Buckley (1969)

Table I. (continued)

Source	RV	Standard	Response criterion	Meth cal	Type diet	Added level, ppm	Reference
Calcium selenate	133	Se, elemental	WB Se	TP	N-.03-.05 ppm	Single ruminal pellet	Kuchel and Buckley (1969)
Calcium selenate	41	Se, elemental	Liv Se	TP	N-.03-.05 ppm	Single ruminal pellet	Kuchel and Buckley (1969)
$3CaSeO_3 \cdot 4H_2O$ RG (41.4% Se)	102	Na_2SeO_3 RG (45.6% Se)	Liv Se	SR	N-.09 ppm	.3	Tarla et al. (1989)
$3CaSeO_3 \cdot 4H_2O$ RG (41.4% Se)	117	Na_2SeO_3 RG	Liv Se	SR	N	6	Henry et al. (1988)
Se, elemental	0	Sodium selenite	WB Se	TP	N	SOD-10, 30 mg	Langlands et al. (1990)
Se, elemental	0	Sodium selenite	GSH-Px	TP	N	SOD-10, 30 mg	Langlands et al. (1990)
Selenomethionine	104	Sodium selenite	WB Se	TP	N-20 µg/day	300 µg/day	Overnes et al. (1986)
Selenomethionine	94	Sodium selenite	GSH-Px	TP	N-20 µg/day	300 µg/day	Overnes et al. (1986)
Selenomethionine	110	Sodium selenite	Liv Se	TP	N-20 µg/day	300 µg/day	Overnes et al. (1986)
Selenomethionine	111	Na_2SeO_3	App abs	MR	N	1	Ehlig et al. (1967)
Selenomethionine	126	Na_2SeO_3	Liv Se	MR	N	1	Ehlig et al. (1967)
Selenomethionine	58	Sodium selenite	Liv GSH-Px	TP	N-.13 ppm	.1	Moksnes and Norheim (1983)
Selenium-yeast (50% L-selenomethionine + selenoglutathione + L-selenocysteine	101	Sodium selenite	WB GSH-Px	MR	N	.1 mg/day	Johansson et al. (1990)

Na$_2$SeO$_4$ (41.8% Se)	117	Na$_2$SeO$_3$ RG (45.6% Se)	Liv Se	SR	N	6	Henry et al. (1988)
Na$_2$SeO$_3$ + fumed amorphous carrier (29.3% Se)	88	Na$_2$SeO$_3$ RG	Liv Se	SR	N	6	Henry et al. (1988)
Timothy, hay, Se-fert 25g/ha (.6 ppm Se)	100	Sodium selenite	WB Se	TP	N-20 µg/day	300 µg/day	Overnes et al. (1986)
Timothy, hay, Se-fert 25g/ha (.6 ppm Se)	86	Sodium selenite	WB GSH-Px	TP	N-20 µg/day	300 µg/day	Overnes et al. (1986)
Timothy, hay, Se-fert 25g/ha (.6 ppm Se)	164	Sodium selenite	Liv Se	TP	N-20 µg/day	300 µg/day	Overnes et al. (1986)
Wheat (9.8 ppm)	283	Sodium selenite	Liv Se	MR	N	1	van Ryssen et al. (1989)
Wheat (9.8 ppm)	101	Sodium selenite	Liv GSH-Px	MR	N	1	van Ryssen et al. (1989)

Rats

Corn	82[c]	-	App abs	-	P	.024-.146	Cary et al. (1973)
Fish, herring	90	Sodium selenite	Liv GSH-Px	SR	SP-.02 ppm	.10,.20	Mutanen et al. (1986b)
Fish, rainbow trout	86	Sodium selenite	App abs	MR	SP-.14 ppm	1.0	Ringdal et al. (1985)
Fish, rainbow trout	119	Sodium selenite	Liv Se	MR	SP-.14 ppm	1.0	Ringdal et al. (1985)
Fish, skipjack, boiled	45	Sodium selenite	Liv GSH-Px	TP	P-.046 ppm	.08	Yoshida et al. (1984)
Fish, skipjack, dried strip	53	Sodium selenite	Liv GSH-Px	TP	P-.046 ppm	.08	Yoshida et al. (1984)
Fish, tuna, raw (1.7 ppm Se)	22	Sodium selenite	Liv GSH-Px	SR	P	.05,.10,.15	Alexander et al. (1983)
Fish, tuna, raw (1.7 ppm Se)	40	Sodium selenite	Kid GSH-Px	SR	P	.05,.10,.15	Alexander et al. (1983)

Table I. (continued)

Source	RV	Standard	Response criterion	Meth cal	Type diet	Added level, ppm	Reference
Fish, tuna, raw (1.7 ppm Se)	43	Sodium selenite	WB GSH-Px	SR	P	.05, .10, .15	Alexander et al. (1983)
Fish, tuna, canned (.16 ppm Se)	32	Sodium selenite	Liv GSH-Px	SR	P	.05, .10, .15	Alexander et al. (1983)
Fish, tuna, canned (.16 ppm Se)	35	Sodium selenite	Kid GSH-Px	SR	P	.05, .10, .15	Alexander et al. (1983)
Fish, tuna, canned (.16 ppm Se)	43	Sodium selenite	WB GSH-Px	SR	P	.05, .10, .15	Alexander et al. (1983)
Fish, tuna, canned (2.9 ppm Se)	57	Sodium selenite	Liv GSH-Px	SR	P	.2	Douglass et al. (1981)
Fish	74[d]	-	Int lab	-	N-.033 ppm	SOD	Richold et al. (1977)
Fish	77[d]	-	Int lab	-	N-.033 ppm	SOD	Richold et al. (1977)
Infant formula, whey-based	95[e]	$Na_2SeO_3 \cdot 5H_2O$	Liv GSH-Px	SR	N-.007 ppm	.025-150	Litov (1987)
Infant formula, casein-based	102[e]	$Na_2SeO_3 \cdot 5H_2O$	Liv GSH-Px	SR	N-.007 ppm	.025-150	Litov (1987)
Infant formula, casein hydrolysate	110[e]	$Na_2SeO_3 \cdot 5H_2O$	Liv GSH-Px	SR	N-.007 ppm	.025-150	Litov (1987)
Infant formula, soy isolate	27[e]	$Na_2SeO_3 \cdot 5H_2O$	Liv GSH-Px	SR	N-.007 ppm	.025-150	Litov (1987)
Kidney	96	Seleno-methionine	Int lab	MR	N-.025 ppm	SOD	Thomson et al. (1975a)
Kidney, beef (5.7 ppm Se)	97	Sodium selenite	Liv GSH-Px	SR	P	.2	Douglass et al. (1981)

Milk, cow's	130	$Na_2SeO_3 \cdot 5H_2O$	Liv GSH-Px	SR	P-.007 ppm	.025-.150	Litov (1987)
Milk, cow's (.43 ppm Se)	87	Sodium selenite	Plasma GSH-Px	SR	P-.015 ppm	.086, .104, .121	Mutanen et al. (1986a)
Milk, cow's (.43 ppm Se)	80	Sodium selenite	Liv GSH-Px	SR	P-.015 ppm	.086, .104, .121	Mutanen et al. (1986a)
Milk, cow's (.67 ppm Se)	74	Sodium selenite	Plasma GSH-Px	SR	P-.015 ppm	.086, .104, .121	Mutanen et al. (1986a)
Milk, cow's (.67 ppm Se)	92	Sodium selenite	Liv GSH-Px	SR	P-.015 ppm	.086, .104, .121	Mutanen et al. (1986a)
Milk, cow's (.28 ppm Se)	66	Sodium selenite	Plasma GSH-Px	SR	P-.015 ppm	.086, .104, .121	Mutanen et al. (1986a)
Milk, cow's (.28 ppm Se)	95	Sodium selenite	Liv GSH-Px	SR	P-.015 ppm	.086, .104, .121	Mutanen et al. (1986a)
Milk (.28 ppm)	144	Sodium selenite	Growth	TP	P	.01	Mathias et al. (1967)
Phenylselenocysteine	34	Sodium selenite	Liv nec	MR	P	.01-10	Schwarz and Foltz (1958)
Potassium selenocyanate	105	Sodium selenite	Liv nec	MR	P	.01-10	Schwarz and Foltz (1958)
Selenic acid	81	Sodium selenite	Liv nec	MR	P	.01-10	Schwarz and Foltz (1958)
Selenium dioxide	69	Sodium selenite	Liv nec	MR	P	.01-10	Schwarz and Foltz (1958)
Selenium, elemental	0	Sodium selenite	Liv nec	MR	P	.01-10	Schwarz and Foltz (1958)
Seleno-amino acid chelate	60	Sodium selenite	WB Se	SR	P	.05, .1, .2	Vinson and Bose (1987)
Seleno-amino acid chelate	88	Sodium selenite	Liv Se	SR	P	.05, .1, .2	Vinson and Bose (1987)
Seleno-DL-cysteine	92	Sodium selenite	Liv nec	MR	P	.01-10	Schwarz and Foltz (1958)
Selenocystine	56	Sodium selenite	Liv GSH-Px	TP	P-.05 ppm	.1, .2	Lane et al. (1991)

Table I. (continued)

Source	RV	Standard	Response criterion	Meth cal	Type diet	Added level, ppm	Reference
Selenocystine	100	Sodium selenite	Liv GSH-Px	TP	P-.035 ppm	.2, 1.0	Sunde et al. (1981a)
Selenocystine	81[c]	-	True abs	-	N-.025	SOD	Thomson et al. (1975b)
Seleno-DL-cystine·HCl	96	Sodium selenite	Liv nec	MR	P	.01-10	Schwarz and Foltz (1958)
Seleno-DL-cystine	93	Sodium selenite	Pla GSH-Px	TP	P-.02 ppm	2	Deagen et al. (1987)
Seleno-DL-cystine	119	Sodium selenite	Liv GSH-Px	TP	P-.02 ppm	2	Deagen et al. (1987)
Selenocystathionine	110	Sodium selenite	Liv nec	MR	P	.01-10	Schwarz and Foltz (1958)
Selenomethionine	76	Sodium selenite	Liv GSH-Px	TP	P-.05 ppm	.1, .2	Lane et al. (1991)
Selenomethionine	89[d]	-	^{75}Se upt	-	P-.16 ppm	SOD	Mason and Weaver (1986)
Selenomethionine	50	Na_2SeO_3	Liv GSH-Px	TP	P-.013 ppm .24% Met	.05, .1, .2, .5	Sunde et al. (1981b)
Selenomethionine	250	$Na_2SeO_3 \cdot 5H_2O$	RBC GSH-Px	SR	P-.025 ppm	.1, .25, .5	Smith and Picciano (1987)
Selenomethionine	87	Sodium selenite	Liv GSH-Px	MR	P-.035 ppm	.2, 1.0	Sunde et al. (1981a)
Selenomethionine	93	Sodium selenite	Liv GSH-Px	TP	P	SOD	Pierce and Tappel (1977)
Selenomethionine	95[c]	-	True abs	-	N-.05 ppm	SOD	Thomson and Stewart (1973)
Selenomethionine	96[c]	-	True abs	-	N-.033 ppm	SOD	Richold et al. (1977)
Selenomethionine	86[c]	-	App abs	-	P	.024-.146	Cary et al. (1973)

Compound	No.	Se source	Tissue	Method	Form	Levels	Reference
Selenomethionine	102	Sodium selenite	Liv GSH-Px	TP	P	2	Yasumoto et al. (1979)
Selenomethionine	58	Sodium selenite	Liv GSH-Px	TP	P	2	Yasumoto et al. 1979
Selenomethionine	86[c]	-	True abs	-	N-.025 ppm	SOD	Thomson et al. (1975b)
Seleno-D-methionine	236	Sodium selenite	Liv Se	TP	N-1 ppm	2.5, 5.0	McAdam and Levander (1987)
Seleno-L-methionine	169	Sodium selenite	Liv Se	TP	P-.1 ppm	2.5, 5.0	McAdam and Levander (1987)
Seleno-L-methionine	151	Na_2SeO_4	Liv Se	MR	P-.3% DL-methionine	.5, 1.5, 2.5	Salbe and Levander (1990)
Seleno-L-methionine	132	Na_2SeO_4	Liv Se	MR	P	.1, .5, 2.5	Salbe and Levander (1990)
Seleno-DL-methionine	202	Sodium selenite	WB GSH-Px	SR	P-.02 ppm	.2, 1.0	Whanger and Butler (1988)
Seleno-DL-methionine	223	Sodium selenite	Liv GSH-Px	SR	P-.02 ppm	.2, 1.0	Whanger and Butler (1988)
Seleno-DL-methionine	96	Sodium selenite	Liv nec	MR	P	.01-10	Schwarz and Foltz (1958)
Seleno-DL-methionine	92	Sodium selenite	Pla GSH-Px	TP	P-.02 ppm	2	Deagen et al. (1987)
Seleno-DL-methionine	101	Sodium selenite	Liv GSH-Px	TP	P-.02 ppm	2	Deagen et al. (1987)
Selenomethionine	86	Sodium selenite	RBC, liv, heart & spleen GSH-Px	SR	P-.03 ppm	.05, .1, .2	L'Abbe and Trick (1991)
Seleno-yeast	120	$Na_2SeO_3 \cdot 5H_2O$	RBC GSH-Px	SR	P-.025 ppm	.1, .25, .5	Smith and Picciano (1987)
Selenoyeast	138	Sodium selenite	WB Se	SR	P	.05, .1, .2	Vinson and Bose (1987)
Selenoyeast	147	Sodium selenite	Liv Se	SR	P	.05, .1, .2	Vinson and Bose (1987)

Table I. (continued)

Source	RV	Standard	Response criterion	Meth cal	Type diet	Added level, ppm	Reference
Shrimp, boiled	73	Sodium selenite	Liv GSH-Px	SR	P-.02 ppm	.10, .20	Mutanen et al. (1986b)
Sodium selenate	122	Sodium selenite	Liv nec	MR	P	.01-10	Schwarz and Foltz (1958)
Sodium selenate	86[d]	-	75Se upt	-	P-.16 ppm	SOD	Mason and Weaver (1986)
Sodium selenate	120	Sodium selenite	Growth	TP	P	5	Ganther and Baumann (1962)
Sodium selenate	83	Sodium selenite	Liver Se	TP	P-.1 ppm	2.5, 5.0	McAdam and Levander (1987)
Sodium selenite	86[d]	-	75Se upt	-	P-.16 ppm	SOD	Mason and Weaver (1986)
Sodium selenite	92[c]	-	True abs	-	N-.05 ppm	SOD	Thomson and Stewart (1973)
Sodium selenite	84[c]	-	True abs	-	N-.033 ppm	SOD	Richold et al. (1977)
Sodium selenite	78[c]	-	App abs	-	P	.024-.146	Cary et al. (1973)
Soy protein isolate	95[d]	-	Int lab	-	P-.16 ppm	SOD	Mason and Weaver (1986)
Soy protein isolate	91[d]	-	Ext lab	-	P-.16 ppm	SOD	Mason and Weaver (1986)
Soy protein isolate	96[d]	-	Ext lab	-	P-.16 ppm	SOD	Mason and Weaver (1986)
Soy protein isolate	92[d]	-	Ext lab	-	P-.16 ppm	SOD	Mason and Weaver (1986)
Wheat	99	Na_2SeO_3	Int lab	MR	P-.2 ppm	4µg	House and Welch (1989)
Wheat (29.3 ppm Se)	83	Sodium selenite	Liv GSH-Px	SR	P	.2	Douglass et al. (1981)
Wheat bran (5.4 ppm Se)	151	Sodium selenite	Liv GSH-Px	SR	P	.05, .10, .15	Alexander et al. (1983)
Wheat bran	134	Sodium selenite	Kid GSH-Px	SR	P	.05, .10, .15	Alexander et al. (1983)

| Wheat bran | 108 | Sodium selenite | WB GSH-Px | SR | P | .05, .10, .15 | Alexander et al. (1983) |

[a]Abbreviations can be found in Appendix I. Chemical formula for a compound given only if provided by the author; RG indicates reagent grade, FG indicates feed grade.

[b]Prevention of exudative diathesis. Calculated as: (Level of Se as Na_2SeO_3 to which test substance corresponds)/(Total level of Se supplied by test substance based on analysis) x 100.

[c]Percentage absorption not relative value.

[d]Percentage of dose not relative value.

[e]Value estimated from figure.

Table II. Relative bioavailability of supplemental selenium sources[a]

Source	Poultry	Swine	Cattle	Sheep	Rats
Sodium selenite	100	100	100	100	100
Calcium selenite	105 (2)	100 (1)	-	110 (2)	-
Cobalt selenite	-	-	105 (1)	-	-
Selenium, elemental	5 (1)[b]	-	-	0 (2)	0 (1)
Selenocystine	110 (9)	-	-	-	95 (6)
Selenodicystine	100 (3)	-	-	-	-
Selenomethionine[c]	80 (12)	120 (2)	-	-	105 (12)
Selenomethionine[d]	115 (17)	150 (1)	245 (1)	-	202 (2)
Selenoyeast	-	-	290 (1)	100 (1)	135 (3)
Sodium selenate	130 (6)	-	-	120 (1)	110 (3)

[a]Average values rounded to nearest "5" and expressed relative to response obtained with sodium selenite. Number of studies or samples involved indicated within parentheses.

[b]One study with liver or kidney selenium accumulation from surfeit dietary levels reported relative values of 95 and 50, respectively, for the two tissues.

[c]From studies in which GSH-Px activity or incidence of exudative diathesis was the response variable.

[d]From studies in which whole body or tissue selenium retention or incidence of pancreatic fibrosis was the response variable.

REFERENCES

Abdel-Ati, K. A., J. D. Latshaw and J. P. Donahoe. 1984. Distribution of selenium in chicken tissues as affected by bursectomy. *Poult. Sci.* **63**:518.

Alexander, A. R., P. D. Whanger and L. T. Miller. 1983. Bioavailability to rats of selenium in various tuna and wheat products. *J. Nutr.* **113**:196.

Ammerman, C. B., H. L. Chapman, G. W. Bouwman, J. P. Fontenot, C. P. Bagley and A. L. Moxon. 1980. Effect of supplemental selenium for beef cows on the performance and tissue selenium concentrations of cows and suckling calves. *J. Anim. Sci.* **51**:1381.

Association of American Feed Control Officials (AAFCO). 1994. Official publication. AAFCO, Atlanta, GA.

Behne, D., A. Kyriakopoulos, H. Gessner, B. Walzog and H. Meinhold. 1992. Type I iodothyronine deiodinase activity after high selenium intake, and relations between selenium and iodine metabolism in rats. *J. Nutr.* **122**:1542.

Beilstein, M. A. and P. D. Whanger. 1986a. Deposition of dietary organic and inorganic selenium in rat erythrocyte proteins. *J. Nutr.* **116**:1701.

Beilstein, M. A. and P. D. Whanger. 1986b. Chemical forms of selenium in rat tissues after administration of selenite or selenomethionine. *J. Nutr.* **116**:1711.

Buckley, W. T., G. Strachan and R. Puls. 1987. Copper and selenium supplementation to calves by means of a soluble glass bolus. *Can. J. Anim. Sci.* **67**:877.

Bunk, M. J. and G. F. Combs, Jr. 1980. Effect of selenium on appetite in the selenium-deficient chick. *J. Nutr.* **110**:743.

Burk, R. F. and P. E. Gregory. 1982. Some characteristics of ^{75}Se-P, a selenoprotein found in rat liver and plasma, and comparison of it with seleno-glutathione peroxidase. *Arch. Biochem. Biophys.* **213**:73.

Byers, F. M. and A. L. Moxon. 1980. Protein and selenium levels for growing and finishing beef cattle. *J. Anim. Sci.* **50**:1136.

Cantor, A. H., M. L. Langevin, T. Noguchi and M. L. Scott. 1975b. Efficacy of selenium compounds and feedstuffs for prevention of pancreatic fibrosis in chicks. *J. Nutr.* **105**:106.

Cantor, A. H., P. D. Moorhead and M. A. Musser. 1982. Comparative effects of sodium selenite and selenomethionine upon nutritional muscular dystrophy, selenium-dependent glutathione peroxidase, and tissue selenium concentrations of turkey poults. *Poult. Sci.* **61**:478.

Cantor, A. H. and M. L. Scott. 1974. The effect of selenium in the hen's diet on egg production, hatchability, performance of progeny and selenium concentration in eggs. *Poult. Sci.* **53**:1870.

Cantor, A. H., M. L. Scott and T. Noguchi. 1975a. Biological availability of selenium in feedstuffs and selenium compounds for prevention of exudative diathesis in chicks. *J. Nutr.* **105**:96.

Cantor, A. H., C. D. Sutton and T. H. Johnson. 1983. Biological availability of selenodicysteine in chicks. *Poult. Sci.* **62**:2429.

Cantor, A. H. and J. Z. Tarino. 1982. Comparative effects of inorganic and organic dietary sources of selenium on selenium levels and selenium-dependent glutathione peroxidase activity in blood of young turkeys. *J. Nutr.* **112**:2187.

Care, A. D., P. J. B. Anderson, D. V. Illingworth, G. Zervas and S. B. Telfer. 1985. The effect of soluble-glass on the copper, cobalt and selenium status of Suffolk cross lambs. *In* "Trace Elements in Man and Animals - 5" (C. F. Mills, I. Bremner and J. K. Chesters, Eds.), p. 717. Commonwealth Agricultural Bureaux, Slough, UK.

Carlos, G., G. Zervas, P. M. Driver, P. J. B. Anderson, D. V. Illingworth S. A. Al-Tekrity and S. B. Telfer. 1985. The effect of soluble-glass boluses on the copper, cobalt and selenium status of Scottish Blackface ewes. *In* "Trace Elements in Man and Animals - 5" (C. F. Mills, I. Bremner and J. K. Chesters, Eds.), p. 714. Commonwealth Agricultural Bureaux, Slough, UK.

Cary, E. E., W. H. Allaway and M. Miller. 1973. Utilization of different forms of dietary selenium. *J. Anim. Sci.* **36**:285.

Chansler, M. W., M. Mutaneu, V. C. Morris and O. A. Levander. 1986. Nutritional bioavailability to rats of selenium in Brazil nuts and mushrooms. *Nutr. Res.* **6**:1419.

Combs, G. F., Jr., S. A. Barrows and F. N. Swader. 1980. Biologic availability of selenium in corn grain produced on soil amended with fly ash. *J. Agric. Food Chem.* **28**:406.

Combs, G. F., Jr. and S. B. Combs. 1986. "The Role of Selenium in Nutrition." Academic Press, New York.

Combs, G. F., Jr. and G. Pesti. 1976. Influence of ascorbic acid on selenium nutrition in the chick. *J. Nutr.* **106**:958.

Combs, G. F., Jr. and M. L. Scott. 1974. Antioxidant effects on selenium and vitamin E function in the chick. *J. Nutr.* **104**:1297.

Combs, G. F., Jr., Q. Su and K. Q. Wu. 1984. Use of the short-term glutathione peroxidase response in selenium-deficient chicks for assessment of bioavailability of dietary selenium. *Fed. Proc.* **43**:473 [Abstract].

Deagen, J. T., J. A. Butler, M. A. Beilstein and P. D. Whanger. 1987. Effects of dietary selenite, selenocystine and selenomethionine on selenocysteine lyase and glutathione peroxidase activities and on selenium levels in rat tissues. *J. Nutr.* **117**:91.

Donald, G. E., J. P. Langlands, J. E. Bowles, A. J. Smith and G. L. Burke. 1993. Selenium supplements for grazing sheep. 3. Development of an intra-ruminal pellet with an extended life. *Anim. Feed Sci. Technol.* **40**:295.

Douglass, J. S., V. C. Morris, J. H. Soares, Jr. and O. A. Levander. 1981. Nutritional availability to rats of selenium in tuna, beef kidney and wheat. *J. Nutr.* **111**:2180.

Echevarria, M. G., P. R. Henry, C. B. Ammerman, P. V. Rao and R. D. Miles. 1988. Estimation of the relative bioavailability of inorganic selenium sources for poultry. 2. Tissue uptake of selenium from high dietary selenium concentrations. *Poult. Sci.* **67**:1585.

Eggert, R. G., E. Patterson, W. T. Akers and E. L. R. Stokstad. 1957. The role of vitamin E and selenium in the nutrition of the pig. *J. Anim. Sci.* **16**:1037 [Abstract].

Ehlig, C. F., D. E. Hogue, W. H. Allaway and D. J. Hamm. 1967. Fate of selenium from selenite or seleno-methionine, with or without vitamin E in lambs. *J. Nutr.* **92**:121.

Gabrielsen, B. O. and J. Opstvedt. 1980a. A biological assay for determination of availability of selenium for restoring blood plasma glutathione peroxidase activity in selenium depleted chicks. *J. Nutr.* **110**:1089.

Gabrielsen, B. O. and J. Opstvedt. 1980b. Availability of selenium in fish meal in comparison with soybean meal, corn gluten meal and selenomethionine relative to selenium in sodium selenite for restoring glutathione peroxidase activity in selenium-depleted chicks. *J. Nutr.* **110**:1096.

Ganther, H. E. and C. A. Baumann. 1962. Selenium metabolism. II. Modifying effects of sulfate. *J. Nutr.* **77**:408.

Groce, A. W., E. R. Miller, J. P. Hitchcock, D. E. Ullrey and W. T. Magee. 1973. Selenium balance in the pig as affected by selenium source and vitamin E. *J. Anim. Sci.* **37**:942.

Harrison, J. H. and H. R. Conrad. 1984. Effect of selenium intake on selenium utilization by the nonlactating dairy cow. *J. Dairy Sci.* **67**:219.

Henry, P. R., M. G. Echevarria, C. B. Ammerman and P. V. Rao. 1988. Estimation of the relative biological availability of inorganic selenium sources for ruminants using tissue uptake of selenium. *J. Anim. Sci.* **66**:2306.

Hidiroglou, M., J. Proulx and J. Jolette. 1985. Intraruminal selenium pellet for control of nutritional muscular dystrophy in cattle. *J. Dairy Sci.* **68**:57.

Hidiroglou, M., J. Proulx and J. Jolette. 1987. Effect of intraruminally administered, selenium soluble-glass boluses on selenium status in cows and their calves. *J. Anim. Sci.* **65**:815.

Hill, C. H. 1976. Mineral interactions. *In* "Trace Elements in Human Health and Disease" (A.S. Prasad, Ed.), Vol. 2. p. 281. Academic Press, New York.

Hogue, D. E. 1958. Vitamin E, selenium and other factors related to nutritional muscular dystrophy in lambs. *In* "Proceedings of the Cornell Nutrition Conference on Feed Manufacturing," p. 32. Ithaca, NY.

House, W. A. and R. M. Welch. 1989. Bioavailability of and interactions between zinc and selenium in rats fed wheat grain intrinsically labeled with ^{65}Zn and ^{75}Se. *J. Nutr.* **119**:916.

Humaloja, T. and H. M. Mykkanen. 1986. Intestinal absorption of ^{75}Se-labeled sodium selenite and selenomethionine in chicks: Effects of time, segment, selenium concentration and method of measurement. *J. Nutr.* **116**:142.

Huque, Q. M. E. and J. Fris Jensen. 1985. Biological availability of selenium and phosphorus in fish meal as affected by condition of fish and type of meal. *Br. Poult. Sci.* **26**:289.

Jenkins, K. J., R. C. Dickson and M. Hidiroglou. 1970. Effects of various selenium compounds on the development of muscular dystrophy and other vitamin E dyscrasias in the chick. *Can. J. Physiol. Pharmacol.* **48**:192.

Jensen, L. S. 1975. Precipitation of a selenium deficiency by high dietary levels of copper and zinc. *Proc. Soc. Exp. Biol. Med.* **149**:113.

Johansson, E., S. O. Jacobsson, J. Luthman and U. Lindh. 1990. The biological response of selenium in individual erythrocytes and GSH-Px in lambs fed sodium selenite or selenium yeast. *J. Vet. Med. A* **37**:463.

Judson, G. J., T-S. Koh, J. D. McFarlane, R. K. Turnbull and B. R. Kempe. 1985. Copper and selenium supplements for cattle: Evaluation of the selenium bullet, copper oxide and the soluble glass bullet. *In* "Trace Elements in Man and Animals - 5" (C. F. Mills, I. Bremner and J. K. Chesters, Eds.), p. 725. Commonwealth Agricultural Bureaux, Slough, UK.

Koh, T-S. and G. J. Judson. 1987. Copper and selenium deficiency in cattle: An evaluation of methods of oral therapy and an observation of a copper-selenium interaction. *Vet. Res. Commun.* **11**:133.

Kuchel, R. E. and R. A. Buckley. 1969. The provision of selenium to sheep by means of heavy pellets. *Aust. J. Agric. Res.* **20**:1099.

L'Abbe, M. R. and K. D. Trick. 1991. Organic selenium is more bioavailable than Na_2SeO_3 for short term glutathione peroxidase (SeGSHPX) activity in rats fed adequate methionine but is less bioavailable in the long term. *FASEB J.* **5**:A715 [Abstract].

Lane, H. W., R. Strength, J. Johnson and M. White. 1991. Effect of chemical form of selenium on tissue glutathione peroxidase activity in developing rats. *J. Nutr.* **121**:80.

Langlands, J. P., G. E. Donald, J. E. Bowles and A. J. Smith. 1990a. Selenium supplements for grazing sheep. 1. A comparison between soluble salts and other forms of supplement. *Anim. Feed Sci. Technol.* **28**:1.

Langlands, J. P., J. E. Bowles, G. E. Donald and A. J. Smith. 1990b. Selenium supplements for grazing sheep. 2. Effectiveness of intra-ruminal pellets. *Anim. Feed Sci. Technol.* **28**:15.

Latshaw, J. D. and M. Osman. 1975. Distribution of selenium in egg white and yolk after feeding natural and synthetic selenium compounds. *Poult. Sci.* **54**:1244.

Laws, J. E., J. D. Latshaw and M. Biggert. 1986. Selenium bioavailability in foods and feeds. *Nutr. Rep. Int.* **33**:13.

Lawson, D. C., N. S. Ritchie and J. J. Parkins. 1991. The use of a multiple trace element and vitamin bolus in cattle under conditions of low selenium or low copper status. *In* "Trace Elements in Man and Animals - 7" (B. Momcilovic, Ed.), p.15-8. Institute for Medical Research and Occupational Health, University of Zagreb, Croatia.

Lawson, D. C., N. S. Ritchie, J. J. Parkins, R. G. Hemingway and H. R. Gresham. 1990. Use of a sustained release bolus for enhancing selenium status in cattle. *Vet. Rec.* **127**:67.

Litov, R. E. 1987. Evaluating the bioavailability of selenium from nutritional formulas for enteral use. *In* "Selenium in Biology and Medicine, Part A" (G.F. Combs, Jr., J.E. Spallholz, O.A. Levander and J.E. Oldfield, Eds.), p. 426. Van Nostrand Reinhold, New York.

Madison, T. C. 1860. Sanitary report - Fort Randell. *In* "Statistical Report on the Sickness and Mortality in the Army in the United States" (R.H. Cooldge, Ed.). Senate Exchange Doc. **52**:37.

Mahan, D. C. and P. L. Magee. 1991. Efficacy of dietary sodium selenite and calcium selenite provided in the diet at approved, marginally toxic and toxic levels to growing swine. *J. Anim. Sci.* **69**:4722.

Mahan, D. C. and A. L. Moxon. 1978. Effects of adding inorganic and organic selenium sources to the diets of young swine. *J. Anim. Sci.* **47**:456.

Mandisodza, K. T., W. G. Pond, D. J. Lisk, D. E. Hogue, L. Krook, E. E. Cary and W. H. Gutenmann. 1979. Tissue retention of Se in growing pigs fed fly ash or white sweet clover grown on fly ash. *J. Anim. Sci.* **49**:535.

Martello, M. A. and J. D. Latshaw. 1982. Utilization of dietary selenium as indicated by prevention of selenium deficiency and by retention in eggs. *Nutr. Rep. Int.* **26**:43.

Mason, A. C. and C. M. Weaver. 1986. Metabolism in rats of selenium from intrinsically and extrinsically labeled isolated soy protein. *J. Nutr.* **116**:1883.

Mathias, M. M., W. H. Allaway, D. E. Hogue, M. V. Marion and R. W. Gardner. 1965. Value of selenium in alfalfa for the prevention of selenium deficiencies in chicks and rats. *J. Nutr.* **86**:213.

Mathias, M. M., D. E. Hogue and J. K. Loosli. 1967. The biological value of selenium in bovine milk for the rat and chick. *J. Nutr.* **93**:14.

McAdam, P. A. and O. A. Levander. 1987. Chronic toxicity and retention of dietary selenium fed to rats as D- of L- selenomethionine, selenite, or selenate. *Nutr. Res.* **7**:601.

Miller, D., J. H. Soares, Jr., P. Bauersfeld, Jr. and S. L. Cuppett. 1972. Comparative selenium retention by chicks fed sodium selenite, selenomethionine, fish meal and fish solubles. *Poult. Sci.* **51**:1669.

Moksnes, K. and G. Norheim. 1983. Selenium and glutathione peroxidase levels in lambs receiving feed supplemented with sodium selenite or selenomethionine. *Acta Vet. Scand.* **24**:45.

Mutanen, M., P. Aspila and H. M. Mykkanen. 1986a. Bioavailability to rats of selenium in milk of cows fed sodium seleniteor selenited barley. *Ann. Nutr. Metab.* **30**:183.

Mutanen, M., P. Koivistoinen, V. C. Morris and O. A. Levander. 1986b. Nutritional availability to rats of selenium in four seafoods: Crab (*Callinectes sapidus*), oyster (*Crassostrea virginica*), shrimp (*Penaeus duorarum*) and Baltic herring (*Clupea harengus*). *Br. J. Nutr.* **55**:219.

Muth, O. H., J. E. Oldfield, L. F. Remmert and J. R. Schubert. 1958. Effects of selenium and vitamin E on white muscle disease. *Science* **128**:1090.

Mykkanen, H. and T. Humaloja. 1984. Effect of lead on the intestinal absorption of sodium selenite and selenomethionine (^{75}Se) in chicks. *Biol. Trace Element Res.* **6**:11.

Mykkanen, H. M. and M. L. Mutanen. 1986. Intestinal interactions of ascorbic acid with different selenium compounds in chicks. *Nutr. Rep. Int.* **33**:575.

Noguchi, T., A. H. Cantor and M. L. Scott. 1973. Mode of action of selenium and vitamin E in prevention of exudative diathesis in chicks. *J. Nutr.* **103**:1502.

National Research Council (NRC). 1989. "Recommended Dietary Allowances." 10th ed. National Academy Press, Washington, DC.

Omaye, S. T. and A. L. Tappel. 1974. Effect of dietary selenium on glutathione peroxidase in the chick. *J. Nutr.* **104**:747.

Osman, M. and J. D. Latshaw. 1976. Biological potency of selenium from sodium selenite, selenomethionine and selenocystine in the chick. *Poult. Sci.* **55**:987.

Overnes, G., K. Moksnes, E. M. Okland and A. Froslie. 1986. The efficacy of hay from selenized soil as a source of selenium in ruminant nutrition. *Acta Agric. Scand.* **36**:332.

Parsons, M. J., P. K. Ku, D. E. Ullrey, H. D. Stowe, P. A. Whetter and E. R. Miller. 1985. Effects of riboflavin supplementation and selenium source on selenium metabolism in the young pig. *J. Anim. Sci.* **60**:451.

Patterson, E. L., R. Milstrey and E. L. R. Stokstad. 1957. Effect of selenium in preventing exudative diathesis in chicks. *Proc. Soc. Exp. Biol. Med.* **95**:617.

Pehrson, B., M. Knutsson and M. Gyllensward. 1989. Glutathione peroxidase activity in heifers fed diets supplemented with organic and inorganic selenium compounds. *Swed. J. Agric. Res.* **19**:53.

Peterson, R. P. and L. S. Jensen. 1975. Induced exudative diathesis in chicks by dietary silver. *Poult. Sci.* **54**:795.

Petterson, D. S., R. H. Casey, H. G. Masters and P. E. Wilson. 1985. Observations on intraruminal glass pellets for trace mineral supplementation of sheep. *In* "Trace Elements in Man and Animals - 5" (C.F. Mills, I. Bremner and J.K. Chesters, Eds.), p. 722. Commonwealth Agricultural Bureaux, Slough, UK.

Pierce, S. and A. L. Tappel. 1977. Effects of selenite and selenomethionine on glutathione peroxidase in the rat. *J. Nutr.* **107**:475.

Rahim, A. G. A., J. R. Arthur and C. F. Mills. 1986. Effects of dietary copper, cadmium, iron, molybdenum and manganese on selenium utilization by the rat. *J. Nutr.* **116**:403.

Richold, M., M. F. Robinson and R. D. H. Stewart. 1977. Metabolic studies in rats of ^{75}Se incorporated in vivo into fish muscle. *Br. J. Nutr.* **38**:19.

Ringdal, O., E. Ø. Bjørnestad and K. Julshamn. 1985. Comparative utilization of fish selenium and inorganic selenite by rats of normal selenium status. *Ann. Nutr. Metab.* **29**:297.

Rotruck, J. T., A. L. Pope, H. E. Ganther, A. B. Swanson, D. G. Hafemen and W. G. Hoekstra. 1973. Selenium: Biochemical role as a component of glutathione peroxidase. *Science* **179**:588.

Salbe, A. D. and O. A. Levander. 1990. Effect of various dietary factors on the deposition of selenium in the hair and nails of rats. *J. Nutr.* **120**:200.

Sankari, S. 1985. Plasma glutathione peroxidase and tissue selenium response to selenium supplementation in swine. *Acta Vet. Scand. Suppl.* **81**:11.

Schwarz, K. and C. M. Foltz. 1957. Selenium as an integral part of Factor 3 against dietary necrotic liver degeneration. *J. Am. Chem. Soc.* **79**:3292.

Schwarz, K. and C. M. Foltz. 1958. Factor 3 activity of selenium compounds. *J. Biol. Chem.* **233**:245.

Schwarz, K. and A. Fredga. 1969. Biological potency of organic selenium compounds. Aliphatic monoseleno-and diseleno- dicarboxylic acids. *J. Biol. Chem.* **244**:2103.

Schwarz, K. and A. Fredga. 1972a. Biological potency of organic selenium compounds: II. Aliphatic selena-carboxylic acids and acid amides. *Bioinorg. Chem.* **2**:47.

Schwarz, K. and A. Fredga. 1972b. Biological potency of organic selenium compounds. III. Phenyl-, benzyl-, and phenylethylseleno-carboxylic acids, and related compounds. *Bioinorg. Chem.* **2**:171.

Schwarz, K. and A. Fredga. 1974. Biological potency of organic selenium compounds. V. Diselenides of alcohols and amines, and some selenium-containing ketones. *Bioinorg. Chem.* **3**:153.

Schwarz, K., L. A. Porter and A. Fredga. 1974. Biological potency of organic selenium compounds. IV. Straight-chain dialkylmono- and diselenides. *Bioinorg. Chem.* **3**:145.

Scott, M. L. and A. H. Cantor. 1971. Tissue selenium levels in chicks receiving graded amounts of dietary selenium. *Fed. Proc.* **30**:237 [Abstract].

Seier, L. and D. B. Bragg. 1973. Influence of vitamin E and antioxidant on the response of dietary selenium by the chick and the biological activity of selenium in feed grain. *Can. J. Anim. Sci.* **53**:371.

Smith, A. M. and M. F. Picciano. 1987. Relative bioavailability of seleno-compounds in the lactating rat. *J. Nutr.* **117**:725.

Sunde, R. A., J. A. Dyer, T. V. Moran, J. K. Evenson and M. Simoto. 1993. Phospholipid hydroperoxide glutathione peroxidase: Full length pig blastocyst cDNA sequence and regulation by selenium status. *Biochem. Biophys. Res. Commun.* **193**:905.

Sunde, R. A., G. E. Gutzke and W. G. Hoekstra. 1981b. Effect of dietary methionine on the biopotency of selenite and selenomethionine in the rat. *J. Nutr.* **111**:76.

Sunde, R. A. and W. G. Hoekstra. 1980. Incorporation of selenium from selenite and selenocystine into glutathione peroxidase in the isolated perfused rat liver. *Biochem. Biophys. Res. Commun.* **93**:1181.

Sunde, R. A., W. K. Sonnenburg, G. E. Gutzke and W. G. Hoekstra. 1981a. Biopotency of selenium for glutathione peroxidase synthesis. *In* "Trace Element Metabolism in Man and Animals-4" (J. McC. Howell, J. W. Gawthorne and C. L. White, Eds.), p. 165. Aust. Academy of Science, Canberra.

Symonds, H. W., B. F. Sansom, D. L. Mather and M. J. Vagg. 1981. Selenium metabolism in the dairy cow: The influence of the liver and the effect of the form of Se salt. *Br. J. Nutr.* **45**:117.

Tarla, F. N., P. R. Henry, C. B. Ammerman and P. V. Rao. 1989. Effect of time on tissue deposition of selenium in sheep fed calcium selenite or sodium selenite. *Nutr. Rep. Int.* **39**:943.

Thomson, C. D., B. A. Robinson, R. D. H. Stewart and M. F. Robinson. 1975b. Metabolic studies of [^{75}Se] selenocystine and [^{75}Se] selenomethionine in the rat. *Br. J. Nutr.* **34**:501.

Thomson, C. D. and R. D. H. Stewart. 1973. Metabolic studies of [^{75}Se] selenomethionine and [^{75}Se] selenite in the rat. *Br. J. Nutr.* **30**:139.

Thomson, C. D., R. D. H. Stewart and M. F. Robinson. 1975a. Metabolic studies in rats of [^{75}Se] selenomethionine and of [^{75}Se] incorporated in vivo into rabbit kidney. *Br. J. Nutr.* **33**:45.

Ursini, F., M. Maiorinoand C. Gregolin. 1985. The selenoenzyme phospholipid hydroperoxide glutathione peroxidase. *Biochim. Biophys. Acta* **839**:62.

van Ryssen, J. B .J., J. T. Deagen, M. A. Beilstein and P. D. Whanger. 1989. Comparative metabolism of organic and inorganic selenium by sheep. *J. Agric. Food Chem.* **37**:1358.

Vinson, J. A. and P. Bose. 1987. Relative bioavailability of inorganic and natural selenium. In: "Selenium in Biology and Medicine, Part A" (G. F. Combs, Jr., J. E. Spellholz, O. A. Levander and J. E. Oldfield, Eds.), p. 445. Van Nostrand Reinhold , New York.

Waschulewski, I. H. and R. A. Sunde. 1988. Effect of dietary methionine on utilization of tissue selenium from dietary selenomethionine for glutathione peroxidase in the rat. *J. Nutr.* **118**:367.

Whanger, P. D. and J. A. Butler. 1988. Effects of various dietary levels of selenium as selenite or selenomethionine on tissue selenium levels and glutathione peroxidase activity in rats. *J. Nutr.* **118**:846.

Whitacre, M. and J. D. Latshaw. 1982. Selenium utilization from menhaden fish meal as affected by processing. *Poult. Sci.* **61**:2520.

Yasumoto, K., K. Iwami and M. Yoshida. 1979. Vitamin B$_6$ dependence of selenomethionine and selenite utilization for glutathione peroxidase in the rat. *J. Nutr.* **109**:760.

Yoshida, M., K. Iwami and K. Yasumoto. 1984. Determination of nutritional efficiency of selenium contained in processed skipjack meat by comparison with selenite. *J. Nutr. Sci. Vitaminol.* **30**:395.

Zhou, Y. P. and G. F. Combs, Jr. 1984. Effects of dietary protein level and level of feed intake on the apparent bioavailability of selenium for the chick. *Poult. Sci.* **63**:294.

15

SODIUM AND CHLORINE BIOAVAILABILITY

Pamela R. Henry

Department of Animal Science
University of Florida
Gainesville, Florida

I. INTRODUCTION

The importance of dietary salt (NaCl) for animals was known for hundreds of years before the metabolic effects of the compound were studied scientifically. Sodium and chlorine along with potassium function to maintain osmotic pressure, acid-base balance, and fluid balance in body tissues. Signs of sodium deficiency include pica, weight loss, inappetence, increased water consumption, reduced milk yield not accompanied by a decrease in milk sodium concentration, decreased egg production, and decreased sodium concentration in feces, urine, and saliva in ruminants (Morris, 1980; Underwood, 1981). Signs of chlorine deficiency in ruminants include inappetence, weight loss, decreased milk production, weakness, decreased concentration of chloride in urine, saliva, and plasma, but not feces, and metabolic alkalosis (Neathery *et al.*, 1981; Fettman *et al.*, 1984a,b). Signs of chlorine deficiency in chicks include inappetence, growth retardation, and decreased serum chloride concentration, as well as mortality, dehydration, and nerve dysfunction (Leach and Nesheim, 1963).

Sodium generally occurs in lower concentrations than chlorine in the majority of forages and concentrates fed to livestock with the exception of some processed feeds such as soybean meal, corn gluten, and brewers and distillers grains (Neathery, 1980). Values for chlorine are unavailable for many feedstuffs. Due to the widespread practice by nutritionists and livestock and poultry producers in the United States of ignoring the contribution of sodium and chlorine from primary dietary ingredients and drinking water and adding supplemental salt to diets, there is generally little concern for a practical sodium or chlorine deficiency to occur. Sodium deficiency is a frequent problem in unsupplemented grazing ruminants. Even when sodium bicarbonate, sodium phosphates, or sodium sulfate are supplemental to diets, sodium chloride is also added, as much from tradition as from

BIOAVAILABILITY OF NUTRIENTS FOR ANIMALS:
AMINO ACIDS, MINERALS, AND VITAMINS

337

need (Coppock, 1986). Unnecessary oversupplementation with sodium and chlorine can cause elevated concentrations of these elements in animal wastes that are used as fertilizers and may cause toxicity to plants and a buildup of these elements in the environment. With some areas of the United States already burdened with saline soils and water supplies, further research on bioavailability and requirements of sodium and chlorine is justified. Considerable attention has been given to salt toxicosis in all species as well as to acid-base balance and ruminal buffering capacity of minerals. Although various sources and levels of sodium and/or chlorine are found in many of these studies, the experimental designs do not allow comparisons of availability. Little research has been conducted to measure bioavailability of sources of either element due to the widespread commercial availability, palatability, and low cost of sodium chloride.

II. BIOAVAILABILITY STUDIES

A. *In Vivo* Estimates of Bioavailability

Feed intake and growth have been used to assess the requirement or toxic level of sodium and/or chlorine for broiler chicks (Leach and Nesheim, 1963; Proudfoot *et al.*, 1985), turkeys (Harms, 1982), Bobwhite quail (Ingram *et al.*, 1984), swine (Alcantara *et al.*, 1980), calves (Neathery *et al.*, 1981), and sheep (de Waal *et al.*, 1989).

In experiments with broilers (Table I), it appeared that the sodium and chlorine in rock salt were somewhat more available for growth than that in evaporated salt; however, additional experiments indicated that the somewhat larger size particles of rock salt were responsible for the growth effect. When samples of the two sources with equal particle sizes were compared, availability was similar (Dilworth *et al.*, 1970a,b).

Damron *et al.* (1986) supplemented sodium-deficient diets for broiler chicks with 196, 392, and 588 ppm added sodium as sodium chloride or sodium bicarbonate in one trial and the lower two added amounts as either source in a second trial. Relative bioavailability values based on growth for sodium in sodium bicarbonate were 105 and 100% compared with sodium chloride in trial one and two, respectively. Based on growth, Damron and Johnson (1986) reported no difference in the availability of sodium from sodium chloride, sodium bicarbonate, or sodium acetate supplemented at 75 ppm sodium in drinking water for broiler chicks fed a low-sodium diet. There was no difference in growth or feed conversion of chicks fed .1% added sodium from sodium chloride or sodium sulfate (Ross, 1977).

Growth was similar in broilers fed sodium chloride or ammonium chloride added to a chlorine-deficient diet (Summers *et al.*, 1967). When 1% chlorine was added to a basal diet (.45% Cl) for chicks, growth was depressed more in those fed calcium chloride ($CaCl_2 \cdot 2H_2O$) than in those fed glutamic·HCl (Nesheim *et al.*, 1964). The chlorine in $CaCl_2 \cdot 2H_2O$ seemed to be more available and, thus, more toxic than that in glutamic·HCl.

A series of experiments was conducted with growing swine that compared availability of sodium from sodium chloride, sodium sulfate, and sodium bicarbonate (Cromwell *et al.*, 1981). Sodium as sulfate appeared to be 85% as available for growth as that in sodium chloride in the first experiment; however, the diet containing sodium sulfate did not contain added chlorine. Growth was also greater in pigs fed sodium chloride than in those fed sodium bicarbonate without supplemental chlorine. When chlorine was added to diets containing sodium bicarbonate, gain averaged 110% of that for sodium chloride in one experiment and 96% in another study.

There was no difference in feed intake or body weight of sheep when sodium sulfate was substituted for sodium chloride at equal sodium levels in drinking water for 15 months (Peirce, 1960).

Availability of sodium in various phosphorus sources has been determined with broilers. Nott and Combs (1969) reported sodium in defluorinated rock phosphate to be 83% as available for growth as that in sodium chloride. Damron *et al.* (1985) compared availability of sodium in three defluorinated phosphates and reagent grade monobasic and dibasic sodium phosphates with that in sodium chloride and reported average values that ranged from 84 to 97%. Damron (1982) reported relative values of 100, 99, 104, and 102% for availability of sodium in sodium chloride, sodium acetate, sodium sulfate, and sodium bicarbonate, respectively, based on chick growth.

The availability of sodium in sodium aluminosilicate (Ethacal®, synthetic sodium zeolite A, 12.6% Na) was 100% of that in sodium chloride to support growth in broilers (Fethiere *et al.*, 1988) and egg production in laying hens (Miles *et al.*, 1988).

Sodium or chlorine deficiency will result in decreased milk production (Smith and Aines, 1959; Fettman *et al.*, 1984a; Link and Olson, 1985), but few researchers have used this criterion as a comparison among sources of either element. Generally, experiments with sodium bicarbonate in dairy cattle have concentrated upon the compound's buffering capacity and not the availability of its sodium (Staples and Lough, 1989). Production of 4% fat corrected milk and actual milk yield (both corrected for feed intake) increased when either sodium chloride or sodium bicarbonate was fed to dairy cows at .55% added sodium with chlorine equalized between diets (Schneider *et al.*, 1986). Relative values, however, could not be estimated from the data presented.

There were no differences in wool production when sodium as sodium sulfate was substituted for sodium chloride in drinking water for sheep (Peirce, 1960); nor were there differences when chlorine as calcium chloride or magnesium chloride was substituted for sodium chloride (Peirce, 1959, 1962).

Summers and Leeson (1985) reported that sodium availability was greater from canola meal than from soybean meal. Broiler performance was maximized when .08% sodium was added to soybean meal diets or .06% sodium was added to diets containing 20% canola meal.

Dietary sodium and chloride are highly available and freely absorbed (Underwood, 1981). The ARC (1980) gives coefficients of absorption of .91 for sodium and .85 for chlorine for both sheep and cattle.

Fecal excretion is not an integral part of sodium or chlorine regulation in ruminants; thus, measurement of apparent absorption yields values very similar to those representing true absorption. Urinary excretion increases with increasing intake (Nelson et al., 1955; Paquay et al., 1969; Neathery, 1980; Morris, 1980). Similar excretion pathways were observed in horses (Schryver et al., 1987) and swine. Apparent absorption of sodium was about 75% in horses (Schryver et al., 1987) and from 82 to 96% in swine (Hagsten and Perry, 1976; Alcantara et al., 1980). Sheep fed ryegrass or white clover had average apparent sodium absorption of 95 and 91%, respectively (Grace et al., 1974). Apparent absorption of sodium in dairy cows fed fresh herbage ranged from 77 to 95% and averaged 85% (Kemp, 1964). Cows fed hay plus oatmeal had apparent sodium absorption values of 81% and values for cows fed hay, corn, and beet pulp averaged 69% (Kemp, 1964). Apparent chlorine absorption in lactating dairy cows fed fresh herbage ranged from 71 to 95% and averaged 88% (Kemp, 1966).

Apparent absorption of sodium from high concentrate diets for sheep was 68% when .2% added sodium was fed as sodium chloride and 63% when .2% added sodium was fed as sodium bicarbonate. Urinary sodium excretion averaged 29 and 63%, respectively, but did not differ significantly (James and Wohlt, 1985). Renal reabsorption of filtered sodium was 97% when beef heifers were given water containing .16% sodium as either sodium chloride or sodium sulfate (Weeth and Hunter, 1971). Fecal and urinary excretions of sodium were similar when sodium from sodium bicarbonate replaced sodium chloride to create chloride-deficient diets for dairy cows and calves (Burkhalter et al., 1979; Coppock et al., 1979).

Martz et al. (1988) fed dairy heifers either semipurified (solka floc or corn cobs as the main fiber source) or conventional (corn silage) diets and measured apparent absorption and retention of sodium. Apparent sodium absorption was 86, 91, and 74% for solka floc, corn cob, and corn silage diets, respectively. Urinary sodium excretion averaged 6.1, 7.8, and 4.4% of intake, respectively.

Serum sodium concentrations tend to remain constant regardless of dietary sodium concentration; however, serum chloride decreases with decreasing intake and may be a useful indicator of availability (Leach and Nesheim, 1963; Morris and Murphy, 1972; Coppock et al., 1979; Neathery et al., 1981; Fettman et al., 1984a,c). Fettman et al. (1984d) reported a significant decline in serum chloride concentration within 3 days of changing cows from a diet containing .42 to .10% chlorine, while serum sodium remained constant whether sodium chloride or bicarbonate was the source of sodium.

There were no differences in plasma sodium concentration of laying hens fed .04, .12 or .24% sodium as sodium chloride or bicarbonate (Cohen et al., 1972). Also, hens fed .31 to .36% sodium from sodium bicarbonate, acetate, sulfate or disodium phosphate had similar plasma sodium concentrations. Although dietary chlorine ranged from .10 to .67%, mature hens fed the element as sodium, calcium, potassium, ferrous or choline chloride had similar plasma chloride concentrations in the same study.

The ratio of salivary Na:K may be a useful measure of sodium availability (Morris and Peterson, 1975; Morris, 1980). Although salivary chloride tends to decline with lower chlorine intake, the response is somewhat variable and, thus, unreliable (Neathery, 1980; Fettman et al., 1984a,c).

III. FACTORS INFLUENCING BIOAVAILABILITY

A. Dietary Factors

Decreasing ruminal pH decreased net transport of sodium and chlorine (Gaebel et al., 1987, 1989), but addition of monensin or lasalocid to a high concentrate diet for steers increased apparent absorption of sodium from 64 to 77 and 73%, respectively (Starnes et al., 1984). Nitrate has also been reported to decrease mucosal to serosal chloride flux but not change sodium flux in isolated sheep ruminal epithelium (Wurmli et al., 1987). Feeding sheep diets containing either 64 or 90% concentrates substituted for hay alone increased the surface area of ruminal papillae by 200 and 400%, respectively, which led to increased net absorption of sodium and chlorine (Gaebel et al., 1987).

Elevated dietary potassium decreased ruminal sodium concentration and absorption in sheep and steers (Scott, 1967; Buchan et al., 1986; Spears and Harvey, 1987). Feeding lambs .18% magnesium oxide also decreased apparent sodium absorption (James and Wohlt, 1985). Growth and mortality of turkey poults fed as much as 4% sodium chloride were not affected by the addition of 1% potassium chloride (Matterson *et al.*, 1948). Bromine (676 to 1352 ppm) partially counteracted signs of chlorine deficiency in chicks, but iodine (537 to 1074) increased deficiency signs and mortality (Leach and Nesheim, 1963). In the same study, fluorine at 268 ppm had no effect.

B. Animal Factors

Although many factors, such as heat stress, lactation, pregnancy, and growth, alter the amount of sodium and chlorine required by animals, these factors do not appear to alter the rate of absorption of the elements and, hence, the bioavailability of sources.

IV. SUMMARY

Sodium and chlorine have been supplied to animals for centuries in the form of common salt, sodium chloride. Requirements for the two elements seem to be met when the salt is consumed in accordance with taste. Because of ease of providing sodium chloride in amounts needed to meet the animal's requirements for sodium and chlorine, there has been little research concerning the bioavailability of other supplemental sources of the two elements (Table II). Also, studies on absorption of sodium and chlorine from feedstuffs are few in number. Research with poultry suggests that sodium in chemically pure compounds is 90 to 100% as well utilized as that in sodium chloride. Sodium present in defluorinated phosphate, however, is about 85% as available for poultry as that in sodium chloride. One study with swine indicated that sodium in sodium bicarbonate was 95% as available as that in sodium chloride. Chlorine either in ammonium chloride for poultry or in potassium chloride for swine was 95% as well utilized as that in sodium chloride.

Sodium and chlorine in feedstuffs are considered to be well absorbed by animals. Apparent absorption of sodium from feedstuffs measured in cattle, sheep, swine, and horses ranged from about 70 to 95% with an average of 85% apparently absorbed. The ARC (1980) estimates absorption to be 91% for sodium and 85% for chlorine for cattle and sheep.

Table I. Bioavailability of sodium and chlorine sources for domestic animals[a]

SODIUM

Poultry

Source	RV	Standard	Response criterion	Meth cal	Type diet	Added level, ppm	Reference
Phosphate, defluorinated FG	83	Sodium chloride RG (NaCl)	Growth	SR	N-200 ppm	120, 200, 350, 610	Nott and Combs (1969)
Phosphate, defluorinated FG	84	NaCl FG	Growth	SR	N-217 ppm	197-983	Damron et al. (1985)
Phosphate, defluorinated FG	84	NaCl FG	Growth	SR	N-217 ppm	197-983	Damron et al. (1985)
Phosphate, defluorinated FG	90	NaCl FG	Growth	SR	N-217 ppm	197-983	Damron et al. (1985)
Sodium acetate (NaC₂H₃O₂)	99	NaCl	Growth	SR	N-180 ppm	196-981	Damron (1982)
Sodium acetate	95	NaCl FG	Growth	MR	N-105, 202 ppm	25, 75 in water	Damron and Johnson (1986)
Sodium aluminosilicate[b]	100	NaCl	Growth	SR	N	200, 400, 600, 800, 1600	Fethiere et al. (1988)
Sodium aluminosilicate[b]	100	NaCl	Egg prod	SR	N	400, 800, 1200, 1700	Miles et al. (1988)
Sodium bicarbonate (NaHCO₃)	102	NaCl	Growth	SR	N-180 ppm	196-981	Damron (1982)
Sodium bicarbonate	105	NaCl FG	Growth	MR	N-300 ppm	196, 392, 588	Damron et al. (1986)
Sodium bicarbonate	100	NaCl FG	Growth	MR	N-300 ppm	196, 392	Damron et al. (1986)
Sodium bicarbonate	96	NaCl FG	Growth	MR	N-105, 202 ppm	25, 75 in water	Damron and Johnson (1986)
Sodium phosphate, dibasic RG (Na₂HPO₄)	97	NaCl FG	Growth	SR	N-217 ppm	197-983	Damron et al. (1985)

Table I. (continued)

Source	RV	Standard	Response criterion	Meth cal	Type diet	Added level, ppm	Reference
Sodium phosphate, monobasic RG (NaH_2PO_4)	92	NaCl FG	Growth	SR	N-217 ppm	197-983	Damron et al. (1985)
Na_2SO_4 RG	100	NaCl FG	Growth	MR	N-1300 ppm	1000	Ross (1977)
Na_2SO_4	104	NaCl	Growth	SR	N-180 ppm	196-981	Damron (1982)
Swine							
$NaHCO_3$	93	NaCl	Growth	MR	N	500, 1000	Cromwell et al. (1981)
CHLORINE							
Poultry							
Ammonium chloride (NH_4Cl)	96	NaCl	Growth	MR	N-730 ppm	1500	Summers et al. (1967)
Swine							
Potassium chloride (KCl)	96	NaCl	Growth	MR	N	1500	Cromwell et al. (1981)

[a]Abbreviations can be found in Appendix I. Chemical formula for a compound given only if provided by the author; RG indicates reagent grade, FG indicates feed grade.
[b]Ethacal®, synthetic sodium zeolite A.

Table II. Relative bioavailability of supplemental sodium and chlorine sources[a]

	Species	
Source	Poultry	Sheep
Sodium		
Sodium chloride	100	100
Phosphate, defluorinated	85 (4)	-
Sodium acetate	100 (2)	-
Sodium aluminosilicate	100 (2)	-
Sodium bicarbonate	100 (4)	95 (1)
Sodium phosphate, dibasic	100 (1)	-
Sodium phosphate, monobasic	90 (1)	-
Sodium sulfate	100 (1)	-
Chlorine		
Ammonium chloride	95 (1)	-
Potassium chloride	-	95 (1)

[a]Average values rounded to nearest "5" and expressed relative to response obtained with sodium chloride. Number of studies or samples involved indicated within parentheses.

REFERENCES

ARC. 1980. "The Nutrient Requirements of Ruminant Livestock". Commonwealth Agricultural Bureaux, Slough, UK.

Alcantara, P. F., L. E. Hanson and J. D. Smith. 1980. Sodium requirements, balance and tissue composition of growing pigs. *J. Anim. Sci.* **50**:1092.

Buchan, W., R. N. B. Kay, Y. Sasaki and D. Scott. 1986. Effects of abrupt changes in food and potassium intake on the rumen sodium reservoir in sheep. *J. Physiol.* **381**:84P.

Burkhalter, D. L., M. W. Neathery, W. J. Miller, R. H. Whitlock and J. C. Allen. 1979. Effects of low chloride intake on performance, clinical characteristics, and chloride, sodium, potassium, and nitrogen metabolism in dairy calves. *J. Dairy Sci.* **62**:1895.

Cohen, I., S. Hurwitz and A. Bar. 1972. Acid-base balance and sodium-to-chloride ratio in diets of laying hens. *J. Nutr.* **102**:1.

Coppock, C. E. 1986. Mineral utilization by the lactating cow - chlorine. *J. Dairy Sci.* **69**:595.

Coppock, C. E., R. A. Aguirre, L. E. Chase, G. B. Lake, E. A. Oltenacu, R. E. McDowell, M. J. Fettman and M. E. Woods. 1979. Effect of a low chloride diet on lactating Holstein cows. *J. Dairy Sci.* **62**:723.

Cromwell, G. L., T. S. Stahly and H. J. Monegue. 1981. Effects of source of sodium and chloride on performance of pigs. *J. Anim. Sci.* **53** (Suppl. 1):237 [Abstract].

Damron, B. L. 1982. Availability of sodium in various feedstuffs. *In* "Proceedings of the Florida Nutrition Conference," p. 127. University of Florida, Gainesville.

Damron, B. L., R. H. Harms and L. F. Stepp. 1985. Sodium availability from phosphate sources. *Poult. Sci.* **64**:1772.

Damron, B. L., and W. L. Johnson. 1986. Response of chicks to two drinking water sodium levels supplied from three different salts. *Florida Acad. Sci.* **49**:116.

Damron, B. L., W. L. Johnson and L. S. Kelly. 1986. Utilization of sodium from sodium bicarbonate by broiler chicks. *Poult. Sci.* **65**:782.

de Waal, H. O., M. A. Baard and E. A. N. Engles. 1989. Effects of sodium chloride on sheep. 1. Diet Composition, body mass changes and wool production of young merino wethers grazing native pasture. *S. Afr. J. Anim. Sci.* **19**:27.

Dilworth, B. C., C. D. Schultz and E. J. Day. 1970a. Salt utilization studies with poultry. 1. Effect of salt sources, particle size and insolubles on broiler performance. *Poult. Sci.* **49**:183.

Dilworth, B. C., C. D. Schultz, and E. J. Day. 1970b. Salt utilization studies with poultry. 2. Optimum particle size of salt for the young chick. *Poult. Sci.* **49**:188.

Fethiere, R., R. D. Miles, R. H. Harms and S. M. Laurent. 1988. Bioavailability of sodium in Ethacal® feed component. *Poult. Sci.* **67** (Suppl. 1):15 [Abstract].

Fettman, M. J., L. E. Chase, J. Bentinck-Smith, C. E. Coppock and S. A. Zinn. 1984a. Nutritional chloride deficiency in early lactation Holstein cows. *J. Dairy Sci.* **67**:2321.

Fettman, M. J., L. E. Chase, J. Bentinck-Smith, C. E. Coppock and S. A. Zinn. 1984b. Effects of dietary chloride restriction in lactating dairy cows. *J. Am. Vet. Med. Assoc.* **185**:167.

Fettman, M. J., L. E. Chase, J. Bentinck-Smith, C. E. Coppock and S. A. Zinn. 1984c. Restricted dietary chloride with sodium bicarbonate supplementation for Holstein cows in early lactation. *J. Dairy Sci.* **67**:1457.

Fettman, M. J., L. E. Chase, J. Bentinck-Smith, C. E. Coppock and S. A. Zinn. 1984d. Restricted dietary chloride and sodium bicarbonate supplementation in early lactation Holstein cows: Cerbrospinal fluid electrolyte alterations. *Am. J. Vet. Res.* **45**:1403.

Gaebel, G., M. Bell and H. Martens. 1989. The effect of low mucosal pH on sodium and chloride movement across the isolated rumen mucosa of sheep. *Q. J. Exp. Physiol.* **74**:35.

Gaebel, G., H. Martens, M. Suendermann and P. Galfi. 1987. The effect of diet, intraruminal pH and osmolarity on sodium, chloride and magnesium absorption from the temporarily isolated and washed reticulo-rumen of sheep. *Q. J. Exp. Physiol.* **72**:501.

Grace, N. D., M. J. Ulyatt, and J. C. Macrae. 1974. Quantitative digestion of fresh herbage by sheep. III. The movement of Mg, Ca, P, K and Na in the digestive tract. *J. Agric. Sci. Camb.* **82**:321.

Hagsten, I. and T. W. Perry. 1976. Evaluation of dietary salt levels for swine. II. Effect on blood and excretory patterns. *J. Anim. Sci.* **42**:1191.

Harms, R. H. 1982. Chloride requirement of young turkeys. *Poult. Sci.* **61**:2447.

Ingram, D. R., H. R. Wilson, W. G. Nesbeth, B. L. Beane and C. R. Douglas. 1984. Sodium chloride requirement of Bobwhite quail chicks. *Poult. Sci.* **63**:1837.

James, L. G. and J. E. Wohlt. 1985. Effect of supplementing equivalent cation amounts from NaCl, MgO, NaHCO₃ and CaCO₃ on nutrient utilization and acid-base status of growing Dorset lambs fed high concentration diets. *J. Anim. Sci.* **60**:307.

Kemp, A. 1964. Sodium requirement of milking cows: Balance trials with cows on rations of freshly mown herbage and on winter rations. *Neth. J. Agric. Sci.* **12**:263.

Kemp, A. 1966. Mineral balance in dairy cows fed on grass, with special reference to magnesium and sodium. *In* "Proceedings of the X International Grassland Congress," p. 411.

Leach, R. M., Jr. and M. C. Nesheim. 1963. Studies on chloride deficiency in chicks. *J. Nutr.* **81**:193.

Link, K. R. J. and W. G. Olson. 1985. The effects of deleting supplemental sodium chloride from the diet on milk production and electrolyte concentrations in serum and urine. *J. Dairy Sci.* **68** (Suppl. 1):135 [Abstract].

Martz, F. A., R. Nieto Ordaz, M. F. Weiss and R. L. Belyea. 1988. Mineral balance for growing dairy heifers fed semipurified diets. *Nutr. Rep. Int.* **38**:665.

Matterson, L. D., H. M. Scott and E. Jungherr. 1948. Salt tolerance of turkeys. *Poult. Sci.* **25**:539.

Miles, R. D., R. Fethiere and R. H. Harms. 1988. The availability of the sodium in Ethacal® feed component for laying hens. *Poult. Sci.* **67** (Suppl. 1):120 [Abstract].

Morris, J. G. 1980. Assessment of sodium requirements of grazing beef cattle: A review. *J. Anim. Sci.* **50**:145.

Morris, J. G. and G. W. Murphy. 1972. The sodium requirements of beef calves for growth. *J. Agric. Sci. Camb.* **78**:105.

Morris, J. G. and G. R. Peterson. 1975. Sodium requirements of lactating ewes. *J. Nutr.* **105**:595.

Neathery, M. W. 1980. Chloride metabolism in cattle. *In* "Proceedings of the Georgia Nutrition Conference," p. 137.

Neathery, M. W., D. M. Blackmon, W. J. Miller, S. Heinmiller, S. McGuire, J. M. Tarabula, R. P. Gentry and J. C. Allen. 1981. Chloride deficiency in Holstein calves from a low chloride diet and removal of abomasal contents. *J. Dairy Sci.* **64**:2220.

Nelson, A. B., R. W. MacVicar, W. Archer, Jr. and J. C. Meiske. 1955. Effect of a high salt intake on the digestibility of ration constituents and on nitrogen, sodium, and chloride retention by steers and wethers. *J. Anim. Sci.* **14**:825.

Nesheim, M. C., R. M. Leach, Jr., T. R. Zeigler and J. A. Serafin. 1964. Interrelationships between dietary levels of sodium, chlorine and potassium. *J. Nutr.* **84**:361.

Nott, H. and G. F. Combs. 1969. Availability of sodium in defluorinated rock phosphate. *Poult. Sci.* **48**:482.

Paquay, R. F. Lomba, A. Lousse and V. Bienfet. 1969. Statistical research on the fate of dietary mineral elements in dry and lactating cows. IV. Chloride. *J. Agric. Sci. Camb.* **73**:223.

Peirce, A. W. 1959. Studies on salt tolerance of sheep. II. The tolerance of sheep for mixtures of sodium chloride and magnesium chloride in the drinking water. *Aust. J. Agric. Res.* **10**:725.

Peirce, A.W. 1960. Studies on salt tolerance of sheep. III. The tolerance of sheep for mixtures of sodium chloride and sodium sulphate in the drinking water. *Aust. J. Agric. Res.* **11**:548.

Peirce, A. W. 1962. Studies on salt tolerance of sheep. IV. The tolerance of sheep for mixtures of sodium chloride and calcium chloride in the drinking water. *Aust. J. Agric. Res.* **3** :479.

Proudfoot, F. G., H. W. Hulan and D. M. Nash. 1985. Effects of a wide range of dietary salt levels on the performance of broiler chicks. *Can. J. Anim. Sci.* **65**:773.

Ross, E. 1977. Apparent inadequacy of sodium requirement in broiler chickens. *Poult. Sci.* **56**:1153.

Schneider, P. L., D. K. Beede and C. J. Wilcox. 1986. Responses of lactating cows to dietary sodium source and quantity and potassium quantity during heat stress. *J. Dairy Sci.* **69**:99.

Schryver, H. F., M. T. Parker, P. D. Daniluk, K. I. Pagan, J. Williams, L. V. Soderholm and H. F. Hintz. 1987. Salt consumption and the effect of salt on mineral metabolism in horses. *Cornell Vet.* **77**:122.

Scott, D. 1967. The effects of potassium supplements upon the absorption of potassium and sodium from the sheep rumen. *Q. J. Exp. Physiol.* **52**:382.

Smith, S. E. and P. D. Aines. 1959. Salt requirements for dairy cattle. *Cornell Agric. Exp. Stn. Bull.*, **938**.

Spears, J. W. and R. W. Harvey. 1987. Lasalocid and dietary sodium and potassium effects on mineral metabolism, ruminal volatile fatty acids and performance of finishing steers. *J. Anim. Sci.* **65**:830

Staples, C. R. and D. S. Lough. 1989. Efficacy of supplemental dietary neutralizing agents for lactating dairy cows. A review. *Anim. Feed Sci. Technol.* **23**:277.

Starnes, S. R., J. W . Spears, M. A. Froetschel and W. J. Croom, Jr. 1984. Influence of monensin and lasalocid on mineral metabolism and ruminal urease activity in steers. *J. Nutr.* **114**:518.

Summers, J. D. and S. Leeson. 1985. Available sodium and potassium in canola and soybean meal. *Can. J. Anim. Sci.* **65**:211.

Summers, J. D., E. T. Moran, Jr. and W. F. Pepper. 1967. A chloride deficiency in a practical diet encountered as a result of using a common sodium sulfate antibiotic potentiating procedure. *Poult. Sci.* **46**:1557.

Underwood, E. J. 1981. " The Mineral Nutrition of Livestock," 2nd ed. Commonwealth Agricultural Bureaux, Slough, U.K.

Weeth, H. J. and J. E. Hunter. 1971. Drinking of sulfate-water by cattle. *J. Anim. Sci.* **32**:277.

Wurmli, R., S. Wolffram and E. Scharrer. 1987. Inhibition of chloride absorption from the sheep rumen by nitrate. *J. Vet. Med.* **34**:476.

16
SULFUR BIOAVAILABILITY

Pamela R. Henry
Clarence B. Ammerman

Department of Animal Science
University of Florida
Gainesville, Florida

I. INTRODUCTION

Sulfur is distributed widely in nature as a component of proteins and numerous other organic compounds and, consequently, it has many structural and regulatory functions in common with nitrogen. Sulfur is a constituent of the amino acids methionine, cysteine, cystine, homocysteine, taurine, and cystathionine, and disulfide bonds are responsible for maintaining the tertiary structure of protein molecules. Microorganisms in the ruminant digestive tract are capable of synthesizing sulfur-containing amino acids and vitamins from inorganic sulfur sources. Nonruminant animals have few assimilatory microorganisms so that the major proportion of their sulfur requirement must be in the form of amino acids. Diets for ruminants that are low in protein or that contain a large proportion of the nitrogen requirement as nonprotein nitrogen may be deficient in sulfur.

II. BIOAVAILABILITY STUDIES

A. *In Vitro* and Ruminal Microflora Estimates of Bioavailbility

Loosli *et al.* (1949) first demonstrated that ruminal microorganisms of sheep fed urea as the sole nitrogen source were able to synthesize methionine from inorganic sulfur and that the sheep grew and remained in positive nitrogen balance. Shortly thereafter, researchers showed that dietary radiolabeled sulfur as sodium sulfate (Na_2SO_4) was incorporated into cystine and methionine in the rumen and utilized to form milk protein (Block and Stekol, 1950; Block *et al.*, 1951). Ruminal synthesis

BIOAVAILABILITY OF NUTRIENTS FOR ANIMALS:
AMINO ACIDS, MINERALS, AND VITAMINS

349

of cystine and its incorporation into wool was eight times greater in a sheep fed labeled sodium sulfate than in one given elemental sulfur; however, there was only one animal per treatment (Hale and Garrigus, 1953).

Emery *et al.* (1957b) reported that synthesis of cystine was about twice as great as that of methionine during a 3-hr *in vitro* culture with labeled sulfur as inorganic sulfate. Microautoradiographs indicated that the majority of organisms did not incorporate radiolabeled sulfur regardless of whether they came from donors fed roughage or concentrate. However, incorporation of sulfate-sulfur into organic compounds was faster with ruminal liquor from cattle fed high-concentrate diets. In further studies, Emery *et al.* (1957a) reported that only 3 (*Butyrivibrio fibrisolvens, Lachnospira multiparous* and *Bacteroides strain B_I-4*) of 10 cultures of ruminal bacteria synthesized organic sulfur compounds from inorganic sulfate when cysteine was present in the media. *Desulphovibrio desulphuricans*, which has been isolated from sheep's rumen (Huisingh *et al.*, 1974), was able to utilize sulfate, sulfite, thiosulfate, tetrathionate, metabisulfite and dithionite, but not elemental sulfur for growth (Postgate, 1951; Ishimoto *et al.*, 1954). Sulfite was a normal intermediate of sulfate reduction. In a review, Bryant (1973) indicated that of the predominant ruminal cellulolytic bacteria, *Bacteroides succinogenes* could utilize cysteine or sulfide but not sulfate. Sulfide sulfur was essential for some strains of *Ruminococcus flavefaciens*. Many strains of both *Ruminococcus flavefaciens* and. *Ruminococcus albus* grew in media containing only sulfide and sulfate sulfur. Lewis (1954) also reported that sulfate, sulfite, and thiosulfate were reduced to sulfide in the rumen of sheep and in *in vitro* cultures.

Labeled [^{35}S]-sulfide-sulfur was absorbed rapidly from the rumen of sheep; only 6 to 9% remained 2 to 3 hr after dosing, and 60 to 73% of the dose appeared in urine within 4 days of dosing. However, more than 90% of a dose of labeled [^{35}S]-sulfate-sulfur was recovered from the rumen after 2 to 3 hr and only 8 to 10% was excreted in urine within 4 days (Bray, 1969). Anderson (1956) and Gawthorne and Nader (1976) also reported the reduction of sulfate to sulfide by ruminal microorganisms and either subsequent utilization in microbial protein synthesis or absorption by the ruminal epithelium. About 55% of the sulfur amino acid content of microbial protein was synthesized *de novo* from the sulfide pool (Gawthorne and Nader, 1976). Sulfate-sulfur was absorbed by the small intestine of sheep rather than the rumen (Bird and Moir, 1971). An average of 74% of ^{35}S ruminally infused as [^{35}S]-methionine in sheep was recovered in omasal digesta and approximately 69% was in an organic form, while 6% of the ^{35}S was inorganic (Bird and Moir, 1972).

The concentration of sulfide in ruminal fluid and the body sulfide pool were greater in sheep fed cystine than in those fed inorganic sulfate, but additional sulfur increased microbial protein synthesis regardless of the sulfur source (Hume and Bird,

1970). Apparent absorption from the rumen of ingested sulfur as either sulfate or cystine was 35% (Bird and Hume, 1971).

Sulfur sources have also been compared with regard to their ability to improve cellulose digestion (Hunt *et al.*, 1954; Trenkle *et al.*, 1958; Gil *et al.*, 1973; Bull and Vandersall, 1973; Spears *et al.*, 1976, 1977, 1978; Guardiola *et al.*, 1980, 1983; Patterson and Kung, 1988). Cellulose digestion generally improves with sulfur supplementation but with no significant difference among sources (Table I). Fertilization of orchardgrass with sulfur improved digestibility of NDF, ADF, and permanganate lignin, but sulfur fertilization had no effect on tall fescue (Spears *et al.*, 1985; Chestnut *et al.*, 1986). Sulfur fertilization also improved these characteristics in corn silage (Buttrey *et al.*, 1986).

Kahlon and Chow (1989) investigated methods to intrinsically label samples of wheat with ^{35}S, and this may prove useful for future bioavailability studies.

B. *In Vivo* Estimates of Bioavailability

1. Ruminants

Utilization of absorbed inorganic sulfur has been demonstrated in avian species and probably occurs in most other species. The predominant need for the element, however, is in the form of sulfur-bearing amino acids which must be provided preformed for the nonruminant or either provided preformed or synthesized by ruminal microflora for the ruminant. Thus, animal growth and nitrogen retention may be the most critical indicators of sulfur bioavailability. Studies are limited, however, in which these criteria were used specifically to determine relative bioavailability among sulfur sources. Many comparisons of sources in ruminants have been based on absorption of the element, implying that absorbability of sulfur is indicative of the element's availability for protein synthesis by ruminal microflora.

Growth responses in ruminants have been used to assess the adequacy of dietary sulfur, especially in diets containing a nonprotein nitrogen source such as urea. With diets for sheep and goats that contained 4 to 5% urea, increased growth has been reported with sulfur supplementation as methionine (Weir and Rendig, 1952; Noble *et al.*, 1955; Mowat and Deelstra, 1970; Bird and Moir, 1972) sulfates (Thomas *et al.*, 1951), and elemental sulfur (Starks *et al.*, 1953; Albert *et al.*, 1955; Onwuka and Akinsoyinu, 1989). Garrigus *et al.* (1950) reported a greater growth response in lambs fed methionine than in those fed elemental sulfur, but the dietary ingredients were not reported.

Supplementation of a purified diet containing urea with inorganic sulfates increased wool production (Thomas *et al.*, 1951). Addition of elemental sulfur to low sulfur diets also tended to improve wool production (Starks *et al.*, 1953; Albert *et al.*, 1955). Supplementation of a purified diet containing urea with elemental sulfur, sodium sulfate and methionine increased wool production and no differences were noted among sources (Starks *et al.*, 1954). Supplementation of sheep fed a purified diet containing urea with methionine hydroxy analog resulted in greater wool production than feeding elemental sulfur; DL-methionine, calcium sulfate, and sodium sulfate gave intermediate responses (Kahlon *et al.*, 1975b).

There was no difference in milk production when .08% sulfur as either sodium sulfate or methionine hydroxy analog was added to a basal diet containing .10% sulfur (Bouchard and Conrad, 1973a). In a second experiment, sodium sulfate or Dynamate® (K_2SO_4+$MgSO_4$) (Pitman-Moore inc., Mundelein, IL) was added to a basal diet (.06% sulfur) for a total of either .18 or .24% sulfur. Milk production was 14% greater in cows supplemented with sulfur, but there was no difference between sources (Bouchard and Conrad, 1973a). There was no difference in milk production when molasses and sodium sulfate contributed .09 and .24% sulfur to a diet containing .06% of the element (Bouchard and Conrad, 1973b). In the same series of studies, feed intake and milk production decreased when lignin-sulfonate provided .24% sulfur to the diet but not when calcium sulfate ($CaSO_4$) was the source. Feeding methionine hydroxy analog, Dynamate, or sodium sulfate did not alter milk production (Bouchard and Conrad, 1974; Wallenius and Whitchurch, 1975).

Apparent absorption of sulfur by calves fed a purified diet ranged from 60 to 63% when elemental sulfur was supplemented at .34 to 1.72% added sulfur (Slyter *et al.*, 1988). Supplementation of sheep diets with elemental sulfur did not alter apparent sulfur absorption from fall-accumulated fescue hay, which averaged 66% (Muntifering *et al.*, 1984). However, sulfur supplementation increased apparent sulfur absorption in sheep from 63 to 66% when early vegetative fescue hay was fed (Muntifering *et al.*, 1984) and from 70 to 85% when early to midbloom hay was fed (Glenn and Ely, 1981).

Fertilization of fescue with 132 kg/ha of sulfur increased apparent sulfur absorption from 52 to 61%, while similar fertilization of orchardgrass resulted in an increase in apparent absorption from 56 to 60% (Spears *et al.*, 1985). Langlands *et al.* (1973) reported an average apparent sulfur absorption of 50% for eight species of temperate forages and three species of tropical forages. Apparent sulfur absorption values in mature sheep were 52% for subterranean clover hay, 37% for mature annual ryegrass hay, and 7% for a low quality grass-clover mixture (Doyle and Egan, 1983).

Supplementation of a low sulfur purified diet (.06% sulfur) with .66% elemental sulfur increased apparent sulfur absorption in sheep from -36% to 40% (Starks *et al.*, 1953). Supplementation of natural diets containing urea for lactating cows with sodium sulfate has also improved sulfur absorption (Jacobson *et al.*, 1969; Grieve *et al.*, 1973). Apparent absorption of sulfur by sheep supplemented with sodium sulfate has ranged from 11% at lower levels of added sulfur to 90% with greater levels of the element (Bird, 1971, 1972; L'Estrange *et al.*, 1972; Kennedy and Siebert, 1972a,b). Sulfur as sulfuric acid (H_2SO_4) was also well absorbed by ruminants and the excess was excreted in urine (L'Estrange and Murphy, 1972; Kennedy and Siebert, 1972b).

True absorption of sulfur in dairy steers fed a concentrate containing urea (.21% sulfur) and corn silage (.20% sulfur) was 68%. When 25 g/day of Na_2SO_4 or an isosulfurous amount of DL-methionine or methionine hydroxy analog was supplemented to diets, true absorption increased to 81, 81, and 77%, respectively (Bull and Vandersall, 1973). The apparent absorption by sheep of sulfur from sulfate was greater than that from elemental sulfur when either urea or soy isolate was the primary source of nitrogen (Goodrich and Tillman, 1966). Kahlon *et al.* (1975a) also reported lower apparent sulfur absorption by sheep supplemented with 1.4 g/day of sulfur as elemental sulfur compared with DL-methionine, methionine hydroxy analog, calcium sulfate, and sodium sulfate. True absorption of ^{35}S in sheep fed a natural diet containing urea was lower for those fed elemental sulfur (36%) than for those fed sodium sulfate (78%) or L-methionine (78%) (Johnson *et al.*, 1971). True ^{35}S retention averaged 27, 56, and 70%, respectively. Steinacher *et al.* (1970) were the only researchers to report greater apparent absorption and retention of sulfur from elemental sulfur than methionine in a study with steers fed a high roughage diet.

Thomas *et al.* (1951) conducted three experiments in which sheep were fed either a low sulfur purified diet or the same diet in which sulfate forms of calcium, magnesium, copper, and manganese were used in the mineral mixture. Apparent sulfur absorption did not differ among diets but retention was negative for the deficient diet.

Supplementation of lactating dairy cows with sulfur as sodium sulfate, methionine hydroxy analog, or Dynamate increased apparent and true sulfur absorption (Bouchard and Conrad, 1973a). From 65 to 77% of sulfur in molasses was apparently absorbed by lactating dairy cows compared with 77 to 87% for sulfur as sodium sulfate (Bouchard and Conrad, 1973b). Sulfur from lignin-sulfonate was only 42 to 53% absorbed, but sulfur from calcium sulfate (agricultural gypsum) was 81 to 87% absorbed (Bouchard and Conrad, 1973b).

Apparent absorption of sulfur was similar when either sodium or calcium sulfate was supplemented to lactating dairy cattle (Bouchard and Conrad, 1973c). Apparent absorption of sulfur was lower in cows fed methionine hydroxy analog than in those fed Dynamate, although total sulfur intake was also greater in the latter group (Bouchard and Conrad, 1974). When methionine hydroxy analog replaced part of the $MgSO_4+K_2SO_4$ and diets were made isosulfurous, apparent absorption of sulfur did not differ. Supplementation of diets for sheep with 1% sulfur as sodium sulfate, sodium bisulfate ($NaHSO_4$), ammonium sulfate [$(NH_4)_2SO_4$], ammonium bisulfate (NH_4HSO_4), or sulfuric acid increased apparent sulfur absorption from 49% in the control diet to 83, 80, 81, 80, and 83%, respectively (Upton *et al.*, 1970).

Weir and Rendig (1954) reported increased serum sulfate sulfur when methionine or elemental sulfur was added to sulfur-deficient diets. Serum sulfate sulfur also increased when 1% sulfur as ammonium sulfate, ammonium bisulfate, sodium bisulfate, sodium sulfate, or sulfuric acid was added to diets for sheep, but there were no differences among sources (L'Estrange et al., 1969). When lambs were dosed orally with radiolabeled sulfur as elemental sulfur, sodium sulfate, or L-methionine, those given sodium sulfate had greater radioactivity in plasma during the first 36 hr after dosing. After 36 hr, those given L-methionine had greater plasma activity than lambs given the other sources (Johnson et al., 1970).

2. Nonruminants

Early studies with nonruminant animals failed to show a response to inorganic sulfur (Daniels and Rich, 1918; Lewis and Lewis, 1927; Kellerman, 1936; Tarver and Schmidt, 1939). Machlin (1955) and Gordon and Sizer (1955), however, reported a growth response in chicks when sodium sulfate was added to a diet containing 15% casein and 10% gelatin as protein sources. Radiolabeled sulfur was rapidly taken up into taurine and other compounds, but was not used to synthesize cystine and methionine. Since then, several researchers have reported a growth response in poultry supplemented with inorganic sulfur (Ross and Harms, 1970; Sloan and Harms, 1972; Ross et al., 1972; Sasse and Baker, 1974a,b; Miles and Harms, 1983; Carew et al., 1986; Harms and Buresh, 1987). Radiolabeled sulfur studies in pigs, rats, and poultry have indicated that inorganic sulfur can be incorporated into taurine but not methionine or cystine (Machlin et al., 1953; Kulwich et al., 1958; Martin et al., 1966; Huovinen and Gustafsson, 1967). Rabbits, like ruminants, have shown some ^{35}S (from $^{35}SO_4$) incorporation into methionine, but this is the result of coprophagy (Kulwich et al., 1954).

Button et al. (1965) reported that sulfur from either calcium sulfate dihydrate ($CaSO_4 \cdot 2H_2O$) or sodium sulfate dihydrate ($Na_2SO_4 \cdot 2H_2O$) was well absorbed by rats and incorporated into cartilage mucopolysaccharides. Sasse and Baker (1974a) reported a marked growth response to potassium sulfate (K_2SO_4) but not taurine in chicks fed a cystine-deficient diet (Table I). Other growth studies with poultry have indicated similar availability of sulfur from inorganic sources including sodium sulfate, $CaSO_4$, sodium thiosulfate ($Na_2S_2O_3$), sodium bisulfite ($NaHSO_3$), magnesium sulfate ($MgSO_4$), potassium sulfate, and Dynamate (Ross and Harms, 1970; Sasse and Baker, 1974b; Miles and Harms, 1983; Carew et al., 1986). The minimal level of sulfate required to elicit a maximal growth response in chicks (Sasse and Baker, 1974a,b) and rats (Smith, 1973) fed a cystine-deficient diet has been reported to be 200 ppm. Sasse and Baker (1974a), Soares (1974), and Anderson et al. (1975) have suggested that inorganic sulfur as sulfate is capable of sparing 15%

of the dietary requirement for cystine. With practical diets for poultry, dicalcium phosphate, fish products and drinking water generally provide significant quantities of sulfur as sulfate, thereby often precluding a response to the element.

III. FACTORS INFLUENCING BIOAVAILABILITY

A. Dietary Factors

Dietary proteins with their sulfur containing amino acids provide a major dietary source of sulfur for animals. Thus, factors that affect protein digestion can, in turn, influence sulfur utilization. In the ruminant animal, for example, protection of protein and amino acids from breakdown in the rumen can result in less sulfur being available for use by ruminal microflora.

Interactions among mineral elements including the copper, molybdenum, and sulfur relationship and that involving sulfur and selenium influence the utilization of sulfur. Also, oxalate has been shown to inhibit sulfate and selenate uptake by the small intestine of sheep (Wolffram *et al.*, 1987). Other dicarboxylate anions including oxaloacetate and fumarate also reduced mucosal sulfate uptake. Generally, inorganic sulfur or methionine has been shown to reduce absorption and utilization of selenium (Combs and Combs, 1986). The reverse is not generally a problem because of the vast difference in requirements. Postgate (1952) did, however, report that selenate ion was a powerful competitive antagonist of sulfate reduction by *Desulphovibrio desulphuricans.*

The interaction among copper, molybdenum, and sulfur is also not generally considered from the standpoint of potential detrimental effects on sulfur utilization because of the large differences in dietary requirements for the three elements. Rather, sulfur inhibits absorption and utilization of copper or molybdenum (Underwood, 1981). However, sodium molybdate (50 ppm molybdenum) inhibited reduction of sulfate as inorganic sulfate to sulfide but enhanced production of sulfide from methionine (Huisingh *et al.*, 1975). Gawthorne and Nader (1976) also reported inhibition of sulfate reduction by molybdate. Molybdenum (8 ppm) and nitrate-nitrogen (.4 or .8%) inhibited *in vitro* cellulose digestion in the presence of .1 to .4% added sulfur as sulfate or sulfide (Spears *et al.*, 1977).

B. Animal Factors

Factors that change the population of ruminal microflora may also affect the availability of inorganic sulfur (Garrigus, 1970). Age, growth rate, and protein synthesis are related to sulfur metabolism. There may be breed differences among sheep with regard to wool production and sulfur content of wool that involve sulfur metabolism (Garrigus, 1970). Apparent absorption of sulfur from three hays was similar in weanling *vs* mature sheep when expressed as a percentage of intake, but weanling lambs incorporated less sulfur into wool and more into tissue than mature sheep (Doyle and Egan, 1983).

IV. SUMMARY

Sulfur is a more critical nutrient for ruminants than nonruminants from the standpoint of potential deficiency. Thus, most bioavailability experiments have been conducted with either sheep or cattle in growth or absorption studies or with *in vitro* ruminal fermentation techniques (Table I). Assuming these criteria, including sulfur absorption, are valid indicators of bioavailability, most sources of sulfur have been well utilized when compared with sodium sulfate as the standard. Organic forms including the isomers of methionine and methionine hydroxy analog have provided sulfur equal in availability to that in sodium sulfate. One *in vitro* study with cystine suggested that the sulfur in this compound was not readily utilized. Inorganic compounds including ammonium bisulfate, ammonium sulfate, calcium sulfate, sodium bisulfate, and sulfuric acid were generally equal to sodium sulfate as a source of sulfur. Elemental sulfur was not utilized as well as sodium sulfate when tested in both cattle and sheep. One *in vitro* study suggested that elemental sulfur was completely unavailable for support of ruminal cellulose digestion. Sodium sulfide was examined *in vitro* only and was not as well utilized as sodium sulfate. In general, apparent absorption of sulfur from plant materials has varied from about 50 to 70%.

Table I. Relative bioavailability of sulfur sources for animals[a]

Source	RV	Standard	Response criterion	Meth cal	Type diet	Added level	Reference
In vitro							
Ammonium sulfate	93	L-Methionine	Prot syn	TP	PM	43 ppm inoculum	Kahlon et al. (1975a)
Calcium sulfate ($CaSO_4 \cdot 2H_2O$)	117	Sodium sulfate (Na_2SO_4)	Cell dig	TP	PM	.12-.24% substrate DM	Bull and Vandersall (1973)
Calcium sulfate	94	L-Methionine	Prot syn	TP	PM	43 ppm inoculum	Kahlon et al. (1975a)
Cystine	35	Na_2SO_4	Cell dig	TP	NG	50 mg/flask	Hunt et al. (1954)
Methionine	109	Na_2SO_4	Cell dig	TP	NG	50 mg/flask	Hunt et al. (1954)
Methionine hydroxy analog	68	Na_2SO_4	Prot syn	TP	PM	10 µg/ml medium	Gil et al. (1973)
Methionine hydroxy analog	124	Na_2SO_4	Cell dig	TP	PM	10 µg/ml medium	Gil et al. (1973)
Methionine hydroxy analog	81	Na_2SO_4	Lcell dig	TP	N	.32% substrate DM	Bull and Vandersall (1973)
Methionine hydroxy analog	29	L-Methionine	Prot syn	TP	PM	43 ppm inoculum	Kahlon et al. (1975a)
Methionine hydroxy analog	113	Na_2SO_4	NDF dig	TP	P	.39% substrate DM	Patterson and Kung (1988)
DL-Methionine	77	Na_2SO_4	Cell dig	TP	PM	10 µg/ml medium	Gil et al. (1973)
DL-Methionine	117	Na_2SO_4	Cell dig	TP	PM	.12-.24% substrate DM	Bull and Vandersall (1973)

Table 1. (continued)

Source	RV	Standard	Response criterion	Meth cal	Type diet	Added level	Reference
DL-Methionine	77	Na_2SO_4	Lcell dig	TP	N	.32% substrate DM	Bull and Vandersall (1973)
DL-Methionine	63	L-Methionine	Prot syn	TP	PM	43 ppm inoculum	Kahlon et al. (1975a)
DL-Methionine	113	Na_2SO_4	Cell dig	TP	N	.15% substrate DM	Guardiola et al. (1983)
DL-Methionine	106	Na_2SO_4	Cell dig	TP	N	.15% substrate DM	Guardiola et al. (1983)
DL-Methionine	111	Na_2SO_4	NDF dig	TP	P	.3% substrate DM	Patterson and Kung (1988)
Sodium sulfate	55	L-Methionine	Prot syn	TP	PM	43 ppm inoculum	Kahlon et al. (1975a)
Sodium sulfide	43	L-Methionine	Prot syn	TP	PM	43 ppm inoculum	Kahlon et al. (1975a)
Sodium sulfide (Na_2S)	102	Na_2SO_4	Cell dig	TP	P	.1-4% substrate DM	Spears et al. (1970)
Sulfur, elemental	0	Na_2SO_4	Cell dig	TP	NG	50 mg/flask	Hunt et al. (1954)
Sulfur, elemental	36	L-Methionine	Prot syn	TP	PM	43 ppm inoculum	Kahlon et al. (1975a)
Sulfur, elemental	17	L-Methionine	Cell dig	TP	P	.085-.680%	Spears et al. (1976)

Cattle

Source	RV	Standard	Response criterion	Meth cal	Type diet	Added level	Reference
Methionine hydroxy analog	83	Na_2SO_4	App abs	MR	N-.20%	.12%	Bull and Vandersall (1973)

Compound							
Methionine hydroxy analog	95	Na_2SO_4	True abs	MR	N-.20%	.12%	Bull and Vandersall (1973)
Methionine hydroxy analog	97	Na_2SO_4	App abs	MR	N-.10%	.08%	Bouchard and Conrad (1973a)
Methionine hydroxy analog	100	Na_2SO_4	True abs	MR	N-.10%	.08%	Bouchard and Conrad (1973a)
DL-Methionine	102	Na_2SO_4	App abs	MR	N-.20%	.12%	Bull and Vandersall (1973)
DL-Methionine	100	Na_2SO_4	True abs	MR	N-.20%	.12%	Bull and Vandersall (1973)
DL-Methionine	101	Na_2SO_4	App abs	TP	N-.21%	.15%	Fron et al. (1990)
DL-Methionine	109	Na_2SO_4	Ur S exc	TP	N-.21%	.15%	Fron et al. (1990)
Molasses	84	Na_2SO_4	App abs	MR	N-.06%	.09, .24%	Bouchard and Conrad (1973b)
Molasses	86	Na_2SO_4	True abs	MR	N-.06%	.09, .24%	Bouchard and Conrad (1973b)
Potassium sulfate + magnesium sulfate[b]	99	Na_2SO_4	App abs	MR	N-.06%	.12, .18%	Bouchard and Conrad (1973a)
Potassium sulfate + magnesium sulfate[b]	97	Na_2SO_4	True abs	MR	N-.06%	.12, .18%	Bouchard and Conrad (1973a)
Sulfur, elemental	44	Na_2SO_4	App abs	TP	N-.21%	.15%	Fron et al. (1990)
Sulfur, elemental	28	Na_2SO_4	Ur S exc	TP	N-.21%	.15%	Fron et al. (1990)

Sheep

Compound							
Ammonium bisulfate (NH_4HSO_4)	98	Na_2SO_4	App abs	MR	N-.45%	1.0%	Upton et al. 1970
Ammonium sulfate [$(NH_4)_2SO_4$]	95	Na_2SO_4	App abs	MR	N-.45%	1.0%	Upton et al. 1970
Calcium sulfate	111	Na_2SO_4	Growth	MR	SP-.034%	1.4 g/day	Kahlon et al. 1975b
Calcium sulfate	102	Na_2SO_4	App abs	MR	SP-.034%	1.4 g/day	Kahlon et al. (1975b)

Table I. (continued)

Source	RV	Standard	Response criterion	Meth cal	Type diet	Added level	Reference
Methionine hydroxy analog	101	Na_2SO_4	Growth	MR	SP-.034%	1.4 g/day	Kahlon et al. (1975b)
Methionine hydroxy analog	105	Na_2SO_4	App abs	MR	SP-.034%	1.4 g/day	Kahlon et al. (1975b)
DL-Methionine	120	Na_2SO_4	Growth	MR	SP-.034%	1.4 g/day	Kahlon et al. (1975b)
DL-Methionine	94	Na_2SO_4	App abs	MR	SP-.034%	1.4 g/day	Kahlon et al. (1975b)
DL-Methionine	102	Na_2SO_4	App abs	MR	N-.26%	.15%	Guardiola et al. (1980)
L-Methionine	100	Na_2SO_4	True abs	MR	N-.12%	NG	Johnson et al. (1971)
Sodium bisulfate ($NaHSO_4$)	96	Na_2SO_4	App abs	MR	N-.45%	1.0%	Upton et al. (1970)
Sulfur, elemental	73	Na_2SO_4	Growth	MR	P-.054%	.2%	Starks et al. (1954)
Sulfur, elemental	45	$MgSO_4+Na_2SO_4$	App abs	MR	P	.2%	Goodrich and Tillman (1966)
Sulfur, elemental	69	$MgSO_4+Na_2SO_4$	App abs	MR	P	.2%	Goodrich and Tillman (1966)
Sulfur, elemental	46	Na_2SO_4	Tru abs	MR	N-.12%	NG	Johnson et al. (1971)
Sulfur, elemental	102	Na_2SO_4	Growth	MR	SP-.034%	1.4 g/day	Kahlon et al. (1975b)
Sulfur, elemental	67	Na_2SO_4	App abs	MR	SP-.034%	1.4 g/day	Kahlon et al. (1975b)
Sulfuric acid (H_2SO_4)	100	Na_2SO_4	App abs	MR	N-.45%	1.0%	Upton et al. (1970)

[a]Abbreviations can be found in Appendix I. Chemical formula for a compound given only if provided by the author.
[b]Dynamate; Pitman-Moore Inc., Mundelein, IL (double sulfate of potassium and magnesium).

Table II. Relative bioavailability of supplemental sulfur sources[a]

Source	In vitro[b]	Species[c] Cattle	Sheep
Sodium sulfate	100	100	100
Ammonium bisulfate	-	-	100 (1)
Ammonium sulfate	-	-	95 (1)
Calcium sulfate	115 (1)	-	105 (1)
Cystine	35 (1)	-	-
Methionine	110 (1)	-	-
Methionine hydroxy analog	95 (3)	95 (2)	-
DL-Methionine	100 (4)	100 (2)	105 (2)
L-Methionine	-	-	100 (1)
Molasses	-	85 (1)	-
Potassium sulfate + magnesium sulfate[d]	-	100 (2)	-
Sodium bisulfate	-	-	95 (1)
Sodium sulfide	70 (2)	-	-
Sulfur, elemental	0 (1)	35 (1)	65 (3)
Sulfuric acid	-	-	100 (1)

[a]Average values rounded to nearest "5" and expressed relative to response obtained with sodium sulfate. Number of studies or samples involved indicated within parentheses.

[b]Either protein synthesis or cellulose digestion served as criterion for most in vitro comparisons.

[c]Based on absorption of sulfur.

[d]Dynamate; Pitman-Moore Inc., Mundelein, IL (double sulfate of potassium and magnesium).

REFERENCES

Albert, W. W., U. S. Garrigus, R. M. Forbes and W. H. Hale. 1955. Modified urea supplements with corn silage for wintering ewe lambs. *J. Anim. Sci.* **14**:143.

Anderson, C. M. 1956. The metabolism of sulphur in the rumen of the sheep. *N.Z. J. Sci. Technol.* **37**:379.

Anderson, J. O., R. E. Warnick and R. K. Dalaic. 1975. Replacing dietary methionine and cystine in chick diets with sulfate or other sulfur compounds. *Poult. Sci.* **54**:1122.

Bird, P. R. 1971. Sulphur metabolism and excretion studies in ruminants. II. Organic and inorganic sulphur excretion by sheep after intraruminal or intraduodenal infusions of sodium sulphate. *Aust. J. Biol. Sci.* **24**:1329.

Bird, P. R. 1972. Sulphur metabolism and excretion studies in ruminants. IX. Sulphur, nitrogen, and energy utilization by sheep fed a sulphur-deficient and a sulphate-supplemented, roughage-based diet. *Aust. J. Biol. Sci.* **25**:1073.

Bird, P. R. and I. D. Hume. 1971. Sulphur metabolism and excretion studies in ruminants. IV. Cystine and sulphate effects upon the flow of sulphur from the rumen and upon sulphur excretion by sheep. *Aust. J. Agric. Res.* **22**:443.

Bird, P. R. and R. J. Moir. 1971. Sulphur metabolism and excretion studies in ruminants. I. The absorption of sulphate in sheep after intraruminal or intraduodenal infusions of sodium sulphate. *Aust. J. Biol. Sci.* **24**:1319.

Bird, P. R. and R. J. Moir. 1972. Sulphur metabolism and excretion studies in ruminants. VIII. Methionine degradation and utilization in sheep when infused into the rumen or abomasum. *Aust. J. Biol. Sci.* **25**:835.

Block, R. J. and J. A. Stekol. 1950. Synthesis of sulfur amino acids from inorganic sulfate by ruminants. *Proc. Soc. Exp. Biol. Med.* **73**:391.

Block, R. J., J. A. Stekol and J. K. Loosli. 1951. Synthesis of sulfur amino acids from inorganic sulfate by ruminants. II. Synthesis of cystine and methionine from sodium sulfate by the goat and by the microorganisms of the rumen of the ewe. *Arch. Biochem. Biophys.* **33**:353.

Bouchard, R. and H. R. Conrad. 1973a. Sulfur requirement of lactating dairy cows. I. Sulfur balance and dietary supplementation. *J. Dairy Sci.* **56**:1276.

Bouchard, R. and H. R. Conrad. 1973b. Sulfur requirement of lactating dairy cows. II. Utilization of sulfates, molasses, and lignin-sulfonate. *J. Dairy Sci.* **56**:1429.

Bouchard, R. and H. R. Conrad. 1973c. Sulfur requirement of lactating dairy cows. III. Fate of sulfur-35 from sodium and calcium sulfate. *J. Dairy Sci.* **56**:1435.

Bouchard, R. and H. R. Conrad. 1974. Sulfur metabolism and nutritional changes in lactating cows associated with supplemental sulfate and methionine hydroxy analog. *Can. J. Anim. Sci.* **54**:587.

Bray, A. C. 1969. Sulphur metabolism in sheep. II. The absorption of inorganic sulphate and inorganic sulphide from the sheep's rumen. *Aust. J. Agric. Res.* **20**:739.

Bryant, M. P. 1973. Nutritional requirements of the predominant rumen cellulolytic bacteria. *Fed. Proc.* **32**:1809.

Bull, L. S. and J. H. Vandersall. 1973. Sulfur source for in vitro cellulose digestion and in vivo ration utilization, nitrogen metabolism, and sulfur balance. *J. Dairy Sci.* **56**:106.

Button, G. M., R. G. Brown, F. G. Michels and J. T. Smith. 1965. Utilization of calcium and sodium sulfate by the rat. *J. Nutr.* **87**:211.

Buttrey, S. A., V. G. Allen, J. P. Fontenot and R. B. Reneau, Jr. 1986. Effect of sulfur fertilization on chemical composition, ensiling characteristics and utilization of corn silage by lambs. *J. Anim. Sci.* **63**:1236.

Carew, S. N., R. H. Davis and A. H. Sykes. 1986. Methionine, sulphate and thiosulphate as sources of dietary sulphur for chicks chronically intoxicated with cyanide. *Nutr. Rep. Int.* **34**:655.

Chestnut, A. B., G. C. Fahey, Jr., L. L. Berger and J. W. Spears. 1986. Effects of sulfur fertilization on composition and digestion of phenolic compounds in tall fescue and orchardgrass. *J. Anim. Sci.* **63**:1926.

Combs, G. F., Jr. and S. B. Combs. 1986. " The Role of Selenium in Nutrition." Academic Press, New York.

Daniels, A. L. and J. K. Rich. 1918. The role of inorganic sulfates in nutrition. *J. Biol. Chem.* **36**:27.

Doyle, P. T. and J. K. Egan. 1983. The utilization of nitrogen and sulfur by weaner and mature merino sheep. *Aust. J. Agric. Res.* **34**:433.

Emery, R. S., C. K. Smith and L. Fai To. 1957a. Utilization of inorganic sulfate by rumen microorganisms. II. The ability of single strains of rumen bacteria to utilize inorganic sulfate. *Appl. Microbiol.* **5**:363.

Emery, R. S., C. K. Smith and C. F. Huffman. 1957b. Utilization of inorganic sulfate by rumen microorganisms. I. Incorporation of inorganic sulfate into amino acids. *Appl. Microbiol.* **5**:360.

Fron, M. J., J. A. Boling, L. P. Bush and K. A. Dawson. 1990. Sulfur and nitrogen metabolism in the bovine fed different forms of supplemental sulfur. *J. Anim. Sci.* **68**:543.

Garrigus, U. S. 1970. The need for sulfur in the diet of ruminants. *In* "Symposium: Sulfur in Nutrition" (O. H. Muth and J. E. Oldfield, Eds.) p. 126. AVI Publishing, Westport, CT.

Garrigus, U. S., H. H. Mitchell, W. H. Hale and J. S. Albin. 1950. The value of elemental sulfur in a methionine deficient sheep ration. *J. Anim. Sci.* **9**:656 [Abstract].

Gawthorne, T. M. and C. J. Nader. 1976. The effect of molybdenum on the conversion of sulphate to sulphide and microbial-protein-sulfur in the rumen of sheep. *Br. J. Nutr.* **35**:11.

Gil, L. A., R. L. Shirley and J. E. Moore. 1973. Effect of methionine hydroxy analog on bacterial protein synthesis from urea and glucose, starch or cellulose by rumen microbes, *in vitro. J. Anim. Sci.* **37**:159.

Glenn, B. P. and D. G. Ely. 1981. Sulfur, nitrate and starch supplementation of tall fescue for the ovine. *J. Anim. Sci.* **53**:1135.

Goodrich, R. D. and A. D. Tillman. 1966. Effects of sulfur and nitrogen sources and copper levels on the metabolism of certain minerals by sheep. *J. Anim. Sci.* **25**:484.

Gordon, R. S. and I. W. Sizer. 1955. Ability of sodium sulfate to stimulate growth of the chicken. *Science* **122**:1270.

Grieve, D. G., W. G. Merrill and C. E. Coppock. 1973. Sulfur supplementation of urea-containing silages and concentrates. II. Ration digestibility, nitrogen, and sulfur balances. *J. Dairy Sci.* **56**:224.

Guardiola, C. M., G. C. Fahey, Jr., J. W. Spears and U. S. Garrigus. 1980. Effect of sulfur supplementation on in vitro cellulose digestion and on nutrient utilization and nitrogen metabolism of lambs fed low quality fescue hay. *Can. J. Anim. Sci.* **60**:337.

Guardiola, C. M., G. C. Fahey, Jr., J. W. Spears and U. S. Garrigus. 1983. The effects of sulphur supplementation on cellulose digestion in vitro and on nutrient digestion, nitrogen metabolism and rumen characteristics of lambs fed on good quality fescue and tropical star grass hays. *Anim. Feed Sci. Technol.* **8**:129.

Hale, W. H. and U. S. Garrigus. 1953. Synthesis of cystine in wool from elemental sulfur and sulfate sulfur. *J. Anim. Sci.* **12**:492.

Harms, R. H. and R. E. Buresh. 1987. A comparison of diets with and without supplemented inorganic sulfate and choline for use in comparing relative potencies of various methionine supplements. *Nutr. Rep. Int.* **35**:909.

Huisingh, J., J. J. McNeill and G. Matrone. 1974. Sulfate reduction by a *desulfovibrio* species isolated from sheep rumen. *Appl. Microbiol.* **28**:489.

Huisingh, J., D. C. Milholland, and G. Matrone. 1975. Effect of molybdate on sulfide production from methionine and sulfate by ruminal microorganisms of sheep. *J. Nutr.* **105**:1199.

Hume, I. D. and P. R. Bird. 1970. Synthesis of microbial protein in the rumen. IV. The influence of the level and form of dietary sulphur. *Aust. J. Agric. Res.* **21**:315.

Hunt, C. H., O. G. Bentley, T. V. Hershberger and J. H. Cline. 1954. The effect of carbohydrates and sulfur on B-vitamins synthesis, cellulose digestion, and urea utilization by rumen microorganisms in vitro. *J. Anim. Sci.* **13**:570.

Huovinen, J. A. and B. E. Gustafsson. 1967. Inorganic sulphate, sulphite and sulphide as sulfur donors in the biosynthesis of sulphur amino acids in germ-free and conventional rats. *Biochim. Biophys. Acta* **136**:441.

Ishimoto, M., J. Koyama, T. Omura and Y. Nagai. 1954. Biochemical studies on sulfate-reducing bacteria. III. Sulfate reduction by cell suspension. *J. Biochem.* **41**:537.

Jacobson, D. R., B. Soewardi, J. W. Barnett, R. H. Hatton and S. B. Carr. 1969. Sulfur, nitrogen, and amino acid balance, and digestibility of low-sulfur and sulfur-supplemented diets fed to lactating cows. *J. Dairy Sci.* **52**:472.

Johnson, W. H., R. D. Goodrich and J. C. Meiske. 1970. Appearance in the blood plasma and excretion of 35S from three chemical forms of sulfur by lambs. *J. Anim. Sci.* **31**:1003.

Johnson, W. H., R. D. Goodrich and J. C. Meiske. 1971. Metabolism of radioactive sulfur from elemental sulfur, sodium sulfate and methionine by lambs. *J. Anim. Sci.* **32**:778.

Kahlon, T. S. and F. I. Chow. 1989. A comparison of methods for the intrinsic labeling of wheat protein with ^{35}S. *J. Agric. Food Chem.* **37**:116.

Kahlon, T. S., J. C. Meiske and R. D. Goodrich. 1975a. Sulfur metabolism in ruminants. I. *In vitro* availability of various chemical forms of sulfur. *J. Anim. Sci.* **41**:1147.

Kahlon, T. S., J. C. Meiske and R. D. Goodrich. 1975b. Sulfur metabolism in ruminants. II. *In vivo* availability of various chemical forms of sulfur. *J. Anim. Sci.* **41**:1154.

Kellerman, J. H. 1936. Sulfur metabolism. The effect of flowers of sulfur on the growth of young white rats fed an otherwise well-balance ration. *Onderstepoort J. Vet. Sci. Anim. Ind.* **7**:199.

Kennedy, P. M. and B. D. Siebert. 1972a. The utilization of spear grass (*Heteropogon contortus*). II. The influence of sulphur on energy intake and rumen and blood parameters in cattle and sheep. *Aust. J. Agric. Res.* **23**:45.

Kennedy, P. M. and B. D. Siebert. 1972b. The utilization of spear grass (*Heteropogon contortus*). III. The influence of the level of dietary sulphur on the utilization of spear grass by sheep. *Aust. J. Agric. Res.* **24**:143.

Kulwich, R., L. Struglia, J. T. Jackson and P. B. Pearson. 1954. Synthesis of cystine and methionine from S^{35}-labeled sodium sulfate in the rabbit. *Fed. Proc.* **13**:463 [Abstract].

Kulwich, R., L. Struglia and P. B. Pearson. 1958. Metabolic fate of S^{35}-labeled sulfate in baby pigs. *Proc. Soc. Exp. Biol. Med.* **97**:408.

Langlands, J. P., H. A. M. Sutherland and M. J. Playne. 1973. Sulphur as a nutrient for Merino sheep. 2. The utilization of sulphur in forage diets. *Br. J. Nutr.* **30**:537.

L'Estrange, J. L., J. J. Clarke and D. M. McAleese. 1969. Studies on high intakes of various sulphate salts and sulphuric acid in sheep. 1. Effects on voluntary feed intake, digestibility and acid-base balance. *Irish J. Agric. Res.* **8**:133.

L'Estrange, J. L. and F. Murphy. 1972. Effects of dietary mineral acids on voluntary food intake, digestion, mineral metabolism and acid-base balance of sheep. *Br. J. Nutr.* **28**:1.

L'Estrange, J. L., P. K. Upton and D. M. McAleese. 1972. Effects of dietary sulphate on voluntary feed intake and metabolism of sheep. I. A comparison between different levels of sodium sulphate and sodium chloride. *Irish J. Agric. Res.* **11**:127.

Lewis, D. 1954. The reduction of sulphate in the rumen of the sheep. *Biochem. J.* **56**:391.

Lewis, G. T. and H. B. Lewis. 1927. The metabolism of sulfur. The effect of elemental sulfur on the growth of the young white rat. *J. Biol. Chem.* **74**:515.

Loosli, J. K., H. H. Williams, W. E. Thomas, F. H. Ferris and L. A. Maynard. 1949. Synthesis of amino acids in the rumen. *Science* **110**:144.

Machlin, L. J. 1955. Studies on the growth response in the chicken from the addition of sulfate to a low-sulfur diet. *Poult. Sci.* **34**:1209 [Abstract].

Machlin, L. J., P. B. Pearson, C. A. Denton and H. R. Bird. 1953. The utilization of sulfate sulfur by the laying hen and its incorporation into cystine. *J. Biol. Chem.* **205**:213.

Martin, W. G., R. J. Miraglia, D. G. Spaeth and H. Patrick. 1966. Synthesis of taurine from sulfate by the chick. *Proc. Soc. Exp. Biol. Med.* **122**:841.

Miles, R. D. and R. H. Harms. 1983. Benefit from the supplementation of K_2SO_4 or K_2-$MgSO_4$ to the diet of turkey poults. *Nutr. Rep. Int.* **28**:381.

Mowat, D. N. and K. Deelstra. 1970. Encapsulated methionine supplement for lambs. *J. Anim. Sci.* **31**:1041 [Abstract].

Muntifering, R. B., S. I. Smith and J. A. Boling. 1984. Effect of elemental sulfur supplementation on digestibility and metabolism of early vegetative and fall-accumulated regrowth fescue hay by wethers. *J. Anim. Sci.* **59**:1100.

Noble, R. L., L. S. Pope and W. D. Gallup. 1955. Urea and methionine in fattening rations for lambs. *J. Anim. Sci.* **14**:132.

Onwuka, C. F. I. and A. O. Akinsoyinu. 1989. Effects of elemental sulphur levels on urea-nitrogen utilization by West African dwarf goats and sheep. *Trop. Agric. (Trinidad)* **66**:158.

Patterson, J. A. and L. Kung, Jr. 1988. Metabolism of DL-methionine and methionine analogs by rumen microorganisms. *J. Dairy Sci.* **71**:3292.

Postgate, J. R. 1951. The reduction of sulphur compounds by *Desulphovibrio desulphuricans*. *J. Gen. Microbiol.* **5**:725.

Postgate, J. R. 1952. Competitive and non-competitive inhibitors of bacterial sulphate reduction. *J. Gen. Microbiol.* **6**:128.

Ross, E., B. L. Damron and R. H. Harms. 1972. The requirement for inorganic sulfate in the diet of chicks for optimum growth and feed efficiency. *Poult. Sci.* **51**:1606.

Ross, E. and R. H. Harms. 1970. The response of chicks to sodium sulfate supplementation of a corn-soy diet. *Poult. Sci.* **49**:1605.

Sasse, C. E. and D. H. Baker. 1974a. Sulfur utilization by the chick with emphasis on the effect of inorganic sulfate on the cystine-methionine interrelationship. *J. Nutr.* **104**:244.

Sasse, C. E. and D. H. Baker. 1974b. Factors affecting sulfate-sulfur utilization by the young chick. *Poult. Sci.* **53**:652.

Sloan, D. R. and R. H. Harms. 1972. Utilization of inorganic sulfate by turkey poults. *Poult. Sci.* **51**:1673.

Slyter, L. L., W. Chalupa and R. R. Oltjen. 1988. Response to elemental sulfur by calves and sheep fed purified diets. *J. Anim. Sci.* **66**:1016.

Smith, J. T. 1973. An optimal level of inorganic sulfate for the diet of a rat. *J. Nutr.* **103**:1008.

Soares, J. H. 1974. Experiments on the requirement of inorganic sulfate by the chick. *Poult. Sci.* **53**:246.

pears, J. W., J. C. Burns, and P. A. Hatch. 1985. Sulfur fertilization of cool season grasses and effect on utilization of minerals, nitrogen, and fiber by steers. *J. Dairy Sci.* **68**:347.

Spears, J. W., L. P. Bush and D. G. Ely. 1977. Influence of nitrate and molybdenum on sulfur utilization by rumen microorganisms. *J. Dairy Sci.* **60**:1889.

Spears, J. W., D. G. Ely, L. P. Bush and R. C. Buckner. 1976. Sulfur supplementation and in vitro digestion of forage cellulose by rumen microorganisms. *J. Anim. Sci.* **43**:513.

Spears, J. W., D. G. Ely and L. P. Bush. 1978. Influence of supplemental sulfur on in vitro and in vivo microbial fermentation of Kentucky 31 tall fescue. *J. Anim. Sci.* **47**:552.

Starks, P. B., W. H. Hale, U. S. Garrigus and R. M. Forbes. 1953. The utilization of feed nitrogen by lambs as affected by elemental sulfur. *J. Anim. Sci.* **12**:480.

Starks, P. B., W. H. Hale, U. S. Garrigus, R. M. Forbes and M. F. James. 1954. Response of lambs fed varied levels of elemental sulfur, sulfate sulfur, and methionine. *J. Anim. Sci.* **13**:249.

Steinacher, G., T. J. Devlin and J. R. Ingalls. 1970. Effect of methionine supplementation posterior to the rumen on nitrogen utilization and sulfur balance of steers on a high roughage ration. *Can. J. Anim. Sci.* **50**:319.

Tarver, H. and C. L. A. Schmidt. 1939. The conversion of methionine to cystine: experiments with radioactive sulfur. *J. Biol. Chem.* **130**:67.

Thomas, W. E., J. K. Loosli, H. H. Williams and L. A. Maynard. 1951. The utilization of inorganic sulfates and urea nitrogen by lambs. *J. Nutr.* **43**:515.

Trenkle, A., E. Cheng and W. Burroughs. 1958. Availability of different sulfur sources for rumen microorganisms in in vitro cellulose digestion. *J. Anim. Sci.* **17**:1191 [Abstract].

Underwood, E. J. 1981. "The Mineral Nutrition of Livestock," 2nd ed. Commonwealth Agricultural Bureaux, Slough, U.K.

Upton, P. K., J. L. L'Estrange and D. M. McAleese. 1970. Studies on high intakes of various sulphate salts and sulphuric acid in sheep. 2. Effects on the absorption, excretion and retention of sulphur. *Irish J. Agric. Res.* **9**:151.

Wallenius, R. W. and R. E. Whitchurch. 1975. Methionine hydroxy analog or sulfate supplementation for high producing dairy cows. *J. Dairy Sci.* **58**:1314.

Weir, W. C. and V. V. Rendig. 1952. Studies on the nutritive value for lambs of alfalfa hay grown on a low sulfur soil. *J. Anim. Sci.* **11**:780 [Abstract].

Weir, W. C. and V. V. Rendig. 1954. Serum inorganic sulfate sulfur as a measure of the sulfur intake of sheep. *J. Nutr.* **54**:87.

Wolffram, S., Y. Stingelin and E. Scharrer. 1987. Inhibition of sulphate and selenate transport in sheep jejunum by oxalate and other dicarboxylate anions. *J. Vet. Med. A.* **34**:679.

17

ZINC BIOAVAILABILITY

David H. Baker

Department of Animal Sciences and
Division of Nutritional Sciences
University of Illinois
Urbana, Illinois

Clarence B. Ammerman

Department of Animal Science
University of Florida
Gainesville, Florida

I. INTRODUCTION

It was in 1934 that zinc was shown conclusively to be required for normal growth and health in rats (Todd *et al.*, 1934). The element is considered to be essential for plants, animals, and humans (Hambidge *et al.*, 1986). It activates several enzymes and is a component of many important metalloenzymes. The element is critically involved in cell replication and in the development of cartilage and bone. Signs of zinc deficiency in animals and humans include retarded growth, abnormal skeletal formation, delayed sexual development, alopecia, dermatitis, abnormal feathering, and impaired reproduction in both males and females. Fetal abnormalities occur and hatchability of eggs is reduced.

Many animal diets require supplementation with zinc because of either low dietary levels or the presence of dietary factors which decrease bioavailability of the element. The critical importance of added dietary zinc for domestic animals was shown in 1955 when it was demonstrated that parakeratosis, a condition being observed in swine, was caused by inadequate dietary zinc (Tucker and Salmon, 1955). It was the practice to feed high calcium levels along with plant proteins containing phytate and this apparently reduced the bioavailability of dietary zinc to the point that a severe deficiency of the element occurred. It was soon demonstrated (O'Dell and Savage,

367

1957; O'Dell *et al.*, 1958) that zinc was required for normal growth and development in poultry. Results obtained with swine and poultry probably led to the observations that zinc deficiency can occur in ruminants under grazing conditions in some areas of the world (Hambidge *et al.*, 1986).

In regard to the human population, severe zinc deficiency in men resulting in dwarfism and delayed sexual development has been observed in certain countries in the Middle East, and it is suggested that marginal intakes of zinc may occur in certain segments of the U.S. population (NRC, 1989). The typical mixed diet of North American adults, in which approximately 70% of the zinc comes from meat or other animal products, is considered to provide adequate levels of the element to maintain normal zinc status in healthy young adults.

II. BIOAVAILABILITY STUDIES

Although there are numerous qualitative studies in domestic animals, there are few quantitative bioavailability data for mammalian species. In many cases it is impossible to obtain a specific value from published work, either because there was no response curve or there was no response to the zinc supplements under the conditions used. Zinc salts, such as the sulfate or carbonate, have commonly been used as standards in bioavailability studies. Experiments with growing chicks (Edwards, 1959) and turkey poults (Sullivan, 1961) showed these salts to be of equal and high bioavailability. Values for relative zinc bioavailability in various feedstuffs and supplements are shown in Table I.

A. *In Vitro* Estimates of Bioavailability

1. Isolated Intestinal Segments and Membranes

Perfusion of isolated segments of pig and chick intestine attached to a continuous flow apparatus has been used to estimate zinc absorption (Hill *et al.*, 1987a,b). The authors equated zinc uptake by gut tissue to absorption.

Uptake of [65]Zn-labeled zinc by everted gut sacs and intestinal strips has been used to measure absorption by rat (Pearson *et al.*, 1966; Oberleas *et al.*, 1966) and pig (Hill *et al.*, 1987a,b) mucosa. An extension of the everted sac technique is the use of brush border membrane vesicles to study zinc uptake or transport (Menard and Cousins, 1983). While this method allows assessment of the kinetics of zinc uptake, neither it nor the everted sac has been applied to absorption of zinc from natural products.

2. Zinc-Binding Assays

In view of early observations that the zinc in oilseed meals is of low availability, several investigators have performed *in vitro* zinc binding assays to serve as indicators of zinc bioavailability. Kratzer *et al.* (1961) and Allred *et al.* (1964) equilibrated soybean and other proteins with ^{65}Zn solutions and measured radioactivity in the protein-bound product. Although the method is rapid and reproducible, casein and soybean protein showed no difference in zinc binding. Similar results were obtained by Seth *et al.* (1975) who investigated rapeseed meal. Lease and Williams (1967) found that the zinc in Texas 61 sesame meal is much less available to chicks than that of Texas 71, Mexican, or California meals. *In vitro* binding of ^{65}Zn by Texas 61 was also higher, but the percentage of dialyzable zinc after pepsin and pancreatin digestion did not differ (Lease, 1967). Jones *et al.* (1985) used equilibrium dialysis to determine zinc binding to proteins in the presence and absence of chelators. When dialyzed against a Tris-histidine buffer, soy products labeled with ^{65}Zn released more radioactivity (60%) than did casein (38%) or egg white (22%). In contrast, the *in vivo* retention of zinc by Japanese quail was greater from the animal products. From these papers it is clear that a satisfactory *in vitro* method for assessing zinc bioavailability remains to be developed.

B. *In Vivo* Estimates of Bioavailability

1. Isotope Retention

One method for estimating absorption of zinc is that of whole-body retention of an ingested isotope (Heth and Hoekstra, 1965). The feedstuff to be evaluated is labeled, extrinsically or intrinsically, with ^{65}Zn and an oral dose is administered over a short time period. Whole-body radiation is determined immediately and at intervals over a period which allows determination of the steady-state loss of endogenous zinc. This technique has been used by numerous investigators to evaluate zinc absorption from natural products (Davies, 1980; Meyer *et al.*, 1983; Ketelson *et al.*, 1984; Stuart *et al.*, 1986; Hempe, 1987; Bobilya, 1989). A variation of this method involves measurement of the percentage of a ^{65}Zn oral dose deposited in specific tissues after an equilibrium period. Stuart *et al.* (1986) measured ^{65}Zn retention in rat tibias and intestine 13 days after an oral dose, and Miller *et al.* (1968) measured zinc retention in several tissues from calves. While this variation of isotope retention does not give a quantitative value of absorption, it is useful for qualitative comparisons. Evans and Johnson (1977) estimated absorption in rats by carcass radioactivity after removal of the gastrointestinal tract.

2. Intestinal Segments *In Situ*

Smith *et al.* (1978) developed an *in situ* vascular perfusion system to study zinc absorption by the rat intestine. The lumen of the segment was continuously perfused with a medium containing ^{65}Zn and the attached arterial system with Krebs Ringer buffer containing 5% serum. Transfer of ^{65}Zn to the venous system was enhanced by introducing histidine into the lumen and decreased by phytate. The method has been used to quantitate zinc absorption by a portion of the gut and to study the effect of other cations in the lumen (Smith and Cousins, 1980; Oestreicher and Cousins, 1982). Luminal perfusion of intact intestinal segments without vascular perfusion has also been used to assess intestinal absorption in the rat (Wapnir and Stiel, 1986).

3. Growth

The first attempt to evaluate zinc bioavailability quantitatively used growing chicks and rats fed purified diets supplemented with graded levels of $ZnCO_3$ as the reference (O'Dell *et al.*, 1972). Feedstuffs, including corn, soybean meal, sesame meal, and fish meal, were substituted in the basal diet to supply, by analysis, 5 to 10 ppm zinc. The data were treated as a standard curve assay. Weight gain of animals fed reference zinc was regressed against the logarithm of dietary zinc to establish the slope of the standard curve. Slope ratio assays have also been applied to growth response assays with rats (Forbes and Parker, 1977; Franz *et al.*, 1980a,b) and chicks (Hempe, 1987). Slope ratio assays based on growth rate of rats predict higher bio-availability than those based on bone zinc (Franz et al., 1980a,b). Best fit curves can be calculated and used for estimation of bioavailability (Franz *et al.*, 1980a,b). Some investigators regress rate of gain on total zinc consumed rather than on dietary concentration (Lo *et al.*, 1981; Forbes *et al.*, 1983) although this generally has little effect on the value derived.

4. Tissue Concentration

Although the zinc concentration in most soft tissues varies little with zinc status, plasma and bone zinc are low in animals deprived of zinc. This has been observed in chicks (Savage *et al.*, 1964), Japanese quail (Fox and Harrison, 1964), calves (Miller *et al.*, 1968), and rats (Huber and Gershoff, 1970). Momcilovic *et al.* (1975) first used total femur zinc for quantitative evaluation of zinc bioavailability in rats. They introduced the slope ratio method to zinc bioavailability by regressing log of femur zinc against the dietary zinc concentration. The log function provided a linear response over a wider range than that occurring with weight gain. This is possibly due to the fact that bone stores zinc to a greater extent than soft tissues. Storage may also account for the lower bioavailability value obtained with the bone zinc assay, as observed by several investigators (Forbes and Parker, 1977; Franz et al., 1980a; Shah and Belonge, 1984). Rat bone seems to serve as a zinc sink and stores surges of readily absorbed zinc. The plasma zinc flux probably increases markedly after a meal of readily available zinc, and a high proportion finds its way into bone since only a limited proportion can be used for growth. Thus, when bone zinc serves as the response criterion, less readily available zinc sources have lower bioavailabilities than is the case when growth rate is the criterion. For dietary concentrations of zinc that slightly exceed the growth requirement, bone zinc content is an acceptable index of bioavailability.

Slope ratios have also been used in chick assays of zinc bioavailability. Hempe (1987) found a linear arithmetic response in tibia zinc as dietary zinc increased over a range of 6 to18 ppm, and the slope ratio of soy flour to $ZnCO_3$ agreed with that obtained when weight gain was the criterion. Henry et al. (1987) analyzed tissues from chicks fed for 1 week a practical-type diet supplemented with graded levels of zinc, ranging from 500 to 1000 ppm. A linear increase in tissue concentration was observed, with bone showing the greatest sensitivity to high levels of dietary zinc.

Hahn and Baker (1993) fed grades doses of various zinc salts to young pigs consuming a basal corn-soybean diet containing 125 ppm zinc. Plasma zinc concentrations were erratic when dietary concentrations were below 1000 ppm added zinc and the reference source was $ZnSO_4 \cdot H_2O$. Between 1000 and 5000 ppm however, excretion routes apparently became saturated such that plasma zinc concentration increased fourfold in a dose-dependent manner. The increase in plasma zinc was twice as great for the sulfate as for zinc oxide, and zinc-methionine produced a response greater than that of the sulfate. Feeding zinc-lysine resulted in plasma zinc concentrations similar to those in pigs fed the sulfate. These results were similar to those reported by Wedekind and Baker (1990) and Wedekind et al. (1992) in which chicks were fed supplemental zinc at low dietary concentrations and weight gain and tibia zinc were the response variables.

Additions of a zinc isotope to test materials as a tracer may augment the precision of a bioavailability estimation (Stuart et al., 1986). In general, the addition of ^{65}Zn to natural products or diets is absorbed and retained to the same extent as that physiologically incorporated into the product, i.e., intrinsically labeled. Tibia zinc concentration in rats fed labeled soy flour was less than that of rats fed reference zinc, but the specific activity of the zinc was not different. This lends credence to the use of isotope retention as a measure of absorption. Evans and Johnson (1977) first compared food extrinsically and intrinsically labeled with ^{65}Zn and found no difference in bioavailablility to the rat.

5. Metalloprotein Concentration and Enzymatic Activities

Several of zinc metalloenzymes have been identified in nature (Vallee, 1988), but most of the metalloenzymes bind zinc so tightly that their activities do not change during nutritional deprivation. Plasma angiotensin converting enzyme activity was low in zinc deprived rats (Reeves and O'Dell, 1986), but it was readily activated *in vitro*. Thus, it is no better as an index than plasma zinc concentration. One promising indicator of zinc status is the plasma concentration of metallothionein (Sato *et al.*, 1984). This protein is induced in tissues by zinc and released proportionally into blood and urine where its concentration can be determined by radioimmunoassay. It may prove to be a useful index of status and, thus, of value in bioavailability measurement (Bremner *et al.*, 1987). Sandoval *et al.* (1992) observed increased liver metallothionine with elevated levels of dietary zinc in chicks and indicated this response may be a useful indicator of zinc bioavailability.

6. Chemical Balance

Zinc balance has been used widely in human studies, but few animal balance trials have been reported. This method is tedious and fraught with lack of precision. There are problems of contamination and difficulty of making total collections as well as that of analytical error. Nevertheless, without a good biochemical index of utilization, zinc balance is probably the method of choice for estimating zinc bioavailability in mature animals. Seal and Heaton (1983) used metabolic balance in mature rats to determine the effect of other dietary components on absorption and retention. Zinc balance, while useful in assessing status, is not a good measure of zinc absorption. Fecal zinc comprises not only unabsorbed zinc, but also endogenous zinc (i.e., inevitable losses) and absorbed zinc that is reexcreted into the gut via intestinal, pancreatic, and biliary secretions.

III. FACTORS INFLUENCING BIOAVAILABILITY

A. Dietary Factors

Two major dietary factors affect zinc bioavailability: (a) chelating agents and (b) metal ion interactions. Other diet components, including both essential and nonessential nutrients, may also be involved.

1. Organic Chelating Agents

Depending upon their chemical nature and complexation constants, organic chelators may affect bioavailability either positively or negatively. Phytate, inositol hexaphosphate, is a common component of plant seeds and is particularly high in oilseeds and cereals. That it decreases the absorption and utilization of zinc in monogastric animals was first demonstrated in chicks (O'Dell and Savage, 1960; Likuski and Forbes, 1964) and confirmed in rats (Likuski and Forbes, 1965; Oberleas et al.,1966; Davies and Nightingale, 1975; Atwal et al., 1980). The detrimental effect of phytate is exaggerated by excess dietary calcium as observed in chicks (O'Dell et al., 1958; Likuski and Forbes, 1965) and rats (Oberleas et al., 1966; Forbes et al., 1983). The effect of phytate depends on its concentration and, thus, on the dietary phytate:zinc ratio (Oberleas and Prasad, 1976: Morris and Ellis, 1980a,b; Lo et al., 1981). In general, molar phytate:zinc ratios above 12 to 15 are detrimental to zinc status when the zinc intake is near the required level. This ratio is affected by dietary calcium so that the ratio of (phytate x calcium):zinc serves as a better predictor of zinc bioavailability than the simple phytate:zinc ratio (Fordyce et al., 1987).

Soon after it was observed that the zinc in soybean protein was poorly absorbed by chicks, Kratzer et al. (1959) found that both autoclaving the protein and addition of EDTA to the diet improved zinc bioavailability for turkey poults. Autoclaving partially destroys phytate (Boland et al., 1975), but it is not a practical procedure because phytate is a relatively stable compound. The EDTA competes with phytate in the binding of zinc, forming a soluble complex. When zinc was near its required level, EDTA improved the performance of chicks fed diets containing phytate but not in diets without phytate (O'Dell et al., 1964). Not all chelating agents are beneficial. As shown by Vohra and Kratzer (1964), the efficacy of chelators was related to their stability constants. Maximal growth stimulation in turkey poults was obtained using compounds whose stability constants ($-\log K_d$) were near 15; EDTA has a constant of 16.5. It was found that 100 mg of EDTA was equivalent to 8 mg of zinc when added to 1 kg of diet (Kratzer and Starcher, 1963).

It is important to recognize that naturally occurring zinc chelators improve zinc bioavailability. Scott and Zeigler (1963) showed that several feedstuffs, including distillers dried solubles and liver extract, improve the availability of zinc in soybean protein. In vitro studies (Lease, 1967) also showed that a soluble fraction of soybean meal increased the dialyzability of zinc in sesame meal and presumably its bioavailability. While the chemical identity of these natural chelators is unknown, peptides and amino acids form complexes with zinc. Both cysteine and histidine bind zinc strongly ($-\log K = 18.2$ and 12.9, respectively) and improve bioavailability in chicks (Nielsen et al., 1966; Hortin et al., 1991).

Other chelators occur in foodstuffs or are derived metabolically from food components. Citrate and picolinic acid, found in milk, have been suggested to improve zinc bioavailability (Lonnerdal et al., 1980; Evans and Johnson, 1980). In one study (Evans and Johnson, 1980), picolinic acid increased absorption, but in another neither chelator affected zinc utilization by rats (Roth and Kirchgessner, 1985). In genetically deficient cattle, picolinate had no effect on zinc absorption, whereas diodoquin was beneficial (Flagstad, 1981). Picolinate impaired zinc uptake by the everted gut sacs (Hill et al., 1987b). Despite their zinc chelating potential, citrate and picolinate do not appear to play a major role in zinc bioavailability. Ascorbic acid is another compound that is thought to enhance zinc bioavailability (Solomons et al., 1979; Aoyagi and Baker, 1994).

2. Metal-Ion Interactions

Hill and Matrone (1970) discussed some of the basic principles that relate the interaction of zinc with metal ions, particularly the cationic transition elements. Probably the strongest and most studied antagonism is that between copper and zinc. In this case, the effect of zinc on copper bioavailability is much more significant than vice versa, but there is evidence that excess copper interferes with zinc absorption (van Campen, 1969). When the Cu:Zn ratio in intestinal segments was increased to 50:1, ^{65}Zn uptake was impaired. Similarly, in the vascularly perfused rat intestine, high concentrations of Cu in the perfusion buffer decreased transfer to the portal perfusate (Oestreicher and Cousins, 1985). Iron and cobalt decreased both uptake and transfer of luminal zinc in perfused intestinal loops from normal mice (Flanagan et al., 1984). In this study, copper increased zinc uptake but decreased transfer to the carcass.

Solomons (1986) has reviewed the literature relating iron and zinc absorption in man. The effect of excess iron was most evident when the Fe:Zn ratio was greater than 2, total iron dose was greater than 25 mg, iron was in the Fe(II) form, and the dose was given without food. Iron deficiency in laboratory animals enhanced both zinc and iron absorption (Flanagan et al., 1980; Hamilton et al., 1978), suggesting that the two elements are absorbed by a common pathway. The effect of excess dietary iron on zinc bioavailability is controversial. Gordon (1987) found that excess iron impaired zinc bioavailability while Fairweather-Tait et al. (1984) and Bafundo et al. (1984) observed no effect. Zinc was not limiting in the latter study.

Of the nonessential or "toxic" elements, cadmium and lead interact most strongly with zinc to decrease its bioavailability. Dietary cadmium was antagonistic to zinc in turkey poults (Supplee, 1961) and chicks (Supplee, 1963; Hill et al., 1963; Lease, 1968). Similar observations have been made in laboratory animals (Bunn and Matrone, 1966) and calves (Powell et al., 1964). Lead interacts with zinc at the level of δ-aminolevulinate dehydratase, an enzyme involved in heme synthesis (Finelli *et al.*, 1975).

Tin is toxic to rats and induces pathology analogous to that of iron, copper, and zinc deficiencies. Rats fed a diet containing 200 ppm tin for 3 weeks retain less zinc in their tissues than controls (Greger and Johnson, 1981). Tibia zinc was sensitive to as low as 100 ppm tin in diets containing 50 ppm zinc (Johnson and Greger, 1984). At 500 ppm tin, zinc absorption was decreased.

3. Other Dietary Components

Fiber has been reported to decrease zinc bioavailability in man, but experiments with rodents have shown little or no effect (Davies *et al.*, 1977; McKenzie and Davies, 1981; Caprez and Fairweather-Tait, 1982). Van der Aar *et al.* (1983) found no detrimental effect of wood cellulose, lignin, pectin, or gum arabic on zinc status of chicks when fed as 8% of the diet. Miller *et al.* (1968) found no difference in ^{65}Zn deposition in tissues of calves fed purified and practical type diets; specific activities were not different. However, zinc deficiency increased ^{65}Zn retention and specific activities in soft tissues suggesting exchange with smaller zinc pools.

IV. SUMMARY

Standard sources of zinc used in bioavailability assays have included the sulfate, carbonate, chloride, oxide and acetate forms of the element with zinc sulfate having been used most frequently (Table II). Zinc from animal products was generally more available than that from plant products. The relative bioavailability of zinc in meat, milk, and milk products as determined with chickens and rats was about 100%. Similar values, determined mainly with rats, for zinc utilization in grains and legume seeds, or in products produced from them, were highly variable but averaged about 60 to 70% depending on source of zinc. The average relative bioavailability for zinc from corn was approximately 45%. Supplemental sources of zinc were generally well utilized and their relative bioavailability was about 100% regardless of source of the element. Earlier research gave a similar value for the utilization of zinc in zinc oxide and zinc sulfate. Some recent research, however, has indicated that the relative bioavailability for zinc in feed grade zinc oxide may be nearer to 50% that of feed grade zinc sulfate. Bone zinc accumulation and growth rate in rapidly growing animals appear to be reliable indicators of relative zinc bioavailability. Liver zinc uptake and metallothionine synthesis have been used to estimate bioavailability, especially when high dietary concentrations were fed.

Table I. Bioavailability of zinc sources for animals[a]

Source	RV	Standard	Response criterion	Meth cal	Type diet	Added level, ppm	Reference
Chickens							
Beef	97	$ZnCO_3$	Growth	SR	P	24	Hempe (1987)
Beef	117	$ZnCO_3$	Plas Zn	SR	P	24	Hempe (1987)
Beef	102	$ZnCO_3$	Tibia Zn	SR	P	24	Hempe (1987)
Beef	100	$ZnSO_4$	Tibia Zn	SR	P	8-22	Hortin et al. (1991)
Corn	63	$ZnCO_3$	Growth	MR	P	5-10	O'Dell et al. (1972)
Corn, high lysine	65	$ZnCO_3$	Growth	MR	P	5-10	O'Dell et al. (1972)
Corn germ	54	$ZnCO_3$	Growth	MR	P	5-10	O'Dell et al. (1972)
Corn germ, high lysine	56	$ZnCO_3$	Growth	MR	P	5-10	O'Dell et al. (1972)
Egg yolk	79	$ZnCO_3$	Growth	MR	P	5-10	O'Dell et al. (1972)
Fish meal	75	$ZnCO_3$	Growth	MR	P	5-10	O'Dell et al. (1972)
Franklinite (Fe, Mn, Zn, $FeO_2)_2$ (16.3% Zn)	70	$ZnSO_4 \cdot 7H_2O$ RG (22.7% Zn)	Growth	MR	SP	10, 20	Edwards (1959)
Hemimorphite ($2ZnO \cdot SiO_2 \cdot H_2O$)	98	$ZnSO_4 \cdot 7H_2O$ RG	Growth	MR	SP	10, 20	Edwards (1959)
Milk, defatted	82	$ZnCO_3$	Growth	MR	P	5-10	O'Dell et al. (1972)
Ore - franklinite + willemite + calcite (16.8% Zn)	95	$ZnSO_4 \cdot 7H_2O$ RG	Growth	MR	SP	10, 20	Edwards (1959)
Oysters	95	$ZnCO_3$	Growth	MR	P	5-10	O'Dell et al. (1972)
Rice	62	$ZnCO_3$	Growth	MR	P	5-10	O'Dell et al. (1972)
Sesame meal	59	$ZnCO_3$	Growth	MR	P	5-10	O'Dell et al. (1960)

Source	Rel. value	Standard	Response	Assay	Stat.	Level (mg/kg)	Reference
Smithsonite (ZnCO₃) (46.8% Zn)	96	ZnSO₄·7H₂O RG	Growth	MR	SP	10, 20	Edwards (1959)
Soybean meal	67	ZnCO₃	Growth	MR	P	5–10	O'Dell et al. (1972)
Sphalerite (ZnS) (64.2% Zn)	60	ZnSO₄·7H₂O RG	Growth	MR	SP	10, 20	Edwards (1959)
Wheat	59	ZnCO₃	Growth	MR	P	5–10	O'Dell et al. (1972)
Willemite Zn₂SiO₄ (46.7%)	103	ZnSO₄·7H₂O RG	Growth	MR	SP	10, 20	Edwards (1959)
ZnCO₃ RG (52.1% Zn)	100	ZnSO₄·7H₂O RG	Growth	MR	SP	10, 20	Edwards (1959)
Zinc carbonate	100	Zinc chloride	Growth	MR	P-6 ppm	20, 40	Pensack et al. (1958)
Zinc carbonate	107	Zinc sulfate	Growth	TP	P-10 ppm	10, 20	Roberson and Schaible (1960a)
Zinc carbonate	123	Zinc sulfate	Decreased growth	TP	N	1000, 2000, 3000	Roberson and Schaible (1960b)
Zinc chloride	99	Zinc sulfate	Growth	TP	P-10 ppm	100	Roberson and Schaible (1958)
Zinc, elemental powder (100.0% Zn)	102	ZnSO₄·7H₂O RG	Growth	MR	SP	10, 20	Edwards (1959)
Zincite ZnO (65.3% Zn)	97	ZnSO₄·7H₂O RG	Growth	MR	SP	10, 20	Edwards (1959)
Zinc-methionine FG	124	ZnSO₄·H₂O FG	Growth	SR	P	7.5, 15	Wedekind et al. (1992)
Zn-methionine FG	176	ZnSO₄·H₂O FG	Bone Zn	SR	P	7.5, 15	Wedekind et al. (1992)
Zinc-methionine	79	ZnCl₂	⁶⁵Zn abs by gut sacs	MR	NG	10 μCi	Hill et al. (1987b)
Zinc-methionine FG	100	Zinc oxide	Bone Zn	TP	SP-8 ppm	10, 20, 30, 40, 50	Pimentel et al. (1991)
ZnO RG	97	ZnSO₄·7H₂O RG	Growth	MR	SP	10, 20	Edwards (1959)
ZnO (79.6% Zn)	104	ZnSO₄·7H₂O RG	Growth	MR	SP	10, 20	Edwards (1959)
Zinc oxide	100	Zinc chloride	Growth	MR	P-6 ppm	20, 40	Pensack et al. (1958)

Table I. (continued)

Source	RV	Standard	Response criterion	Meth cal	Type diet	Added level, ppm	Reference
Zinc oxide	108	Zinc sulfate	Growth	TP	P-10 ppm	10, 20	Roberson and Schaible (1960a)
ZnO FG (72% Zn)	61	ZnSO$_4$·H$_2$O FG	Growth	SR	P-13 ppm	7.5, 15	Wedekind and Baker (1990)
ZnO FG (72% Zn)	44	ZnSO$_4$·H$_2$O FG	Bone Zn	SR	P-13 ppm	7.5, 15	Wedekind and Baker (1990)
Zinc oxide	61	Zinc sulfate	Decreased growth	MR	N	1000, 2000, 3000	Roberson and Schaible (1960b)
Zinc proteinate	100	Zinc chloride	Growth	MR	P-6 ppm	20, 40	Pensack et al. (1958)
Turkeys							
Zinc carbonate (54.0% Zn)	100	ZnSO$_4$·7H$_2$O RG	Growth	TP	P-14 ppm	20, 30, 40	Sullivan (1961)
ZnCl$_2$ RG (45.6% Zn)	88	ZnSO$_4$·7H$_2$O RG	Growth	TP	P-14 ppm	20, 30, 40	Sullivan (1961)
Zinc citrate [Zn$_3$(C$_6$H$_5$O$_7$)$_2$·2H$_2$O]	128	ZnO	Growth	TP	P-17 ppm	15	Vohra and Kratzer (1966)
1,2- Diaminocyclohexane-tetraacetic acid-Zn (ZnC$_{14}$H$_{20}$O$_8$N$_2$)	108	ZnO	Growth	TP	P-17 ppm	15	Vohra and Kratzer (1966)
Diethylenetriamine-pentaacetic acid-Zn (ZnC$_{14}$O$_{10}$H$_{23}$N$_3$)	118	ZnO	Growth	TP	P-17 ppm	15	Vohra and Kratzer (1966)
Zinc-EDTA (ZnC$_{10}$H$_{14}$O$_8$N$_2$) (19.1% Zn)	118	ZnO	Growth	TP	P-17 ppm	15	Vohra and Kratzer (1966)
Zinc-EDTA	110	Zn	Growth	TP	P-25 ppm	30	Kratzer et al. (1959)
ZnO (71.6% Zn)	78	ZnSO$_4$·7H$_2$O RG	Growth	TP	P-14 ppm	20, 30, 40	Sullivan (1961)
ZnSO$_4$·H$_2$O (36.4% Zn)	75	ZnSO$_4$·7H$_2$O RG	Growth	TP	P-14 ppm	20, 30, 40	Sullivan (1961)

$Zn_2HP_3O_{10}$ (29.7% Zn)	69	ZnO	Growth	TP	P-17 ppm	15	Vohra and Kratzer (1966)
$Zn_3(PO_4)_2 \cdot 4H_2O$ (43.4% Zn)	48	ZnO	Growth	TP	P-17 ppm	15	Vohra and Kratzer (1966)
$Zn_2P_2O_{27} \cdot 4H_2O$ (34.9% Zn)	61	ZnO	Growth	TP	P-17 ppm	15	Vohra and Kratzer (1966)
$Zn_3P_6O_{18}$ (29.8% Zn)	70	ZnO	Growth	TP	P-17 ppm	15	Vohra and Kratzer (1966)
Zn- phytate $[Zn_6C_6H_6O_{24} \cdot 3H_2O]$ (19.1% Zn)	76	ZnO	Growth	TP	P-17 ppm	15	Vohra and Kratzer (1966)

Japanese Quail

Casein (42 ppm Zn)	47[b]	-	^{65}Zn ext lab	-	P-60 ppm	SOD	Jones et al. (1985)
Egg white (.8 ppm Zn)	38[b]	-	^{65}Zn ext lab	-	P-60 ppm	SOD	Jones et al. (1985)
Soy concentrate (37 ppm Zn)	25[b]	-	^{65}Zn ext lab	-	P-60 ppm	SOD	Jones et al. (1985)
Soy flour (48 ppm Zn)	24[b]	-	^{65}Zn ext lab	-	P-60 ppm	SOD	Jones et al. (1985)

Swine

Zinc-lysine	100	$ZnSO_4$	Plas Zn	SR	N	3000, 5000	Hahn and Baker (1993)
Zinc metal dust (99.3% Zn)	133	Zinc oxide	Ser Zn	SR	N-20 ppm	25, 50	Miller et al. (1981)
Zinc-methionine	100	$ZnCl_2$	^{65}Zn abs by gut sacs	MR	--	10 μCi	Hill et al. (1987b)
Zinc-methionine	>100	$ZnSO_4$	Plas Zn	SR	N	3000, 5000	Hahn and Baker (1993)
Zinc oxide	50	$ZnSO_4$	Plas Zn	SR	N	3000, 5000	Hahn and Baker (1993)

Table l. (continued)

Source	RV	Standard	Response criterion	Meth cal	Type diet	Added level, ppm	Reference
Cattle							
Corn forage	100	$^{65}Zn\ Cl_2$	Int lab	MR	N-3 ppm	SOD-35 μCi	Neathery et al. (1972)
Corn forage	139	$^{65}Zn\ Cl_2$	Int lab	MR	N-3 ppm	SOD-35 μCi	Neathery et al. (1972)
Zinc carbonate	58	Zinc sulfate	Plas Zn	MR	N-40 ppm	SOD-20 mg/kg BW	Kincaid (1979)
Zinc chloride	42	Zinc sulfate	Plas Zn	MR	N-40 ppm	SOD-20 mg/kg BW	Kincaid (1979)
Zinc-methionine	103	Zinc oxide	Milk yield	MR	N-50 ppm	400 mg/day	Kincaid et al. (1984)
Zinc-methionine	133	Zinc oxide	Milk somatic cell counts	MR	N-50 ppm	400 mg/day	Kincaid et al. (1984)
Zinc-methionine (4% Zn)	99	Zinc oxide	Growth	MR	N-81 ppm	360 mg/day	Greene et al. (1988)
Zinc-methionine	106	ZnO	Growth	MR	N	25	Spears (1989)
Zinc-methionine	105	Zinc oxide	Growth	MR	N	2500 ppm in mineral supp.	Spears and Kegley (1991)
ZnO	100	$ZnSO_4 \cdot H_2O$	Wound healing	MR	N-30 ppm	400	Miller et al. (1967)
Zinc oxide	98	Zinc sulfate	Liver Zn	MR	N-33 ppm	600	Miller et al. (1970)
Zinc oxide	98	Zinc sulfate	App abs	MR	N-33 ppm	600	Miller et al. (1970)
Zinc oxide	98	Zinc sulfate	Plas Zn	MR	N-40 ppm	SOD-20 mg/kg BW	Kincaid (1979)

Zinc-polysaccharide complex	144	ZnO	Rum fl microbial Zn	MR	N	172	Kennedy et al. (1988)

Sheep

Zinc, chelated	91	$ZnSO_4·H_2O$ RG	Plas Zn	MR	P	25	Ho and Hidiroglou (1977)
Zinc, chelated	125	$ZnSO_4·H_2O$ RG	Growth	MR	P	25	Ho and Hidiroglou (1977)
Zinc EDTA	17	Zinc sulfate	Liv Zn	TP	N	240 mg/kg BW	Smith and Embling (1984)
Zinc-methionine	95	ZnO	Plas Zn	MR	SP-3 ppm	5	Spears (1989)
Zinc-methionine	103	ZnO	App abs	MR	SP-3 ppm	5	Spears (1989)
Zinc oxide	71	Zinc sulfate	Liv Zn	TP	Pasture	3x/wk	Smith and Embling (1984)
Zinc, sequestered	108	$ZnSO_4·H_2O$ RG	Plas Zn	MR	P	25	Ho and Hidiroglou (1977)
Zinc, sequestered	103	$ZnSO_4·H_2O$ RG	Growth	MR	P	25	Ho and Hidiroglou (1977)

Rats

Barley (28 ppm Zn)	18[b]	-	^{65}Zn ext lab	-	-	SOD	Tidehag et al. (1988)
Beans (31 ppm Zn)	77	Zinc sulfate	Growth	SR	SP-45ppm;	3-14	Franz et al. (1980a)
Beans (31 ppm Zn)	50	Zinc sulfate	Bone Zn	SR	SP-45ppm	3-14	Franz et al. (1980a)
Beans, field, high tannin, hulls	108	$ZnSO_4$	App abs	MR	SP < 1 ppm	10	Lantzsch and Scheuermann (1981)
Beans, field, high tannin, kernal	69	$ZnSO_4$	App abs	MR	SP < 1 ppm	10	Lantzsch and Scheuermann (1981)
Beans, field, high tannin, whole	75	$ZnSO_4$	App abs	MR	SP < 1 ppm	10	Lantzsch and Scheuermann (1981)
Beans, field, low tannin, hulls	110	$ZnSO_4$	App abs	MR	SP < 1 ppm	10	Lantzsch and Scheuermann (1981)

Table I. (continued)

Source	RV	Standard	Response criterion	Meth cal	Type diet	Added level, ppm	Reference
Beans, field, low tannin, kernal	48	$ZnSO_4$	App abs	MR	SP < 1 ppm	10	Lantzsch and Scheuermann (1981)
Beans, field (*Vicia faba*), low tannin, whole	48	$ZnSO_4$	App abs	MR	SP < 1 ppm	10	Lantzsch and Scheuermann (1981)
Beans, lima boiled	95	Zinc sulfate	Growth	SR	SP-.45 ppm	6	Franz et al. (1980b)
Beans, lima boiled	80	Zinc sulfate	Bone Zn	SR	SP-.45 ppm	6	Franz et al. (1980b)
Beans, navy	78	$ZnCl_2$	^{65}Zn ret	MR	SP-12 ppm	SOM -.5 μmol	Hunt et al. (1987)
Beans, white, boiled	77	Zinc sulfate	Growth	SR	SP-.45 ppm;	6	Franz et al. (1980b)
Beans, white, boiled	50	Zinc sulfate	Bone Zn	SR	SP-.45 ppm	6	Franz et al. (1980b)
Beef	100	Zinc sulfate	Growth	SR	SP	2, 4, 6	Luhrsen and Rotruck (1979)
Beef (132 ppm Zn)	104	Zinc sulfate	Bone Zn	SR	SP-.7 ppm	3, 6, 12	Shah and Belonje (1981)
Beef	116	$ZnSO_4 \cdot 7H_2O$	Growth	SR	SP < 1 ppm	3, 6, 12	Shah and Belonje (1984)
Beef	104	$ZnSO_4 \cdot 7H_2O$	Bone Zn	SR	SP < 1 ppm	3, 6, 12	Shah and Belonje (1984)
Beef, cooked	101	Zinc carbonate	Growth	SR	SP	2-12	Brown et al. (1985)
Beef, cooked	102	Zinc carbonate	Bone Zn	SR	SP	2-12	Brown et al. (1985)
Beef	83	$ZnCl_2$	^{65}Zn ret	MR	SP-12 ppm	SOM-1.5 μmol	Hunt et al. (1987)
Bread, white, unleavened	78	Zinc sulfate	Bone Zn	SR	SP-.45 ppm	6	Franz et al. (1980b)
Bread, white, leavened	102	Zinc sulfate	Growth	SR	SP-.45 ppm	6	Franz et al. (1980b)
Bread, white, leavened	73	Zinc sulfate	Bone Zn	SR	SP-.45 ppm	6	Franz et al. (1980b)
Bread, whole wheat, leavened	82	Zinc sulfate	Bone Zn	SR	SP-.45 ppm	1-14	Franz et al. (1980b)

Food	Value	Zn source	Response criterion	MR/SR	SP	SOM	Reference
Bread, whole wheat, leavened	85	$ZnCl_2$	^{65}Zn ret	MR	SP-12 ppm	SOM-1.5 μmol	Hunt et al. (1987)
Bread, whole wheat, unleavened	62	Zinc sulfate	Bone Zn	SR	SP-.45 ppm	1-14	Franz et al. (1980b)
Bread, whole wheat, unleavened flat	89	$ZnCl_2$	^{65}Zn ret	MR	SP-12 ppm	SOM-1.5 μmol	Hunt et al. (1987)
Brewers grains (22 ppm Zn)	18.5[b]	-	^{65}Zn ext lab	-	-	SOD	Tidehag et al. (1988)
Cheese	90	$ZnCl_2$	^{65}Zn ret	MR	SP-12 ppm	SOM-1.5μmol	Hunt et al. (1987)
Chicken	94[b]	-	^{65}Zn int lab	-	SP	SOM-8	Stuart et al. (1986)
Chicken	92[b]	-	^{65}Zn ext lab	-	SP	SOM-8	Stuart et al. (1986)
Chicken	121	$ZnCl_2$	^{65}Zn ret	MR	SP-12 ppm	SOM-1.5μmol	Hunt et al. (1987)
Corn, alkali-treated	46	Zinc sulfate	Growth	SR	SP-.45 ppm	1-14	Franz et al. (1980b)
Corn, alkali-treated	30	Zinc sulfate	Bone Zn	SR	SP-.45 ppm	1-14	Franz et al. (1980b)
Corn, raw endosperm flour	51[b]	-	^{65}Zn int & ext lab	-	SOM	20-90 μg/day	Evans and Johnson (1977)
Corn forage	114	$ZnCl_2$	^{65}Zn int lab	MR	SP-5 ppm	SOM	Neathery et al. (1975)
Corn forage	102	$ZnCl_2$	^{65}Zn ext lab	MR	SP-5 ppm	SOM	Neathery et al. (1975)
Corn	57	$ZnCO_3$	Growth	MR	P	5-10	O'Dell et al. (1972)
Corn, high lysine	55	$ZnCO_3$	Growth	MR	P	5-10	O'Dell et al. (1972)
Corn (24 ppm Zn)	52	Zinc sulfate	Growth	SR	SP-.45 ppm	3-14	Franz et al. (1980a)
Corn (24 ppm Zn)	31	Zinc sulfate	Bone Zn	SR	SP-.45 ppm	3-14	Franz et al. (1980a)

Table I. (continued)

Source	RV	Standard	Response criterion	Meth cal	Type diet	Added level, ppm	Reference
Corn	52	Zinc sulfate	Growth	SR	SP-.45 ppm	1-14	Franz et al. (1980b)
Corn	31	Zinc sulfate	Bone Zn	SR	SP-.45 ppm	1-14	Franz et al. (1980b)
Corn	104	$ZnCl_2$	^{65}Zn ret	MR	SP-12 ppm	SOM-1.5 μmol	Hunt et al. (1987)
Egg	86[b]	-	Int lab	-	SP-11 ppm	SOD	Meyer et al. (1983)
Egg	85[b]	-	Ext lab	-	SP-11 ppm	SOD	Meyer et al. (1983)
Egg	115	$ZnCl_2$	^{65}Zn ret	MR	SP-12 ppm	SOM-1.5 μmol	Hunt et al. (1987)
Egg yolk	76	$ZnCO_3$	Growth	MR	P	5-10	O'Dell et al. (1972)
Fish meal	84	$ZnCO_3$	Growth	MR	P	5-10	O'Dell et al. (1972)
Liver, uncooked	32[b]	-	^{65}Zn int & ext lab	-	SOM	20-90 μg/day	Evans and Johnson (1977)
Liver, cooked	33[b]	-	^{65}Zn int & ext lab	-	SOM	20-90 μg/day	Evans and Johnson (1977)
Milk, cow's	15[b]	-	^{65}Zn ext lab	-	N	SOD	Sandstrom et al. (1983)
Milk, cow's	21[b]	-	^{65}Zn ext. lab	-	N	SOD-.5 ml	Lonnerdal et al. (1985)
Milk	111	$ZnCl_2$	^{65}Zn ret	MR	SP-12 ppm	SOM-1.5 μmol	Hunt et al. (1987)
Milk, cow's, 2% fat	43[b]	--	^{54}Zn int & ext lab	--	N	SOM- 20-90 μg/day	Evans and Johnson (1977)
Milk, cow, casein fraction	20[b]	-	^{65}Zn ext lab	-	N	SOD-.5 ml	Lonnerdal et al. (1985)

Sample	Value	Form	Method				Reference
Milk, cow's, defatted (4.1% Zn)	18.5[b]	-	65Zn ext lab	-	N	SOD	Kiely et al. (1988)
Milk, cow's defatted	43[b]	-	65Zn int & ext lab	-	SOM	20-90 µg/day	Evans and Johnson (1977)
Milk, defatted	79	ZnCO$_3$	Growth	MR	P	5-10	O'Dell et al. (1972)
Milk, cow, whey fraction	28[b]	-	65Zn ext lab	-	N	SOD-.5 ml	Lonnerdal et al. (1985)
Milk, cow's infant formula	24[b]	-	65Zn ext lab	-	N	SOD	Sandstrom et al. (1983)
Milk, cow infant formula	86	Zinc sulfate	Bone Zn	SR	P-.8 ppm	3, 6, 9, 12	Momcilovic et al. (1976)
Milk, cow's infant formula (27 ppm Zn)	82	Zinc sulfate	Bone Zn	SR	SP-6 ppm	3-12	Momcilovic and Shah (1976)
Oats (37 ppm Zn)	17[b]	-	65Zn ext lab	-	-	SOD	Tidehag et al. (1988)
Oysters	87	ZnCl$_2$	65Zn ret	MR	SP-12 ppm	SOM-1.5 µmol	Hunt et al. (1987)
Peanut flour, defatted	37	ZnSO$_4$·7H$_2$O	Bone Zn	SR	SP	4, 8, 16	Ali et al. (1981)
Peas, (Pisum sativa), immature	108	Zinc sulfate	65Zn int lab	MR	P-1 ppm	SOD-6-54 µg	Welch et al. (1974)
Peas, mature	86	Zinc sulfate	65Zn int lab	MR	P-1 ppm	SOD-6-54 µg	Welch et al. (1974)
Peas, mature	80	Zinc sulfate	65Zn int lab	MR	P-1 ppm	SOD-6-54 µg	Welch et al. (1974)
Pork	121	ZnCl$_2$	65Zn ret	MR	SP-12 ppm	SOD-1.5 µmol	Hunt et al. (1987)
Rapeseed protein concentrate (129 ppm Zn)	53	Zinc sulfate	Bone Zn	SR	SP-.7 ppm	3, 6, 12	Shah and Belonje (1981)

Table 1. (continued)

Source	RV	Standard	Response criterion	Meth cal	Type diet	Added level, ppm	Reference
Rapeseed protein concentrate	80	$ZnSO_4 \cdot 7H_2O$	Growth	SR	SP < 1 ppm	3, 6, 12	Shah and Belonje (1984)
Rapeseed protein concentrate	53	$ZnSO_4 \cdot 7H_2O$	Bone Zn	SR	SP < 1 ppm	3, 6, 12	Shah and Belonje (1984)
Rice	39	$ZnCO_3$	Growth	MR	P	5-10	O'Dell et al. (1972)
Rice	84	$ZnCl_2$	^{65}Zn ret	MR	SP-12 ppm	SOM-1.5 μmol	Hunt et al. (1987)
Rice, brown (16 ppm Zn)	59	Zinc sulfate	Growth	SR	SP-45 ppm	3-14	Franz et al. (1980a)
Rice, brown Zn-phytate	25	Zinc sulfate	Bone Zn	SR	SP-45 ppm	3-14	Franz et al. (1980a)
Rice, brown	59	Zinc sulfate	Growth	SR	SP-45 ppm	1-14	Franz et al. (1980b)
Rice, brown	25	Zinc sulfate	Bone Zn	SR	SP-45 ppm	1-14	Franz et al. (1980b)
Rice, white (12 ppm Zn)	99	Zinc sulfate	Growth	SR	SP-45 ppm	3-14	Franz et al. (1980a)
Rice, white (12 ppm Zn)	76	Zinc sulfate	Bone Zn	SR	SP-45 ppm	3-14	Franz et al. (1980a)
Rice, white raw	99	Zinc sulfate	Growth	SR	SP-45 ppm	1-14	Franz et al. (1980b)
Rice, white raw	76	Zinc sulfate	Bone Zn	SR	SP-45 ppm	1-14	Franz et al. (1980b)
Rice, white, boiled	92	Zinc sulfate	Growth	SR	SP-45 ppm	1-14	Franz et al. (1980b)
Rice, white, boiled	69	Zinc sulfate	Bone Zn	SR	SP-45 ppm	1-14	Franz et al. (1980b)
Rye forage	120	$ZnCl_2$	^{65}Zn int lab	MR	SP-5 ppm	SOM	Neathery et al. (1975)
Rye (31 ppm)	19.3[b]	-	^{65}Zn ext lab	-	-	SOD	Tidehag et al. (1988)
Soybeans, immature, cooked	99	Zinc sulfate	^{65}Zn ini lab	MR	SP<1 ppm	SOM -11-50 μg	Welch and House (1982)

Food							
Soybeans, mature, cooked	65	Zinc sulfate	^{65}Zn int lab	MR	SP<1 ppm	SOM-11-50 μg	Welch and House (1982)
Soy beverage flour	40	Zinc carbonate	Bone Zn	SR	P	2, 4, 6, 8	Forbes et al. (1979)
Soy concentrate (32 ppm Zn)	20	Zinc carbonate	Bone Zn	SR	P	2, 4, 6, 8	Forbes et al. (1979)
Soy concentrate (34 ppm Zn)	63	$ZnSO_4 \cdot 7H_2O$	Growth	SR	SP < 1 ppm	3, 6, 12	Shah and Belonje (1984)
Soy concentrate (34 ppm Zn)	47	$ZnSO_4 \cdot 7H_2O$	Bone Zn	SR	SP < 1 ppm	3, 6, 12	Shah and Belonje (1984)
Soy concentrate, acid ppt	68[b]	-	Int lab	-	SP-8 ppm	SOD	Ketelsen et al. (1984)
Soy concentrate, acid ppt	74[b]	-	Ext lab	-	SP-8 ppm	SOD	Ketelsen et al. (1984)
Soy concentrate, acid ppt	93	Zinc carbonate	Growth	SR	P	3, 6, 9, 11	Erdman et al. (1980)
Soy concentrate, acid ppt	48	Zinc carbonate	Bone Zn	SR	P	3, 6, 9, 11	Erdman et al. (1980)
Soy concentrate-neutralized	52[b]	-	Int lab	-	SP-8 ppm	SOD	Ketelsen et al. (1984)
Soy concentrate-neutralized	51[b]	-	Ext lab	-	SP-8 ppm	SOD	Ketelsen et al. (1984)
Soy concentrate, neutralized	66	Zinc carbonate	Growth	SR	P	3, 6, 9, 11	Erdman et al. (1980)
Soy concentrate, neutralized	29	Zinc carbonate	Bone Zn	SR	P	3, 6, 9, 11	Erdman et al. (1980)
Soy flour	73[b]	-	Int lab	-	SP-8 ppm	SOD	Meyer et al. (1983)
Soy flour	65[b]	-	Int lab	-	SP-11 ppm	SOD	Meyer et al. (1983)
Soy flour	64[b]	-	Ext lab	-	SP-11 ppm	SOD	Meyer et al. (1983)
Soy flour	75[b]	-	Int lab	-	SP-8 ppm	SOD	Ketelsen et al. (1984)
Soy flour	76[b]	-	Ext lab	-	SP-8 ppm	SOD	Ketelsen et al. (1984)
Soy flour	78	$ZnCl_2$	^{65}Zn ret	MR	SP-12 ppm	SOM-1.5 μmol	Hunt et al. (1987)
Soy flour	80[b]	-	Ext lab	-	SP-8 ppm	SOD	Meyer et al. (1983)

Table I. (continued)

Source	RV	Standard	Response criterion	Meth cal	Type diet	Added level, ppm	Reference
Soy flour, full fat	55	Zinc carbonate	Growth	SR	P	3, 6, 9, 12	Forbes and Parker (1977)
Soy flour, full fat	34	Zinc carbonate	Bone Zn	SR	P	e, 6, 9, 12	Forbes and Parker (1977)
Soy flour, defatted	76[b]	-	^{65}Zn int lab	-	SP	SOM-8	Stuart et al. (1986)
Soy flour, defatted	76[b]	-	^{65}Zn ext lab	-	SP	SOM-8	Stuart et al. (1986)
Soy isolate, acid ppt.	106	Zinc carbonate	Growth	SR	P	3, 6, 9, 11	Erdman et al. (1980)
Soy isolate, acid ppt.	64	Zinc carbonate	Bone Zn	SR	P	3, 6, 9, 11	Erdman et al. (1980)
Soy isolate, neutralized	85	Zinc carbonate	Growth	SR	P	3, 6, 9, 11	Erdman et al. (1980)
Soy isolate, neutralized	46	Zinc carbonate	Bone Zn	SR	P	3, 6, 9, 11	Erdman et al. (1980)
Soy protein isolate (30 ppm Zn)	23	Zinc sulfate	Bone Zn	SR	P	2, 4, 6, 8	Lo et al. (1981)
Soy protein isolate	100	Zinc sulfate	Growth	SR	SP	2, 4, 6	Luhrsen and Rotruck (1979)
Soy protein isolate	65	Zinc sulfate	Bone Zn	SR	SP	2, 4, 6	Luhrsen and Rotruck (1979)
Soy protein, textured (34 ppm)	47	Zinc sulfate	Bone Zn	SR	SP-.7 ppm	3, 6, 12	Shah and Belonje (1981)
Spinach (Spinacia oleracea)	140	Zinc sulfate	^{65}Zn int lab	MR	SP	19-85	Welch et al. (1977)
Wheat	38	ZnCO$_3$	Growth	MR	P	5-10	O'Dell et al. (1972)
Wheat (37 ppm Zn)	13[b]	-	^{65}Zn ext lab	-	N	SOD	Tidehag et al. (1988)
Wheat	56[b]	-	^{65}Zn int lab	-	SP <1 ppm	SOM-33-35 μg	House and Welch (1989)

Compound	Value	Form	Endpoint			Dose	Reference
Wheat	64[b]	-	^{65}Zn ext lab	-	SP <1 ppm	SOM-33-35 μg	House and Welch (1989)
Wheat bran (124 ppm Zn)	34	$ZnSO_4 \cdot 7H_2O$	Growth	MR	SP <1 ppm	18.5	Davies et al. (1977)
Wheat bran (85 ppm Zn)	51	$ZnSO_4 \cdot 7H_2P$	Bone Zn	MR	SP	6, 12	Morris and Ellis (1980b)
Wheat bran	31	$ZnSO_4 \cdot 7H_2O$	Bone Zn	SR	SP	4, 8, 16	Ali et al. (1981)
Wheat bran, low phytate (85 ppm Zn)	80	$ZnSO_4 \cdot 7H_2O$	Bone Zn	MR	SP	6, 12	Morris and Ellis (1980b)
Wheat, dehulled, flour	83	Zinc sulfate	Growth	SR	SP-.45 ppm	6	Franz et al. (1980b)
Wheat, dehulled, flour (24 ppm Zn)	19[b]	-	^{65}Zn ext lab	-	-	SOD	Tidehag et al. (1988)
Wheat, whole, flour	79	Zinc sulfate	Growth	SR	SP-.45 ppm	1-14	Franz et al. (1980b)
Wheat, whole, flour	60	Zinc sulfate	Bone Zn	SR	SP-.45 ppm	1-14	Franz et al. (1980b)
Zinc acetate	13[b]	-	^{65}Zn liv	-	N	SOD	Lonnerdal et al. (1985)
Zinc aspartate	96	Zinc acetate	Pup liver Zn	TP	P-9 ppm	10 ppm in water	Lonnerdal et al. (1985)
Zinc citrate	106	Zinc acetate	Pup liver Zn	TP	P-9 ppm	10 ppm in water	Lonnerdal et al. (1985)
Zinc citrate	16[b]	-	^{65}Zn liv	-	N	SOD	Lonnerdal et al. (1985)
Zinc citrate	99	Zinc sulfate	Growth	MR	P	10	Roth and Kirchgessner (1985)
Zinc citrate	113	Zinc sulfate	Bone Zn	MR	P	10	Roth and Kirchgessner (1985)
Zinc citrate	106	Zinc sulfate	Growth	MR	P	10	Roth and Kirchgessner (1985)
Zinc citrate	99	Zinc sulfate	Bone Zn	MR	P	10	Roth and Kirchgessner (1985)
Zinc citrate	101	Zinc sulfate	Growth	MR	P	10	Roth and Kirchgessner (1985)
Zinc citrate	97	Zinc sulfate	Bone Zn	MR	P	10	Roth and Kirchgessner (1985)

Table I. (continued)

Source	RV	Standard	Response criterion	Meth cal	Type diet	Added level, ppm	Reference
Zinc EDTA	44[b]	-	^{65}Zn liv	-	N	SOD	Lonnerdal et al. (1985)
Zinc nitrilotriacetate	101	Zinc acetate	Pup liver Zn	TP	P-9 ppm	10 ppm in water	Lonnerdal et al. (1985)
Zn$_3$ phytate (16.6% Zn)	93	ZnSO$_4$·7H$_2$O	Growth	MR	P <1 ppm	3, 6, 9	Morris and Ellis (1980a)
Zn$_6$ phytate (30.4% Zn)	98	ZnSO$_4$·7H$_2$O	^{65}Zn liv	-	N	SOD	Lonnerdal et al. (1985)
Zinc phytate	8[b]	-	^{65}Zn liv	-	N	SOD	Lonnerdal et al. (1985)
Zinc picolinate	15[b]	-	^{65}Zn liv	-	N	SOD	Lonnerdal et al. (1985)
Zinc picolinate	84	Zinc acetate	Pup liver Zn	TP	P-9 ppm	10 ppm in water	Lonnerdal et al. (1985)
Zinc picolinate	125	Zinc acetate	Liver Zn	MR	P-8.5 ppm	10 ppm	Evans and Johnson (1980)
Zinc picolinate	136	Zinc acetate	Kidney Zn	MR	P-8.5 ppm	10 ppm	Evans and Johnson (1980)
Zinc picolinate	101	Zinc sulfate	Growth	MR	P	10	Roth and Kirchgessner (1985)
Zinc picolinate	93	Zinc sulfate	Bone Zn	MR	P	10	Roth and Kirchgessner (1985)
Zinc picolinate	102	Zinc sulfate	Growth	MR	P	10	Roth and Kirchgessner (1985)
Zinc picolinate	101	Zinc sulfate	Bone Zn	MR	P	10	Roth and Kirchgessner (1985)
Zinc picolinate	108	Zinc sulfate	Growth	MR	P	10	Roth and Kirchgessner (1985)
Zinc picolinate	94	Zinc sulfate	Bone Zn	MR	P	10	Roth and Kirchgessner (1985)

[a]Abbreviations can be found in Appendix I. Chemical formula for a compound given only if provided by the author; RG indicates reagent grade, FG indicates feed grade.
[b]Percentage absorption, not relative value.

Table II. Relative bioavailability of supplemental zinc sources[a]

Source	Poultry	Swine	Cattle	Sheep	Rats
Standards					
Zinc acetate	-	-	-	-	100
Zinc chloride	100	100	-	-	-
Zinc sulfate	100	-	100	100	100
Zinc aspartate	-	-	-	-	95 (1)
Zinc carbonate	105 (5)	-	60 (1)	-	-
Zinc, chelated				110 (2)	-
Zinc citrate	-	-	-	-	100 (7)
Zinc, elemental	100 (1)	130 (1)	-	-	-
Zinc-lysine	-	100 (1)	-	-	-
Zinc-methionine	125 (3)	100 (2)	-	100 (2)	-
Zinc oxide[b]	100 (5)	-	100 (4)	70 (1)	-
Zinc oxide[b]	55 (2)	50 (1)	-	-	-
Zinc picolinate	-	-	-	-	105 (9)
Zinc proteinate	100 (1)	-	-	-	-
Zinc, sequestered	-	-	-	105 (2)	-

[a]Average values rounded to nearest "5" and expressed relative to response with sulfate, chloride, or acetate forms of zinc. Number of studies or samples involved indicated within parentheses. Terminology for sources is that of the author(s).

[b]Some recent studies have indicated zinc oxide to be less bioavailable than that observed in earlier research.

REFERENCES

Ali, R., H. Staub, G. Coccodrilli, Jr. and L. Schanbacher. 1981. Nutritional significance of dietary fiber: Effect on nutrient bioavailability and selected gastrointestinal functions. *J. Agric. Food Chem.* **29**:465.

Allred, J. B., F. H. Kratzer and J. W. G. Porter. 1964. Some factors affecting the *in vitro* binding of zinc by isolated soya-bean protein and by α-casein. *Br. J. Nutr.* **18**:575.

Aoyagi, S. and D. H. Baker. 1994. Copper-amino acid complexes are partially protected against inhibiting effects of L-cysteine and L-ascorbate on copper absorption in chicks. *J. Nutr.* **124**:388.

Atwal, A. S., N. A. M. Eskin, B. E. McDonald and M. Vaisey-Genser. 1980. The effects of phytate on nitrogen utilization and zinc metabolism in young rats. *Nutr. Rep. Int.* **21**:257.

Bafundo, K. W., D. H. Baker and P. R. Fitzgerald. 1984. The iron-zinc interrelationship in the chick as influenced by *Eimeria acervulina* infection. *J. Nutr.* **114**:1306.

Bobilya, D. J. 1989. Assessment of the nutritional status and bioavailability of zinc for neonatal pigs. Ph.D. Dissertation, University of Missouri, Columbia.

Boland, A. R. de, G. B. Garner and B. L. O'Dell. 1975. Identification and properties of "phytate" in cereal grains and oilseed products. *J. Agric. Food Chem.* **23**:1186.

Bremner, I., J. N. Morrison, A. M. Wood and J. R. Arthur. 1987. Effects of changes in dietary zinc, copper and selenium supply and of endotoxin administration on metallothionein I concentrations in blood cells and urine in the rat. *J. Nutr.* **117**:1595.

Brown, C. R., P. J. Bechtel, R. M. Forbes and R. S. Vogel. 1985. Bioavailability of zinc derived from beef and the effect of low dietary zinc intake on skeletal muscle zinc concentration. *Nutr. Res.* **5**:117.

Bunn, C. R. and G. Matrone. 1966. *In vivo* interactions of cadmium, copper, zinc and iron in the mouse and rat. *J. Nutr.* **90**:395.

Caprez, A. and S. J. Fairweather-Tait. 1982. The effect of heat treatment and particle size of bran on mineral absorption in rats. *Br. J. Nutr.* **48**:467.

Davies, N.T. 1980. Studies on the absorption of zinc by rat intestine. *Br. J. Nutr.* **43**:189.

Davies, N. T., V. Hristic and A. A. Flett. 1977. Phytate rather than fibre as the major determinant of zinc bioavailability to rats. *Nutr. Rep. Int.* **15**:207.

Davies, N. T. and R. Nightingale. 1975. The effects of phytate on intestinal absorption and secretion of zinc, and whole-body retention of Zn, copper, iron and manganese in rats. *Br. J. Nutr.* **34**:243.

Edwards, H. M., Jr. 1959. The availability to chicks of zinc in various compounds and ores. *J. Nutr.* **69**:306.

Erdman, J. W., Jr., K. E. Weingartner, G. E. Mustakas, R. D. Schmutz, H. M. Parker and R. M. Forbes. 1980. Zinc and magnesium bioavailability from acid-precipitated and neutralized soybean protein products. *J. Food Sci.* **45**:1193.

Evans, G. W. and E. C. Johnson. 1980. Zinc absorption in rats fed a low-protein diet and a low-protein diet supplemented with tryptophan or picolinic acid. *J. Nutr.* **110**:1076.

Evans, G. W., E. C. Johnson and P. E. Johnson. 1979. Zinc absorption in the rat determined by radioisotope dilution. *J. Nutr.* **109**:1258.

Evans, G. W. and P. E. Johnson. 1977. Determination of zinc availability in foods by the extrinsic label technique. *Am. J. Clin. Nutr.* **30**:873.

Fairweather-Tait, S. J., V. Payne and C. M. Williams. 1984. The effect of iron supplements on pregnancy in rats given a low-zinc diet. *Br. J. Nutr.* **52**:79.

Finelli, V. N., D. S. Klauder, M. A. Karaffa and H. G. Petering. 1975. Interaction of zinc and lead on δ-aminolevulinate dehydratase. *Biochem. Biophys. Res. Commun.* **65**:303.

Flagstad, T. 1981. Zinc absorption in cattle with a dietary picolinic acid supplement. *J. Nutr.* **111**:1996.

Flanagan, P. R., J. Haist, I. MacKenzie and L. S. Valberg. 1984. Intestinal absorption of zinc: Competive interactions with iron, cobalt, and copper in mice with sex-linked anemia. *Can. J. Physiol. Pharmacol.* **62**:1124.

Flanagan, P. R., J. Haist and L. S. Valberg. 1980. Comparative effects of iron deficiency induced by bleeding and a low-iron diet on the intestinal absorptive interactions of iron, cobalt, manganese, zinc, lead and cadmium. *J. Nutr.* **110**:1754.

Forbes, R. M., J. W. Erdman, Jr., H. M. Parker, H. Kondo and S. M. Ketelsen. 1983. Bioavailability of zinc in coagulated soy protein (Tofu) to rats and effect of dietary calcium at a constant phytate:zinc ratio. *J. Nutr.* **113**:205.

Forbes, R. M. and H. M. Parker. 1977. Biological availability of zinc in and as influenced by whole fat soy flour in rat diets. *Nutr. Rep. Int.* **15**:681.

Forbes, R. M., K. E. Weingartner, H. M. Parker, R. R. Bell and J. W. Erdman, Jr. 1979. Bioavailability to rats of zinc, magnesium and calcium in casein-, egg- and soy protein-containing diets. *J. Nutr.* **109**:1652.

Fordyce, E. J., R. M. Forbes, K. R. Robbins and J. W. Erdman, Jr. 1987. Phytate x calcium/zinc molar ratios: Are they predictive of zinc bioavailability? *J. Food Sci.* **52**:440.

Fox, M. R. S. and B. N. Harrison. 1964. Use of Japanese quail for the study of zinc deficiency. *Proc. Soc. Exp. Biol. Med.* **116**:256.

Franz, K. B., B. M. Kennedy and D. A. Fellers. 1980a. Relative bioavailability of zinc using weight gain of rats. *J. Nutr.* **110**:2263.

Franz, K. B., B. M. Kennedy and D. A. Fellers. 1980b. Relative bioavailability of zinc from selected cereals and legumes using rat growth. *J. Nutr.* **110**:2272.

Gordon, D. T. 1987. Interactions among iron, zinc and copper. *In* "AIN Symposium Proceedings on Nutrition '87" (O. A. Levander, Ed.). p. 27

Greene, L. W., D. K. Lunt, F. M. Byers, N. K. Chirase, C. E. Richmond, R. E. Knutson and G. T. Schelling. 1988. Performance and carcass quality of steers supplemented with zinc oxide or zinc methionine. *J. Anim. Sci.* **66**:1818.

Greger, J. L. and M. A. Johnson. 1981. Effect of dietary tin on zinc, copper and iron utilization by rats. *Food Cosmet. Toxicol.* **19**:163.

Hahn, J. D. and D. H. Baker. 1993. Growth and plasma zinc responses of young pigs fed pharmacologic levels of zinc. *J. Anim. Sci.* **71**:3020.

Hambidge, K. M., C. E. Casey and N. F. Krebs. 1986. Zinc. *In* "Trace Elements in Human and Animal Nutrition" (W. Mertz, Ed.) 5th ed., p. 1. Academic Press, New York.

Hamilton, D. L., J. E. C. Bellamy, J. D. Valberg and L. S. Valberg. 1978. Zinc, cadmium and iron interactions during intestinal absorption in iron-deficient mice. *Can. J. Physiol. Pharmacol.* **56**:384.

Hempe, J. M. 1987. Zinc bioavailability in the chick. Ph.D. Dissertation, University of Missouri, Columbia.

Henry, P. R., C. B. Ammerman and R. D. Miles. 1987. Effect of dietary zinc on tissue mineral concentration as a measure of zinc bioavailability in chicks. *Nutr. Rep. Int.* **35**:15.

Heth, D. A. and W. G. Hoekstra. 1965. Zinc-65 absorption and turnover in rats I. A procedure to determine zinc-65 absorption and the antagonistic effect of calcium in a practical diet. *J. Nutr.* **85**:367.

Hill, C. H. and G. Matrone. 1970. Chemical parameters in the study of *in vivo* and *in vitro* interactions of transition elements. *Fed. Proc.* **29**:1474.

Hill, C. H., G. Matrone, W. L. Payne and C. W. Barber. 1963. *In vivo* interactions of cadmium and copper, zinc and iron. *J. Nutr.* **80**:227.

Hill, D. A., E. R. Peo, Jr. and A. J. Lewis. 1987a. Effect of zinc source and picolinic acid on ^{65}Zn uptake in an *in vitro* continuous flow perfusion system for pig and poultry intestinal segments. *J. Nutr.* **117**:1704.

Hill, D. A., E. R. Peo and A. J. Lewis. 1987b. Influence of picolinic acid on the uptake of ^{65}zinc-amino acid complexes by the everted rat gut. *J. Anim. Sci.* **65**:173.

Ho, S. K. and M. Hidiroglou. 1977. Effects of dietary chelated and sequestered zinc and zinc sulfate on growing lambs fed a purified diet. *Can. J. Anim. Sci.* **57**:93.

Hortin, A. E., P. J. Bechtel and D. H. Baker. 1991. Efficacy of pork loin as a source of zinc and effect of added cysteine on zinc bioavailability. *J. Food Sci.* **56**:1505.

House, W. A. and R. M. Welch. 1989. Bioavailability of and interactions between zinc and selenium in rats fed wheat grain intrinsically labeled with ^{65}Zn and ^{75}Se. *J. Nutr.* **119**:916.

Huber, A. M. and S. N. Gershoff. 1970. Effects of dietary zinc and calcium on the retention and distribution of zinc in rats fed semipurified diets. *J. Nutr.* **100**:949.

Hunt, J. R., P. E. Johnson and P. B. Swan. 1987. Dietary conditions influencing relative zinc bioavailability from foods to the rat and correlations with *in vitro* measurements. *J. Nutr.* **117**:1913.

Johnson, M. A. and J. L. Greger. 1984. Absorption, distribution and endogenous excretion of zinc by rats fed various dietary levels of inorganic tin and zinc. *J. Nutr.* **114**:1843.

Jones, A. O. L., M. R. S. Fox and B. E. Fry, Jr. 1985. *In vitro* assessment of zinc binding to protein foods as a potential index of zinc bioavailability. Comparsion of *in vitro* and *in vivo* data. *J. Agric. Food Chem.* **33**:1123.

Kennedy, D. W., W. M. Craig, L. L. Southern and M. Engstrom. 1988. Ruminal partitioning of zinc in steers fed a polysaccharide complex of zinc or zinc oxide. *J. Anim. Sci.* **66**(Suppl. 1):462 [Abstract].

Ketelson, S. M., M. A. Stuart, C. M. Weaver, R. M. Forbes and J. W. Erdman, Jr. 1984. Bioavaiability of zinc to rats from defatted soy flour, acid-precipitated soy concentrate and neutralized soy concentrate as determined by intrinsic and extrinsic labeling techniques. *J. Nutr.* **114**:536.

Kiely, J., A. Flynn, H. Singh and P. F. Fox. 1988. Improved zinc bioavailability from colloidal calcium phosphate-free cow's milk. *In* " Trace Elements in Man and Animals - 6" (L.S. Hurley, C.L. Keen, B. Lonnerdal and R.B. Rucker, Eds.). Plenum Press, New York.

Kincaid, R. L. 1979. Biological availability of zinc from inorganic sources with excess dietary calcium. *J. Dairy Sci.* **62**:1081.

Kincaid, R. L., A. S. Hodgson, R. E. Riley, Jr. and J. D. Cronrath. 1984. Supplementation of diets for lactating cows with zinc as zinc oxide and zinc methionine. *J. Dairy Sci.* **67**(Suppl. 1):103 [Abstract].

Kratzer, F. H., J. B. Allred, P. N. Davis, B. J. Marshall and P. Vohra. 1959. The effect of autoclaving soybean protein and the addition of ethylenediaminetetracetic acid on the biological availability of dietary zinc for turkey poults. *J. Nutr.* **68**:313.

Kratzer, F. H., J. B. Allred and J. W. G. Porter. 1961. Factors influencing the *in vitro* binding of zinc. *Poult. Sci.* **40**:1421 [Abstract].

Kratzer, F. H. and B. Starcher. 1963. Quantitative relation of EDTA to availability of zinc for turkey poults. *Proc. Soc. Exp. Biol. Med.* **113**:424.

Lantzsch, H.-J. and S.E. Scheuermann. 1981. Effect of dehulling on zinc availability of field beans. *In* "Trace Element Metabolism in Man and Animals - 4" (J. McC. Howell, J. M. Gawthorne and C. L. White, Eds.). Australian Academy of Science, Canberra.

Lease, J. G. 1967. Availability to the chick of zinc-phytate complexes isolated from oil seed meals by an *in vitro* digestion method. *J. Nutr.* **93**:523.

Lease, J. G. 1968. Effect of graded levels of cadinium on tissue uptake of [65]Zn by the chick over time. *J. Nutr.* **96**:294.

Lease, J. G. and W. P. Williams, Jr. 1967. Availability of zinc and comparison of *in vitro* and *in vivo* zinc uptake of certain oil seed meals. *Poult. Sci.* **46**:233.

Likuski, H. J. A. and R. M. Forbes. 1964. Effect of phytic acid on the availability of zinc in amino acid and casein diets fed to chicks. *J. Nutr.* **84**:145.

Likuski, H. J. A. and R. M. Forbes. 1965. Mineral utilization in the rat. IV. Effect of calcium and phytic acid on the utilization of dietary zinc. *J. Nutr.* **85**:230.

Lo, G. S., S. L. Settle, F. H. Steinke and D. T. Hopkins. 1981. Effect of phytate: zinc molar ratio and isolated soybean protein on zinc bioavailability. *J. Nutr.* **111**:2223.

Lonnerdal, B., C. L. Keen, J. G. Bell and L. S. Hurley. 1985. Zinc uptake and retention from chelates and milk fractions. *In* "Trace Elements in Man and Animals - 5" (C. F. Mills, I. Bremner and J. K. Chesters, Eds.). Commonwealth Agricultural Bureaux, Slough, UK.

Lonnerdal, B., A. G. Stanislowski and L. S. Hurley. 1980. Isolation of a low molecular weight zinc binding ligand from human milk. *J. Inorg. Biochem.* **12**:71.

Luhrsen, K. R. and J. T. Rotruck. 1979. Comparative studies with weanling rats to measure zinc bioavailability from soy protein isolate and beef. *Fed. Proc.* **38**:558 [Abstract].

McKenzie, J. M. and N. T. Davies. 1981. Influence of dietary protein on zinc availability from bread in rats. *In* "Trace Element Metabolism in Man and Animals-4" (J. McC. Howell, J. M. Gawthorne and C. L. White, Eds.), p. 111. Australian Academy of Science, Canberra.

Menard, M. P. and R. J. Cousins. 1983. Effect of citrate, glutathione and picolinate on zinc transport by brush border membrane vesicles from rat intestine. *J. Nutr.* **113**:1653.

Meyer, N. R., M. A. Stwart and C. M. Weaver. 1983. Bioavailability of zinc from defatted soy flour, soy hulls and whole eggs as determined by intrinsic and extrinsic labeling techniques. *J. Nutr.* **113**:1255.

Miller, W. J., D. M. Blackmon, R. P. Gentry and F. M. Pate. 1970. Effects of high but nontoxic levels of zinc in practical diets on [65]Zn and zinc metabolism in Holstein calves. *J. Nutr.* **100**:893.

Miller, W. J., D. M. Blackmon, J. M. Hiers, Jr., P. R. Fowler, C. M. Clifton and R. P. Gentry. 1967. Effects of adding two forms of supplemental zinc to a practical diet on skin regeneration in Holstein heifers and evaluation of a procedure for determining rate of wound healing. *J. Dairy Sci.* **50**:715.

Miller, W. J., Y. G. Martin, R. P. Gentry and D. M. Blackmon. 1968. [65]Zn and stable zinc absorption, excretion and tissue concentrations as affected by type of diet and level of zinc in normal calves. *J. Nutr.* **94**:391.

Momcilovic, B., B. Belonje, A. Giroux and B. G. Shah. 1975. Total femur zinc as the parameter of choice for a zinc bioassay in rats. *Nutr. Rep. Int.* **12**:197.

Momcilovic, B., B. Belonje, A. Giroux and B. G. Shah. 1976. Bioavailability of zinc in milk and soy protein-based infant formulas. *J. Nutr.* **106**:913.

Momcilovic, B. and B. G. Shah. 1976. Bioavailability of zinc in infant foods. *Nutr. Rep. Int.* **14**:717.

Miller, E. R., P. K. Ku, J. P. Hitchcock and W. T. Magee. 1981. Availability of zinc from metallic zinc dust for young swine. *J. Anim. Sci.* **52**:312.

Morris, E. R. and R. Ellis. 1980b. Bioavailability to rats of iron and zinc in wheat bran: Response to low-phytate bran and effect of the phytate/zinc molar ratio. *J. Nutr.* **110**:2000.

Morris, E. R. and R. Ellis. 1980a. Effect of dietary phytate/zinc molar ratio on growth and bone zinc response of rats fed semipurified diets. *J. Nutr.* **110**:1037.

Neathery, M. W., J. W. Lassiter, W. J. Miller and R. P. Gentry. 1975. Absorption, excretion and tissue distribution of natural organic and inorganic zinc-65 in the rat. *Proc. Soc. Exp. Biol. Med.* **149**:1.

Neathery, M. W., S. Rachmat, W. J. Miller, R. P. Gentry and D. M. Blackmon. 1972. Effect of chemical form of orally administered ^{65}Zn on absorption and metabolism in cattle. *Proc. Soc. Exp. Biol. Med.* **139**:953.

Nielsen, F. H., M. L. Sunde and W. G. Hoekstra. 1966. Effect of some dietary synthetic and natural chelating agents on the zinc-deficiency syndrome in the chick. *J. Nutr.* **89**:35.

National Research Council (NRC). 1989. "Recommended Dietary Allowances," 10th ed. National Academy Press, Washington, DC.

Oberleas, D., M. E. Muhrer and B. L. O'Dell. 1966. Dietary metal-complexing agents and zinc availability in the rat. *J. Nutr.* **90**:56.

Oberleas, D. and A. S. Prasad. 1976. Factors affecting zinc homeostasis. *In* "Trace Elements in Human Health and Disease" (A.S. Prasad and D. Oberleas, Eds.), Vol. 1.   p. 155. Academic Press, New York.

O'Dell, B. L., C. E. Burpo and J. E. Savage. 1972. Evaluation of zinc availability in foodstuffs of plant and animal origin. *J. Nutr.* **102**:653.

O'Dell, B. L., P. M. Newberne and J. E. Savage. 1958. Significance of dietary zinc for the growing chicken. *J. Nutr.* **65**:503.

O'Dell, B. L. and J. E. Savage. 1957. Potassium, zinc and distillers dried solubles as supplements to a purified diet. *Poult. Sci.* **36**:459.

O'Dell, B. L. and J. E. Savage. 1960. Effect of phytic acid on zinc availability. *Proc. Soc. Exp. Biol. Med.* **103**:304.

O'Dell, B. L., J. M. Yohe and J. E. Savage. 1964. Zinc availability in the chick as affected by phytate, calcium and ethylenediaminetetracetate. *Poult. Sci.* **43**:415.

Oestreicher, P. and R. J. Cousins. 1982. Influence of intraluminal constituents on zinc absorption by isolated, vascularly perfused rat intestine. *J. Nutr.* **112**:1978.

Oestreicher, P. and R. J. Cousins. 1985. Copper and zinc absorption in the rat: Mechanism of mutual antagonism. *J. Nutr.* **115**:159.

Pearson, W. N., T. Schwink and M. Reich. 1966. *In vitro* studies of zinc absorption in the rat. *In* "Zinc Metabolism" (A. S. Prasad, Ed.), p. 239. Thomas, Springfield, IL.

Pensack, J. M., J. N. Henson and P. D. Bogdnoff. 1958. The effects of calcium and phosphorus on the zinc requirements of growing chickens. *Poult. Sci.* **37**:1232 [Abstract].

Pimentel. J. L., M. E. Cook and J. L. Greger. 1991. Research note: Bioavailability of zinc-methionine for chicks. *Poult. Sci.* **70**:1637.

Powell, G. W., W. J. Miller, J. D. Morton and C. M. Clifton. 1964. Influence of dietary cadmium level and supplemental zinc on cadmium toxicity in the bovine. *J. Nutr.* **84**:205.

Reeves, P. G. and B. L. O'Dell. 1986. Effects of dietary zinc deprivation on the activity of angiotensin-converting enzyme in serum of rats and guinea pigs. *J. Nutr.* **116**:128.

Roberson, R. H. and P. J. Schaible. 1958. The zinc requirement of the chick. *Poult. Sci.* **37**:1321.

Roberson, R. H. and P. J. Schaible. 1960a. The availability to the chick of zinc as the sulfate, oxide or carbonate. *Poult. Sci.* **39**:835.

Roberson, R. H. and P. J. Schaible. 1960b. The tolerance of growing chicks for high levels of different forms of zinc. *Poult. Sci.* **39**:893.

Roth, H. P. and M. Kirchgessner. 1985. Utilization of zinc from picolinic or citric acid complexes in relation to dietary protein source in rats. *J. Nutr.* **115**:1641.

Sandoval, M., P. R. Henry, C. B. Ammerman, R. D. Miles and R. J. Cousins. 1992. Tissue metallothionine concentration as an estimate of bioavailability of zinc for chicks. *Poult. Sci.* **71**(Suppl. 1):67 [Abstract].

Sandstrom, B., C. L. Keen and B. Lonnerdal. 1983. An experimental model for studies of zinc bioavailability from milk and infant formulas using extrinsic labeling. *Am. J. Clin. Nutr.* **38**:420.

Sato, M., R. K. Mehra and I. Bremner. 1984. Measurement of plasma metallothionein-I in the assessment of the zinc status of zinc-deficient and stressed rats. *J. Nutr.* **114**:1683.

Savage, J. E., J. M. Yohe, E. E. Pickett and B. L. O'Dell. 1964. Zinc metabolism in the growing chick. Tissue concentration and effect of phytate on absorption. *Poult. Sci.* **43**:420.

Scott, M. L. and T. R. Zeigler. 1963. Evidence for natural chelates which aid in the utilization of zinc by chicks. *J. Agric. Food Chem.* **11**:123.

Seal, C. J. and F. W. Heaton. 1983. Chemical factors affecting the intestinal absorption of zinc *in vitro* and *in vivo*. *Br. J. Nutr.* **50**:317.

Seth, P. C. C., D. R. Clandinin and R. T. Hardin. 1975. *In vitro* uptake of zinc by rapeseed meal and soybean meal. *Poult. Sci.* **54**:626.

Shah, B. G. and B. Belonje. 1981. Bioavailability of zinc in beef with and without plant protein. *Fed. Proc.* **40**:855 [Abstract].

Shah, B. G. and B. Belonje. 1984. Bioavailability of zinc in beef with and without plant protein concentrates. *Nutr. Res.* **4**:71.

Smith, B. L. and P. P. Embling. 1984. The influence of chemical form of zinc on the effects of toxic intraruminal doses of zinc to sheep. *J. Appl. Toxicol.* **4**:92.

Smith, K. T. and R. J. Cousins. 1980. Quantitative aspects of zinc absorption by isolated, vascularly perfused rat intestine. *J. Nutr.* **110**:316.

Smith, K. T., R. J. Cousins, B. L. Silbon and M. L. Failla. 1978. Zinc absorption and metabolism by isolated, vascularly perfused rat intestine. *J. Nutr.* **108**:1849.

Solomons, N. W. 1986. Competitive interaction of iron and zinc in the diet: Consequences for human nutrition. *J. Nutr.* **116**:927.

Solomons, N. W., R. A. Jacob, O. Pineda and F. F. Viteri Studies on the bioavailability of zinc in man. III. Effect of ascorbic acid on zinc absorption. *Am. J. Clin. Nutr.* **32**:2495.

Spears, J. W. 1989. Zinc methionine for ruminants: Relative bioavailability of zinc in lambs and effects of growth and performance of growing heifers. *J. Anim. Sci.* **67**:835.

Spears, J. W. and E. B. Kegley. 1991. Effect of zinc and manganese methionine on performance of beef cows and calves. *J. Anim. Sci.* **69**(Suppl. 1):59 [Abstract].

Stuart, S. M., S. M. Ketelsen, C. M. Weaver and J. W. Erdman, Jr. 1986. Bioavailability of zinc to rats as affected by protein source and previous dietary intake. *J. Nutr.* **116**:1423.

Sullivan, T. W. 1961. The availability of zinc in various compounds to broad breasted bronze poults. *Poult. Sci.* **40**:340.

Supplee, W. C. 1961. Production of zinc deficiency in turkey poults by dietary cadmium. *Poult. Sci.* **40**:827.

Supplee, W. C. 1963. Antagonistic relationship between dietary cadmium and zinc. *Science* **139**:119.

Tidehag, P., A. Moberg, B. Sunzel, G. Hallmans, R. Sjostrom and K. Wing. 1988. The availability of zinc, cadmium and iron from different grains measured as isotope absorption and mineral accumulation in rats. *In* "Trace Elements in Man and Animals - 6" (L. S. Hurley, C. L. Keen, B. Lonnerdal and R. B. Rucker, Eds.), p. 507. Plenum Press, New York.

Todd, W. R., C. A. Elvehjem and E. B. Hart. 1934. Zinc in the nutrition of the rat. *Am. J. Physiol.* **107**:146.

Tucker, H. F. and W. D. Salmon. 1955. Parakeratosis or zinc deficiency disease in the pig. *Proc. Soc. Exp. Biol. Med.* **88**:613.

Vallee, B. L. 1988. Zinc: Biochemistry, physiology, toxicology and clinical pathology. *Biofactors* **1**:31.

Van der Aar, P. G., G. C. Fahey, Jr., S. C. Ricke, S. E. Allen and L. L. Berger. 1983. Effects of dietary fibers on mineral status of chicks. *J. Nutr.* **113**:653.

Van Campen, D. R. 1969. Copper interference with the intestinal aborption of zinc-65 by rats. 9 *J. Nutr.* **97**:104.

Vohra, P. and F. H. Kratzer. 1964. Influence of various chelating agents on the availability of zinc. J. Nutr. **82**:249.

Vohra, P. and F. H. Kratzer. 1966. Influence of various phosphates and other complexing agents on the availability of zinc for turkey poults. *J. Nutr.* **89**:106.

Wapnir, R. A. and L. Stiel. 1986. Zinc intestinal absorption in rats: Specificity of amino acids as ligands. *J. Nutr.* **116**:2171.

Wedekind, K. J. and D. H. Baker. 1990. Zinc bioavailability in feed-grade sources of zinc. *J. Anim. Sci.* **68**:684.

Wedekind, K. J., A. E. Hortin and D. H. Baker. 1992. Methodology for assessing zinc bioavailability: Efficacy estimates for zinc-methionine, zinc sulfate and zinc oxide. *J. Anim. Sci.* **70**:178.

Welch, R. M. and W. A. House. 1982. Availability to rats of zinc from soybean seeds as affected by maturity of seed, source of dietary protein, and soluble phytate. *J. Nutr.* **112**:879.

Welch, R. M., W. A. House and W. H. Allaway. 1974. Availability of zinc from pea seeds to rats. *J. Nutr.* **104**:733.

Welch, R. M., W. A. House and D. van Campen. 1977. Effects of oxalic acid on availability of zinc from spinach leaves and zinc sulfate to rats. *J. Nutr.* **107**:929.

18

VITAMIN BIOAVAILABILITY

David H. Baker

Department of Animal Sciences and
Division of Nutritional Sciences
University of Illinois
Urbana, Illinois

I. INTRODUCTION

The available literature on vitamin bioavailability in feed ingredients is very limited. Most of the vitamins present in feedstuffs exist as precursor compounds or coenzymes that are often bound or complexed in some manner. Hence, gut processes are required to either release or convert vitamin precursors or complexes to usable and absorbable chemical entities.

Vitamin bioavailability in formulated diets for livestock and companion animals is dependent on two factors: (a) stability of free vitamins in vitamin and vitamin-mineral premixes as well as in diets and supplements and (b) utilization efficiency from plant- and animal-source feed ingredients. Information on factors affecting the stability of crystalline vitamins in diets and premixes can be found in the reviews of Wornick (1968), Schneider (1986), McGinnis (1986), Zhuge and Klopfenstein (1986), and Coelho (1991). Regarding vitamin bioavailability in feed ingredients for nonruminant animals, virtually no research is available for the pig; even with chicks or rats, few feed ingredients have been evaluated. Sauberlich (1985) has reviewed the subject of vitamin bioavailability in human foods as affected by various food processing procedures. Thus, laboratory animal as well as human data are the primary sources of information that have been used for this review.

Many pitfalls exist in vitamin bioavailability assessment (Baker, 1986a, b). Body stores often preclude development of a distinct deficiency during the course of a conventional growth trial, and even if a frank deficiency can be produced, one must deal with the vexing question of whether the responding criterion (usually weight gain) increases because of the vitamin being supplied or because feed intake of an unpalatable purified diet is increased. With rodents, moreover, coprophagy (fecal recycling) may lead to overestimation of true bioavailability. At least five factors must be carefully considered in order to arrive at meaningful bioavailability estimates: (a) pretest periods to attain desired deficiency states generally are necessary, (b) activity of a key enzyme of which the vitamin is a component or cofactor usually is less desirable as a dependent variable than vitamin-dependent weight gain, (c) precursor materials (e.g., methionine for choline, tryptophan for niacin) must be carefully controlled, (d) effects of coprophagy must be considered, and (e) use of specific vitamin inhibitors or antagonists may assist in establishing veracity of assessed bioavailability values.

In preparing vitamin premixes, whether commercial or experimental, several precautions should be considered. The carrier material should be uniform in texture and particle size. If carbohydrate, it should not contain free aldehyde groups. Thus, dextrose and lactose should be avoided as carriers. Both thiamin and folacin have free amino groups that can react with free carbonyl groups to form Maillard linkages that cannot be broken by digestive enzymes in the upper small intestine. High potency vitamin premixes used for fortification of purified diets generally should not contain either choline or vitamin E activity. Pure choline chloride is extremely hygroscopic and pure DL-α-tocopheryl acetate (all-*rac*-α-tocopheryl acetate) is a liquid. As such, these substances are not suitable components of purified vitamin premixes. All-*rac*-α-tocopheryl acetate can be dissolved in ether or blended with fat, premixed with carbohydrate, screened, and then added directly to the diet. Commercial vitamin premixes generally use choline and vitamin E sources that are already premixed (i.e., diluted) and this makes them suitable as components of a complete (feed grade) vitamin premix. Once prepared, vitamin premixes should be stored in a dark container that is as air-tight and oxygen-free as possible and kept in a cool, dry place. Avoiding heat, light, oxygen, and moisture will minimize loss of potency.

Generally, the fat-soluble vitamins are less heat labile than the water-soluble vitamins, although the former can lose biopotency when subjected to high temperatures in the presence of oxygen. Among the water-soluble vitamins, thiamin, folacin, pantothenic acid, and ascorbic acid are considered the most heat labile.

II. WATER-SOLUBLE VITAMINS

A. Thiamin

Crystalline thiamin is available to the food and feed industries as thiamin·HCl (89% thiamin) or thiamin·NO$_3$ (92% thiamin). These compounds are stable up to 100°C and are readily soluble in water (NRC, 1987). One IU of thiamin activity is equivalent to 3 μg of crystalline thiamin·HCl. The thiamin contained in dietary feed ingredients is present largely in phosphorylated forms, either as protein-phosphate complexes or as thiamin mono-, di-, or triphosphates.

Thiamin is absorbed from the upper part of the small intestine via a saturable, carrier-mediated, sodium-dependent, energy-requiring, active process (Sauberlich, 1985). It is phosphorylated to its esters soon after entering enterocytes. Studies with rats and humans have indicated that folacin deficiency may decrease intestinal absorption of thiamin (Thompson et al., 1971; Howard et al., 1974). Thiamin phosphorylation and transport may also be decreased by the coccidiostat, amprolium (Bauchop and King, 1968; Menon and Sognen, 1971).

Among the vitamins, thiamin is one of the most poorly stored; body stores are exhausted within 1 to 2 weeks. The pig, however, appears to be an exception in that this species can store large quantities of thiamin in skeletal muscle, mostly as thiamin pyrophosphate (NRC, 1987).

Thiamin contains a free amino group which makes it subject to heat processing losses via the Maillard reaction (Farrer, 1955). Any processing procedure that involves alkaline treatment generally leads to loss of thiamin activity. Also, treatment of feed ingredients with sulfur dioxide inactivates thiamin (NRC, 1988).

Some raw ingredients (e.g., shellfish and freshwater fishes) contain heat-labile thiaminases which may destroy thiamin bioactivity in diets to which these ingredients are added (Murata, 1982). Thermostabile antithiamin factors also have been identified in certain plant foodstuffs (Hilker and Somogy, 1982). Plants, such as bracken fern, horsetail, and yellow-star thistle, contain antithiamin activity that has been reported to cause problems in horses (Roberts et al., 1949; Lott, 1951; Martin, 1975). While feeds containing thiaminases are of concern in diet formulation for cats and fur-bearing animals, they are considered of minimal consequence in the nutrition of other livestock species. Thiamin in fish meal is lost to the fish solubles fraction when fish meal is made. Likewise, due to the high-temperature processing, meat meals contain very little bioavailable thiamin.

Pelleting causes some loss of thiamin activity as does storage of crystalline thiamin in the presence of minerals (Gadient, 1986). Adams (1982) found 48 and 95% retention of activity when stored in the form of the HCl and NO_3, respectively, in a premix for 21 days at 40°C and 85% relative humidity. In a complete feed stored under similar conditions, thiamin·HCl retained only 21% of its activity, while thiamin·NO_3 retained 98% of its activity. Thus, the mononitrate form of crystalline thiamin is a more stable form in diets stored in hot environments.

Grains and soybean meal are sufficiently rich in thiamin such that, even with considerable losses due to heat or lengthy storage, swine or poultry fed practical diets seldom respond to supplementation with this vitamin (Easter et al., 1983). However, because raw meat products are commonly fed to cats and fur-bearing animals, thiamin supplementation of diets for these species is commonplace.

Thiamin addition to ruminant diets has been controversial and has mainly centered on prevention or treatment of polioencephalomalacia (Brent and Bartley, 1984). While injected thiamin elicits immediate responses in affected ruminant animals, oral thiamin supplementation has not been tested. Certain individual ruminants appear to have high thiaminase concentrations in digesta which reduce bioavailability of dietary thiamin. Elevated sulfate intakes increase ruminal destruction of thiamin (Goetsch and Owens, 1987). Whenever diets contain high sulfate concentrations (gypsum in feed or water, errors in supplement formulation), ruminants are likely to show signs of polioencephalomalacia. High sulfate levels in the rumen apparently cause cleavage of the thiamin ring. Goetsch and Owens (1987) reported that thiamin flow from the rumen was reduced by 25% upon adding .51% sulfur to the diet.

B. Riboflavin

Crystalline riboflavin is available for addition to feeds or premixes and is considered quite stable (Sauberlich, 1985; Gadient, 1986), although it is easily destroyed by uv light when in solution. In feedstuffs, riboflavin exists primarily as the nucleotide coenzymes, flavin adenine dinucleotide (FAD) and flavin mononucleotide (FMN). Before riboflavin can be absorbed from the gut, FAD and FMN must be hydrolyzed by phosphatases present in the intestinal brush border (Akiyama et al., 1982). Absorption then proceeds throughout the entire small intestine via an active but saturable transport system involving phosphorylation of free riboflavin. The enzyme (flavokinase) which phosphorylates riboflavin is competitively inhibited by chlorpromazine, a compound in the phenothiazine category of antiemetic and antipsychotic drugs.

Riboflavin, even in crystalline form, is not completely absorbed from the gut when administered in the absence of food. Axelson and Gibaldi (1972) estimated that only 20% of a 1000 µg oral dose of crystalline riboflavin was absorbed by the rat. Excess riboflavin in the diet, moreover, may be absorbed less efficiently than lower levels (NRC, 1987). Absorption of riboflavin from the small intestine of ruminant animals has been estimated at about 35% (Miller et al., 1983a,b; Zinn et al., 1987).

Some foods, especially cereals, contain small amounts of riboflavin activity in covalent linkage with protein. The covalent linkage often exists as histidinyl or cysteinyl FAD, and these covalently bound flavins are poorly digested in the gut. Whether these covalently bound flavins exist in feed ingredients used in animal diets is not known, but it is likely that many cereal grains, already low in riboflavin, contain riboflavin in forms that are complexed with protein.

Animal studies dealing with riboflavin bioavailability in feeds or foods are limited. Chung and Baker (1990) performed growth assays with young chicks fed riboflavin-deficient purified (amino acid) diets as well as corn-soybean meal diets. Maximal growth occurred at a dietary riboflavin concentration of 1.8 mg/kg for the purified diet and 2.63 mg/kg for the corn-soybean meal diet. They estimated that riboflavin bioavailability in the corn-soybean meal diet was 59%. For purposes of either requirement or bioavailability assessment, knowledge of "total" riboflavin in the basal assay diet is essential. In the Chung and Baker (1990) report, microbiological assay of their corn-soybean meal diet yielded a value of 2.03 mg riboflavin/kg diet; fluorometric assay, however, gave an estimate of 1.23 mg riboflavin/kg. They suggested that riboflavin analysis done by microbiological assay was more valid than that done by fluorometric methodology.

It would seem reasonable that measurements of growth as well as erythrocyte glutathione reductase (EGR) activity might provide a good basis for estimating riboflavin bioavailability in feedstuffs. In both pigs (Frank *et al.*, 1988) and fish (Lovell, 1989), EGR has been reported to be a sensitive indicator of riboflavin status. Because ingredients such as zinc, iron, copper, ascorbic acid, tetracyclines, caffeine, theophylline, and tryptophan, have been reported to either chelate or form complexes with riboflavin (Jusko and Levy, 1975), their effects on riboflavin bioavailability should be assessed. Likewise, aflatoxin present in feedstuffs decreases riboflavin utilization (Hamilton *et al.*, 1974). Hence, aluminosilicates that bind aflatoxin may improve riboflavin utilization in diets contaminated with aflatoxin (Chung *et al.*, 1990). For humans, alcohol is also a factor of concern for riboflavin status, because ethanol inhibits enzymes required for conversion of FAD to riboflavin in the gut (Sauberlich, 1985).

C. Niacin

The term niacin is the generic descriptive term for pyridine 3-carboxylic acid and other derivatives delivering nicotinamide activity. Thus, pyridine 3-carboxylic acid itself is properly referred to as nicotinic acid (Anonymous, 1979). Nicotinic acid is a very stable compound when added to feed or premixes, being affected little by heat, light, oxygen, or moisture. It is absorbed from the small intestine by a carrier-mediated, N sodium-dependent process at low concentrations, but by passive diffusion at higher concentrations (Sauberlich, 1985). Nicotinamide absorption via simple diffusion occurs at twice the rate of that occurring with niacin (NRC, 1987). As a result, excessive ingestion of nicotinic acid is tolerated better than excess intakes of nicotinamide (Baker *et al.*, 1976). Much of the niacin activity present in feedstuffs exists as nicotinamide nucleotides, which release nicotinamide during the absorptive process. If free nicotinic acid is ingested, it is converted in the mucosa to nicotinamide via the nicotinamide dinucleotide pathway (Henderson and Gross, 1979).

Niacin activity can be purchased as either free nicotinic acid or free nicotinamide. Relative to nicotinic acid, nicotinamide has been observed to be roughly 125% bioavailable in delivering niacin bioactivity to chicks (Baker et al., 1976; Oduho and Baker, 1993); a value of 109% has been estimated for rats (Carter and Carpenter, 1982). Other work, however, has suggested nicotinic acid and nicotinamide to be equal in biopotency for chicks (Bao-Ji and Combs, 1986; Ruiz and Harms, 1988).

In plant-source feed ingredients, a substantial portion of the niacin is bound and therefore unavailable (Kodicek and Wilson, 1960; Luce et al., 1966, 1967; Darby et al., 1975; Yen et al., 1977; Carter and Carpenter, 1982). Ghosh et al. (1963) estimated that 85 to 90% of the niacin present in cereal grains and 40% in oilseeds is in a bound unavailable form. Alkaline hydrolysis is the primary means by which niacin can be effectively released from its bound state in these ingredients. Sweet corn, harvested at the milky stage, has its niacin in fully available forms (Carpenter et al., 1988). Meat and milk products contain essentially no bound niacin, but instead contain unbound forms of niacin, including free nicotinic acid and nicotinamide.

Assessment of nicotinic acid bioavailability in feeds and foods is complicated by the fact that, except in cats (NRC, 1986), mink (Warner et al., 1968), brook trout (Poston and DiLorenzo, 1973), and probably foxes, tryptophan serves as a precursor of nicotinic acid. Thus, all ingredients that contain pyridine forms of niacin also contain tryptophan. In nonruminant meat-producing animals, 50 mg of tryptophan yields roughly 1 mg of nicotinic acid (Baker et al., 1973; NRC, 1988; Czarnecki et al., 1983; Baker, 1986a). Thus, with a dietary niacin requirement in chicks of 20 mg/kg, 900 mg/kg of excess dietary tryptophan can eliminate the dietary need for niacin (Baker et al., 1973). Cats and probably other feline species (NRC, 1986) have a higher level of the enzyme picolinic acid carboxylase than other species that have been studied. This enzyme degrades a key intermediate (α-amino-β-muconic-ϵ-semialdehyde) in the tryptophan to niacin pathway, giving rise to picolinic acid instead of quinolinic acid. Thus, the niacin yield from tryptophan in felids is very low. Because ducks have a three- to four-fold higher level of picolinic acid carboxylase than chickens (Hoffmann-LaRoche, 1989), ducks may be less efficient than chickens in converting tryptophan to niacin.

It has been proposed that the leucine present in corn-soybean meal diets antagonizes tryptophan or niacin, or impairs the metabolic conversion of tryptophan to niacin. This subject has been controversial for some time (Anonymous, 1986; Cook and Carpenter, 1987; Lowry and Baker, 1989). It appears that pellagra is associated with tryptophan/niacin deficiency and not with excess ingestion of leucine. Soybean meal is rich in tryptophan and, because growing chicks and poults are fed diets containing high levels of soybean meal, the excess tryptophan therein contributes significantly to the niacin requirement. Thus, it is often difficult to show growth responses to niacin when it is added to conventional corn-soybean meal poultry diets.

Recent evidence has shown that iron deficiency in chicks impairs the efficacy of tryptophan as a niacin precursor (Oduho et al., 1994). Iron is a required cofactor for two enzymes in the pathway leading to nicotinic acid mononucleotide synthesis from tryptophan. Using purified diets that were just adequate in tryptophan but severely deficient in niacin, Oduho et al. (1994) demonstrated that 63 mg tryptophan were required to yield 1 mg of niacin for chicks fed iron-deficient diets (10 ppm iron), whereas chicks fed iron-adequate diets (40 ppm iron) converted tryptophan to niacin far more efficiently (42:1, wt/wt). Oduho and Baker (1993) also found that nicotinamide adenine dinucleotide (NAD) was fully effective as a niacin precursor, while nicotinamide was 124% active relative to nicotinic acid as a precursor for NAD biosynthesis.

To precisely determine bioavailable niacin activity, free of the niacin activity furnished by tryptophan, one must carefully control a number of dietary variables (Baker, 1986a). Minimal prerequisites involve knowing precisely the tryptophan requirement for maximal growth of noncoprophagic animals fed a diet with excess nicotinic acid. With this information, one can then supplement a niacin-free diet (containing tryptophan at its minimal requirement for tryptophan per se) with graded levels of nicotinic acid (the standard) or tryptophan to produce linear growth responses. Slope ratio analysis would give a value for the efficiency of tryptophan as a nicotinic acid precursor. Knowing this, together with the precise levels of bioavailable tryptophan present in the feed ingredients under study, one can use slope ratio bioassays to predict niacin bioavailability freed of the tryptophan contribution. Hence, the growth contribution provided from the bioavailable tryptophan would need to be subtracted from the total growth response in order to obtain a (corrected) growth response from niacin per se. Even if all these steps are taken, however, one would still need to be concerned with whether the dependent response variable (e.g., growth) was affected only by the niacin and tryptophan furnished by the supplemented feed ingredient. Often, addition of feed ingredients to purified niacin-free diets (e.g., a chemically defined crystalline amino acid diet) will alter food intake and/or growth responses, and such responses may be unrelated to the niacin/tryptophan provided by the feed ingredient in question. Hence, accurate assessment of (tryptophan-free) niacin bioavailability is extremely difficult to accomplish and, in fact, probably never has been done.

Although ruminant animals have long been considered as having more than enough microbial B-vitamin synthesis in the rumen to meet physiological requirements (Hungate, 1966), in certain instances exogenous nicotinic acid has elicited responses in cattle (Brent and Bartley, 1984). Milk production in dairy cattle often is increased when 6 to 12 g nicotinic acid or nicotinamide is fed daily during early lactation (Jaster, 1988). Supplemental niacin is thought to exert effects on carbohydrate and lipid metabolism and thereby to decrease the incidence of ketosis (Waterman et al., 1972, Jaster et al., 1983a,b). Added niacin may enhance microbial protein synthesis and increase propionate production (Riddel et al., 1980, 1981). Although research results with niacin for cattle have not shown consistent benefits, supplemental niacin may prove useful in dairy herds with a high incidence of ketosis or in situations in which cows are excessively fat (NRC, 1989a).

D.   Pantothenic Acid (PA)

This B-vitamin consists of pantoic acid joined to ß-alanine by an amide bond. It is generally sold in crystalline form as either D- or DL-calcium PA, and only the D-isomer has bioactivity (Rosenberg, 1942; Staten et al., 1980). Thus, 1 g of D-calcium PA = .92 g of PA bioactivity. Crystalline PA is relatively stable to heat, oxygen, and light, but it loses activity rapidly when exposed to heat in the presence of moisture. Racemic calcium PA is known to have hygroscopic and electrostatic properties that contribute to handling problems. Through complexing procedures, several manufactures now produce free-flowing, nonhygroscopic D-calcium PA for the feed industry (Hoffman-LaRoche, 1989).

Most of the PA found in feed ingredients is contained in coenzyme A (CoA), acyl CoA synthetase, and acyl carrier protein. Because CoA contains peptide linkages and a free SH group, it seems possible that exposure of foods or feeds containing CoA to an acid or alkaline environment might decrease PA bioavailability. During digestion, PA is released from coenzyme forms of the vitamin and then absorbed into portal blood and transported to tissue cells where it is used for resynthesis of Co-A and its acyl derivatives.

Pantothenic acid is abundant in most feed ingredients, particularly animal by-products, whole grain cereals, and legumes. Thus, practical-type diets for animals contain plethoric levels of total PA. Soybean meal is particularly rich in PA. Southern and Baker (1981) estimated that the PA present in both corn and dehulled soybean meal was 100% bioavailable to chicks relative to crystalline D-PA. The bioavailability of PA in barley, wheat, and sorghum, however, was estimated to be only 60% available based upon chick growth bioassays. Sauberlich (1985) estimated that PA in the typical adult American diet was only 50% bioavailable. Nonetheless, a clinically recognized PA deficiency has never been described for the human, indicative of the plentiful PA supply in most human foods. Excess PA is excreted in the urine (Fox, 1984). Urinary excretion of PA should be evaluated as a means of assessing PA status and/or bioavailability of PA in foods and feeds.

E. Vitamin B_{12}

Plant foodstuffs are devoid of B_{12}. Microorganisms are the sole source of B_{12} in nature and this accounts for the B_{12} activity in animal and fermentation by-products (Seetharam and Alpers, 1982). Cyanocobalamin (i.e., synthetic B_{12}) is available in crystalline form where 1 USP unit is considered equivalent to 1 ug of the vitamin. During the isolation of fermentation-derived crystalline B_{12}, the cyano group is attached to cobalt. This group must be removed by the body before cobalamin can be converted into its active form. In animal and fermentation-based feedstuffs, B_{12} exists bound to protein in the methyl form (methylcobalamin) or the 5'-deoxyadenosyl form (adenosylcobalamin). Crystalline cyanocobalamin is considered very stable when stored in feeds and premixes (Gadient, 1986).

Receptor sites for B_{12} absorption are located in the ileum. Prior to absorption, cobalamin is bound to a glycoprotein, commonly referred to as the intrinsic factor. Intrinsic factor is derived from the parietal cells of gastric mucosa. Some of the ingested cobalamin, however, is bound by R proteins derived from the mouth (salivary glands) and the stomach. The R proteins are largely degraded by pancreatic proteases in the gut lumen, but intrinsic factor is protease insensitive. In pancreatic insufficiency, cobalamin cannot be released from the R proteins for subsequent binding by intrinsic factor. Hence, animals or humans lacking intrinsic factor or with pancreatic disorders are subject to B_{12} absorption problems. Pernicious anemia in humans generally is characterized by a deficiency in the production of intrinsic factor. This condition drastically reduces the bioavailability of dietary vitamin B_{12}.

As the cobalamin-intrinsic factor complex crosses the ileal mucosa, intrinsic factor is released, and the cobalamin is transferred to a plasma-transport protein, transcobalamin II. Other cobalamin-binding proteins exist in plasma and liver. Transcobalamin I, for example, is the form in which B_{12} is stored in the liver. In blood, B_{12} exists primarily as methylcobalamin, while in liver it exists mainly as 5'-deoxyadenosyl cobalamin. Little is known about the bioavailability of orally ingested B_{12} in these forms in products like processed blood and meat meals.

Vitamin B_{12} is stored effectively in the body, principally in the liver (Ellenbogen, 1984). Tissue storage resulting from excess B_{12} ingestion in humans (and from biosynthesis in the large intestine) delays development of B_{12} deficiency signs for many months after a diet devoid of B_{12} is initiated. Signs of folate deficiency almost always accompany B_{12} deficiency because B_{12} is required for folate metabolism. Lack of either folate or B_{12}, therefore, prevents proper transfer of methyl groups in the synthesis of thymidine. This, in turn, produces a defect in DNA synthesis. Adequate quantities of B_{12} are synthesized in the rumen of ruminant animals provided that adequate cobalt is present in the diet. Many B_{12} analogs are also synthesized, however, some of which may antagonize the action of B_{12} (Elliot, 1980).

Methodology for determining vitamin B_{12} bioavailability in foods has not been established. Difficulty in producing B_{12} deficiency in experimental animals is a real problem in establishing a bioavailability assay system. If a deficiency could be produced, growth rate or urinary excretion of methylmalonic acid might be used as criteria for assessment of B_{12} bioavailability. In B_{12} deficiency, propionate conversion to succinate decreases, and this results in excretion of methylmalonate in the urine (NRC, 1987).

F. Choline

In animal nutrition, choline remains in the B-vitamin category, even though the quantity required far exceeds the "trace organic nutrient" definition of a vitamin. Choline is absorbed primarily in the small intestine and is required by the body for (a) phospholipid synthesis, (b) acetyl choline formation, and (c) transmethylation of homocysteine to methionine. When a choline deficit is produced experimentally by feeding a choline-free diet to chicks, functions a and/or b seem to have priority over c in that betaine (the methylated product of choline oxidation) does not elicit a growth response, whereas choline does. When about two-thirds of the dietary choline needed for maximal growth is supplied (as choline), then synthetic choline and betaine are equally efficacious (Lowry et al., 1987).

In mammals, the dietary need for choline can be eliminated by surfeit ingestion of methionine. Three methyl groups from methionine (S-adenosylmethionine) are transferred to phosphatidyl ethanolamine, thereby facilitating choline biosynthesis. In avians, however, methylation of phosphatidyl ethanolamine is limited such that excess methionine has minimal choline-sparing capacity (DuVigneaud et al., 1940; Jukes et al., 1945; Baker et al., 1983; Czarnecki et al., 1983). Moreover, excess levels of dietary protein markedly increase the bird's dietary need for choline (Molitoris and Baker, 1976a; Ketola and Nesheim, 1974), no doubt a reflection of the drain on the methyl pool resulting from increased uric acid excretion.

Both choline (e.g., choline chloride) and betaine are available for supplementation of animal diets. Poultry fed practical-type corn-soybean based diets respond equally to either compound, but Lowry et al. (1987) have suggested that purified diets require preformed choline to satisfy at least two-thirds of the total need for choline/betaine. After the need for choline per se (phospholipid and/or acetyl choline formation) has been satisfied, choline and betaine appear to be interchangeable in meeting the remainder of the requirement (i.e., for transmethylation purposes).

In its crystalline form, choline chloride (87% choline) is hygroscopic, and therefore is considered a stress agent to other vitamins in a vitamin-mineral premix.

Choline itself, however, is quite stable in premixes and feeds. Feed ingredients and crude unprocessed fat sources contain most of the choline as phospholipid-bound phosphatidyl choline. The bioavailability of choline in this form is not known, although early work with expeller (high fat) vs solvent-extracted (low fat) soybean meal would suggest that the former is richer in bioavailable choline than the latter (Berry et al., 1943). This implies that phospholipid-bound choline is at least partially available. Refined plant oils generally have been subjected to alkaline treatment and bleaching, and these processes almost totally remove the phospholipid-bound choline (Reiners and Gooding, 1975; Anderson et al., 1979).

Like niacin, for which tryptophan serves as a precursor, choline deficiency is difficult to produce in mammals consuming diets with excess methionine. Because all common feed ingredients would supply both choline and methionine, it is difficult if not impossible to separate responses from one or the other. Hence, choline bioavailability assessment is difficult in mammals. Use of the transmethylation inhibitors, ethionine or 2-amino-2-methyl-1-propanol, might prove useful in this endeavor (Molitoris and Baker, 1976b; Anderson et al., 1979; Lowry and Baker, 1987; Lowry et al., 1987).

For chick growth and relative to crystalline choline chloride, the choline present in soybean meal has been estimated to be as low as 60 to 75% bioavailable by Molitoris and Baker (1976b) but as high as 85 to 90% bioavailable by Fritz et al. (1967). March and MacMillan (1980) presented evidence that choline bioavailability in rapeseed meal is lower than that in soybean meal. In their work with chicks, production of trimethylamine (resulting from bacterial degradation of choline) in the intestine was greater in chicks fed rapeseed meal than in those fed soybean meal. Concerning betaine, its bioavailability in products like sugar beets and wheat is not known.

Conventional corn-soybean meal swine grower diets generally do not respond to choline supplementation (NCR-42, 1980) but broiler chick diets, despite being higher in choline-rich soybean meal, generally do respond (Lowry et al., 1987). Minimizing liver lipid, and in the case of birds, minimizing perosis, may require higher dietary levels of choline than are required to maximize rate and efficiency of weight gain (Anderson et al., 1979). Swine pregnancy has been shown to benefit from choline addition to corn-soybean meal diets (NCR-42, 1976; Stockland and Blaylock, 1974). In cattle and sheep, orally ingested choline is rapidly degraded in the rumen, but rumen microbes synthesize choline. That microbial choline synthesis may be inadequate to support a high level of milk production is indicated by the work of Sharma and Erdman (1989) who reported milk-yield responses in Holstein cows receiving 30 to 50 g/day of choline via abomasal infusion. Part of the postruminal responses observed for methionine may result from methionine-methyl serving as a precursor for choline biosynthesis.

G. Biotin

Commercial D-biotin is a sulfur-containing imidazole derivative that has no specific unit of activity. Thus, 1 g of D-biotin = 1 g of activity. Much of the biotin in feed ingredients exists in a bound form, ϵ-N-biotinyl-L-lysine (biocytin) which is a component of protein. While crystalline biotin appears to be absorbed well from the small intestine, the bioavailability of biotin in biocytin varies widely and is dependent on the digestibility of the proteins in which it is found. A large portion of the biotin requirement of humans and most animals comes from bacterial synthesis in the gut. Human balance studies have shown that urinary excretion often exceeds biotin intake, while fecal excretion of biotin often is five times greater than biotin intake.

Pelleting or heat has little effect on biotin activity in feeds, but oxidative rancidity severely reduces biotin bioavailability. Avidin, a glycoprotein found in egg albumen, binds biotin and renders it totally unavailable. Proper heat treatment of egg white will denature avidin and prevent it from binding biotin. Commercially available spray-dried egg white has not undergone sufficient heat treatment to totally denature the avidin therein. Additional heat treatment has been shown to markedly improve the growth-promoting efficacy of this product for dogs, partly because of avidin destruction and partly due to destruction of protease inhibitors (Rudnick and Czarnecki-Maulden, 1988).

Tabulated estimates of biotin bioavailability in feedstuffs are shown in Table I. Among the cereal grains, bioavailability of biotin in corn is high (100%) while that in wheat, barley, triticale, and sorghum is only about 50% (Anderson and Warnick 1970; Frigg, 1976; Anderson et al., 1978; Whitehead et al., 1982; Misir and Blair, 1988a,b). Bioavailable biotin concentrations of .11 mg/kg (corn), .08 mg/kg (barley), .09 mg/kg (sorghum) and .04 mg/kg (wheat) were estimated by Anderson et al. (1978). Feedstuff ingredient tables generally list the biotin concentration in soybean meal as .30 mg/kg. Buenrostro and Kratzer (1984) reported that biotin is 100% available in soybean meal and 86% available in meat and bone meal for laying hens. High bioavailabilities of biotin in soybean meal and lower availabilities in other oilseed meals also have been reported by Whitehead et al. (1982) and by Misir and Blair (1988a,b). Hence, with high amounts of bioavailable biotin present in corn-soybean meal diets, growing-finishing pigs generally do not respond to supplemental biotin (Easter et al., 1983). For growing pigs fed wheat-barley-soy diets, however, feed efficiency responses have been observed (Partridge and McDonald, 1990). With sows, Bryant et al. (1985a,b) have provided evidence that under some conditions supplemental biotin may improve conception rate, decrease the weaning-to-estrous interval, and improve both foot health and hair coat, particularly in advanced parities. More recently, Lewis et al. (1989) reported that adding .33 mg biotin/kg diet to a corn-soybean meal diet throughout gestation and lactation increased the number of pigs weaned but did not improve foot health. This result confirms an earlier study by Hamilton and Veum (1984) showing positive effects on numbers of pigs weaned from adding .55 mg biotin/kg to a corn-soybean meal diet during both gestation and lactation.

Biotin is a vitamin where an accurate test exists to assess the veracity of the bioavailability growth assay. Thus, growth responses to ingredients added to a biotin-free purified diet can be measured in the presence and absence of crystalline avidin. Anderson *et al.* (1978) observed that growth rate of biotin-depleted chicks was doubled by supplementation with 20% corn, but growth rate was not increased when the same quantity of corn was fed in the presence of 3.81 mg avidin/kg diet. Similar results occurred with barley. These results, therefore, provide convincing evidence that the growth responses observed from feed-grain supplementation of the biotin-free purified diet resulted from the available biotin *per se* furnished by the grains.

Buenrostro and Kratzer (1984) have suggested that the concentration of biotin in both plasma and egg yolk of laying hens may offer a means of assessing biotin bioavailability in feed ingredients. Subsequent work suggested that liver biotin content was a useful index of biotin status (Kratzer *et al.*, 1988, Misir and Blair, 1988a,b). Hepatic (Anderson *et al.*, 1978) and blood (Whitehead *et al.*, 1982) pyruvate carboxylase activity have also been used successfully to assess biotin bioavailability in feed ingredients.

In the study of Kratzer *et al.* (1988), biotin content of egg yolk was found not high enough to counteract the avidin present in egg white. Thus, most of the biotin present in egg yolk is bound to protein. The two biotin-binding proteins BBP-I and BBP-II are saturated with biotin and account for virtually all of the biotin present in egg yolk (White and Whitehead, 1987).

H. Vitamin B_6

This B vitamin consists of three closely related naturally occurring pyridine derivatives: pyridoxine, pyridoxal, and pyridoxamine. Each can exist in foods either in the free or the phosphorylated form. Plant products generally are rich in pyridoxine, whereas animal products contain primarily phosphorylated pyridoxal (Leklem, 1988). An additional form of B_6 occurs in plant-source feedstuffs, i.e., pyridoxine glucoside (Kabir *et al.*, 1983). This form of B_6 may account for up to 50% of the total vitamin B_6 content of oilseeds such as soybeans and sunflower seeds. The bioavailability of B_6 in pyridoxine glucoside is not known, although Trumbo *et al.* (1988) have presented clear evidence that this compound is poorly utilized as a source of B_6 activity for rats. The most common form of B_6 used for diet supplementation is pyridoxine hydrochloride.

Absorption of vitamin B_6 from the gut occurs via passive diffusion. Chick bioavailability work suggests that vitamin B_6 is about 40% bioavailable in corn and about 60% bioavailable in soybean meal (Yen et al., 1976). Moderate heat treatment (80 to 120°C) of corn enhanced B_6 bioavailability while greater heat treatment (160°C) decreased availability (Yen et al., 1976). Much of the vitamin B_6 activity in corn exists as pyridoxal and pyridoxamine, forms which are more heat labile than pyridoxine (Schroeder, 1971). Even with the reduced bioavailability of vitamin B_6 in commercial corn and soybean meal relative to crystalline pyridoxine·HC1, a surfeit of available B_6 is still present in practical-type diets for most animal species, thus precluding a response to supplemental vitamin B_6 if added to these diets (Easter et al., 1983).

Vitamin B_6 availability studies have been carried out with human foods using laboratory animal models (Sauberlich, 1985). Food processing procedures, such as canning, heating, and freezing, have been shown to decrease the bioavailability of vitamin B_6. Also, B_6 bioavailability in both sterilized evaporated milk and infant formulas is at or below 50% (Tomarelli et al., 1955; Hodson, 1956; Davies et al., 1959). In studies with young men based upon plasma pyridoxal phosphate level or urinary B_6 (i.e., 4-pyridoxic acid) excretion, B_6 bioavailability in the average American diet was estimated to be about 75% (Tarr et al., 1981). Fiber from wheat bran has been shown to have no adverse effects on B_6 bioavailability in rats (Hudson et al., 1988).

In premixes, vitamin B_6 can lose bioactivity, particularly when minerals in the form of carbonates or oxides are present (Verbeeck, 1975). High temperatures enhance loss of activity. Adams (1982) found 76% retention of B_6 activity after 3 months of storage at room temperature, but only 45% retention after 3 months of storage at 37°C. Loss of B_6 activity in pelleted complete feeds averages about 20% during 3 months of storage at room temperature (Gadient, 1986).

Several dietary factors can alter B_6 bioavailability. B_6 antagonists include linatine in linseed. This compound, however, seems to have a systemic effect on B_6 metabolism rather than having an effect on gut absorption of B_6 (Sauberlich, 1985). Also, pyridoxal and pyridoxal phosphate have a free aldehyde group that can react with amino groups present in the diet (i.e., free amino acids, ε-amino groups of lysine in proteins). Heat processing or cooking enhances these Maillard-type reactions and decreases vitamin B_6 bioavailability. Pyridoxallysine products have been reported to have between 0 and 50% B_6 bioavailability (Gregory, 1981).

Vitamin B_6 generally is not included in vitamin or vitamin-mineral premixes designed for supplementation of practical diets for swine and poultry. Cats, dogs, mink, and foxes, however, typically are fed diets higher in animal-source protein, and diets that also are more concentrated in crude protein. High protein intakes are known to increase the need for B_6 (NRC, 1987). Thus, conventional diets for cats, dogs, and carnivorous fur-bearing animals typically contain supplemental B_6.

I. Folic Acid

The term folacin is the accepted generic term for folic acid and related compounds exhibiting "folacin" activity. Chemically, folic acid consists of a pteridine ring, *para*-aminobenzoic acid (PABA), and glutamic acid. Animal cells cannot synthesize PABA, nor can they attach glutamic acid to pteroic acid (i.e., pteridine attached to PABA). Thus, folic acid must be supplied in the diet of nonruminant animals. The folacin present in feeds and foods exists largely as polyglutamates. In plants, folacin exists as a polyglutamate conjugate containing a γ-linked polypeptide chain of (primarily) seven glutamic acid residues. The normal gut proteases do not cleave the glutamate residues from this compound. Instead, a group of intestinal enzymes known as conjugases (folyl polyglutamate hydrolases) removes all but the last glutamate residue. Only the monoglutamyl form is thought to be absorbed into the enterocyte. Most of the folic acid taken up by the brush border is reduced to tetrahydrofolate (FH_4) and then methylated to N^5-methyl-FH_4, the predominant form of folate in blood plasma. The majority of the N^5-methyl-FH_4 in blood is bound to protein.

Like thiamin, folacin has a free amino group (on the pteridine ring), and this makes it very sensitive to losses in activity due to heat treatment, particularly if heat is applied to foods or feeds containing reducing sugars such as lactose or dextrose. Whether the free amino group of folacin (or thiamin) can bind to the free aldehyde moiety of pyridoxal or pyridoxalphosphate is not known. Adams (1982) reported only 38% retention of folacin activity when folic acid was stored for 3 weeks at 45°C in a mineral-free premix. At room temperature, 57% of original activity was present after 3 months of storage. Verbeeck (1975) observed even greater losses when minerals were included in the premix.

Bioavailability estimates are limited for the bound or polyglutamate forms of folacin found in foods. Generally, hematological responses, changes in blood folate levels or urinary folate excretion have been used to assess folate status in humans (Tamura and Stokstad, 1973). Growth assay estimation of folacin bioavailability in laboratory animals has not been done.

Intestinal conjugase inhibitors may be present in certain beans and pulses, and these may impede folacin absorption (Krumdieck *et al.*, 1973; Bailey, 1988). Fiber from a variety of foods extrinsically labeled with tritiated folate has been shown to exhibit only minor effects on hepatic [^{3}H]folate retention or on urinary tritium excretion in rats (Abad and Gregory, 1988).

Growing animals fed conventional corn-soybean meal diets generally do not respond to folacin supplementation. Hence, it is not generally provided at supplemental levels for such diets (Easter *et al.*, 1983). For gestating-lactating sows, however, some workers have observed an increase in live pigs farrowed as a result of folacin supplementation (Thaler, 1988, Lindemann and Kornegay, 1989), while others have observed no response (Pharazyn and Aherne, 1987). Matte *et al.* (1984) reported a response in live pig litter size at birth from 15 mg intramuscular injections at 2-week intervals during breeding and for the first 60 days of gestation.

J. Vitamin C (Ascorbic Acid)

Ascorbic acid is a water-soluble vitamin that is oxidized easily in air to dehydroascorbate. Both forms are physiologically active, but both are heat labile, particularly when heat is applied in the presence of trace metals such as copper, iron, or zinc. Compared to other water-soluble vitamins, large concentrations of ascorbate are present in both plant and animal tissues. Ascorbic acid can be synthesized in most animals. Exceptions include primates, guinea pigs, and most fishes. Fishes, both warm and cold-water and both fresh and saltwater species, lack the enzyme L-gulonolactone oxidase and thus cannot synthesize vitamin C (Tucker and Halver, 1984). Thus, ascorbic acid is of minimal concern in animal nutrition but of considerable concern in human and fish nutrition. Commercial vitamin C is available in several different forms, but only L-ascorbic acid has antiscorbutic properties for animals. Ascorbate-2-sulfate is utilized by trout and catfish and is apparently more stable than ascorbic acid (Lovell, 1989).

Intestinal absorption is an active process in species that require ascorbic acid in the diet but is passive in other species (Hornig *et al.*, 1973; Spenser *et al.*, 1963). Diets high in pectin, zinc, iron, or copper have been reported to decrease ascorbate absorption (Keltz *et al.*, 1978; Solomons and Viteri, 1982). Adams (1982) observed considerable losses of vitamin C activity in stored layer rations. Coating ascorbate with ethylcellulose appeared to minimize the loss of potency. Likewise, Hilton *et al.* (1977) found a 70% loss of supplemental ascorbic acid during (fish) feed preparation; virtually complete destruction occurred after 7 weeks of storage. Gadient (1986) noted that both pelleting and extruding can markedly reduce the bioactivity of supplemental ascorbate added to feeds and premixes. Losses due to oxidation are also well known, as ascorbic acid can be reversibly oxidized to dehydroascorbate (oxidized) which in turn can be irreversibly oxidized to diketogulonic acid. While both reduced and oxidized ascorbate retain scurvy-preventing vitamin C activity, diketogulonic acid has no activity. Because ascorbic acid serves as a reducing agent, it frequently is added at plethoric levels to purified vitamin premixes used in research in an attempt to prevent autooxidation of the other vitamins present therein.

III. FAT-SOLUBLE VITAMINS

A. Vitamin A

Vitamin A nomenclature policy dictates that the term "vitamin A" be used for all β-ionone derivatives, other than provitamin A carotenoids, that exhibit the biological activity of all-*trans* retinol (i.e., vitamin A alcohol or vitamin A_1). Esters of retinol should be referred to as retinyl esters. Vitamin A is present in animal tissues, eggs, and whole milk, while plant materials contain only provitamin A precursors that must be acted upon in the gut or by the liver to form retinol. Both natural vitamin A and synthetic retinol analogs are commonly referred to as retinoids.

Pepsin in the stomach and proteolytic enzymes, lipases, and esterases in the duodenum are required to release vitamin A and carotenoids from foods (Sauberlich, 1985). The resulting retinol and carotenoids pass into the mucosal cells where most of the carotenoids are cleaved by 15,15'-carotenoid dioxygenase to retinaldehyde. Retinaldehyde is then reduced by retinaldehyde reductase to retinol. The retinol is esterified, incorporated into chylomicrons, and then transported to the liver. Carotenoids not cleaved in the small intestine are absorbed as such in association with chylomicrons. β-Carotene and other carotenoids are not efficiently metabolized to retinol in the gut. Thus, on a weight basis, preformed vitamin A has considerably more retinol bioactivity than vitamin A precursors. Potency of β-carotene relative to vitamin A is dependent on a number of factors: level of supplementation, previous nutritional history, the mixture of carotenoid isomers present, digestibility of the diet, presence of antioxidants, and protein as well as fat content of the diet (Ullrey, 1972). While the absorption efficiency of vitamin A is relatively constant over a wide range of doses (Olson, 1984), higher doses of carotenoids are absorbed much less efficiently than lower doses (Erdman *et al.*, 1988). A minimal level of dietary fat is required for gut absorption of both vitamin A and carotenoids.

Based upon rat data, 1 IU of vitamin A = .3 μg crystalline vitamin A alcohol (retinol), .344 μg vitamin A acetate, or .55 μg vitamin A palmitate. Retinol equivalent (RE) is the new nomenclature used to describe vitamin activity in foods and feeds. One RE is defined as 1 mg of all-*trans* retinol, 6 mg of all-trans-β-carotene or 12 mg of other vitamin A-active carotenoids. Thus, 1 RE = 3.3 IU of vitamin A. Also, 1 mg β-carotene is considered equivalent to 1667 IU vitamin A activity for poultry (NRC, 1984a) but only 280 IU vitamin A activity for swine (NRC, 1988; Ullrey, 1972) and 400 IU for cattle and horses (NRC, 1989a,b). Feline species cannot convert β-carotene to vitamin A (NRC, 1986), and mink appear to be in the same category (NRC, 1982). Unlike these species, dogs can convert β-carotene to vitamin A with an estimated efficiency of 1 mg β-carotene = 833 IU vitamin A (NRC, 1985). Corn carotenoids for swine have been found to contain between 123 and 261 IU/mg vitamin A activity (relative to all-*trans*-retinyl palmitate) based upon Ullrey's 1972 calculations. Corn carotenoids consist of about 25% β-carotene (most active), 25% β-zeaecarotene (least active), and 50% cryptoxanthin (intermediate activity). Thus, if one assumes that swine are only 30% as efficient as rats in converting all-*trans*-β-carotene to vitamin A (Braude *et al.*, 1941), and given that corn carotenoids are less efficient precursors of vitamin A than β-carotene itself, Ullrey has calculated that only 15% of the analyzed corn carotenoids would be converted and stored as vitamin A in the liver. Pigs appear to be relatively inefficient in β-carotene absorption from the gut, and this may explain, in part, why vitamin A precursors are inefficient sources of vitamin A for swine.

Vitamin A esters are more stable in feeds and premixes than retinol. The hydroxyl group as well as the four double bonds on the retinol side chain are subject to oxidative losses. Thus, esterification of vitamin A alcohol does not totally protect this vitamin from oxidative losses. Current commercial sources of vitamin A are generally "coated" esters of acetate (1 IU = .344 μg) or palmitate (1 IU = .549 μg) that contain an added antioxidant such as ethoxyquin or butylated hydroxytoluene.

Mosisture in premixes and feedstuffs has a negative effect on vitamin A stability. Water causes vitamin A beadlets to soften and become more permeable to oxygen (Schneider, 1986). Thus, both high humidity and the presence of free choline chloride (hygroscopic) enhance vitamin A destruction. Trace minerals also exacerbate vitamin A losses in premixes exposed to moisture. For maximal retention of vitamin A activity, premixes should be as moisture free as possible and have a pH above 5. Low pH causes isomerization of all-*trans* vitamin A to less potent *cis* forms and also results in deesterification of vitamin A esters to more labile retinol (De Ritter, 1976). Heat processing, especially extrusion, likewise can reduce vitamin A bioavailability (Harper, 1988).

Crystalline β-carotene is absorbed from the gut more efficiently than the ß-carotene existing in foods and feeds. Rao and Rao (1970), for example, found that the β-carotene present in carrots, papayas, and a mixed vegetable was absorbed by humans at 36, 46, and 33% of the efficiency of crystalline β-carotene. Also, proper cooking impacts β-carotene absorption. Rodriquez and Irwin (1972) reported that only 1% of the β-carotene was absorbed from raw carrots, while mild cooking enhanced the absorption efficiency dramatically. Some of the carotenoids in vegetable products are complexed with protein, and mild cooking apparently releases some of the β-carotene from these complexes (Erdman *et al.*, 1988). Overcooking, however, may have the opposite effect, i.e., carotenoid bioavailability may be reduced. This may be due to conversion of all-*trans*-β-carotene to the *cis*-β-carotene isomers during heating. β-Carotene is also known to be rapidly destroyed by sunlight and air.

In terms of nutrient-nutrient interactions that may affect vitamin A bioavailability, zinc deficiency has been reported to reduce utilization of vitamin A by reducing alcohol dehydrogenase activity (Solomons and Russell, 1980), although Smith (1980) concluded that zinc deficiency does not alter vitamin A absorption. Synthetic antioxidants and vitamin E may protect the integrity of vitamin A in the gut, thereby enhancing bioavailability (Sauberlich, 1985). Arnich and Arthur (1980) found that vitamin E deficiency reduced vitamin A utilization, but excess vitamin E was no more beneficial than an adequate level. Inadequate protein ingestion has been associated with reduced absorption of vitamin A (Weber, 1983), and fiber ingestion, especially pectin, has been shown to reduce the efficacy of a crystalline β-carotene supplement (Erdman et al., 1986; Anonymous, 1987). The mycotoxins, aflatoxin and ochratoxin, have also been reported to decrease the absorption of carotenoids (Tung and Hamilton, 1973; Huff and Hamilton, 1975). In forages, carotene in alfalfa hay may be more bioavailable than that in grass hay (NRC, 1989b). Also, ensiling has been reported to preserve β-carotene, but its bioavailability may be low (NRC, 1984b).

Quantification of vitamin A bioavailability is difficult. Accumulation of vitamin A in the liver may be the most acceptable method (Erdman et al., 1988; Chung et al., 1990). In the report of Erdman et al. (1986), neither growth rate nor serum vitamin A was observed to be a definitive measurement of the effectiveness of β-carotene as a source of vitamin A for chicks.

B. Vitamin D

Vitamin D is composed of a group of sterol compounds that occur in nature primarily in animal products. The D vitamins are produced from the provitamins ergosterol in plants and 7-dehydrocholesterol in animals. Ultraviolet radiation spontaneously cleaves the β ring of these sterols to form ergocalciferol (vitamin D_2) from ergosterol in plants and cholecalciferol (vitamin D_3) from 7-dehydrocholesterol in animals. In practice, the term vitamin D is appropriate for all steroids having cholecalciferol biological activity. Commercially, most vitamin D is available as a crystalline spray-dried cholecalciferol, 1 IU being equivalent to .025 μg of cholecalciferol.

Vitamin D is efficiently absorbed along with fat from the upper small intestine. Fat malabsorption problems due to pancreatic insufficiency or a lack of bile salt production will decrease the efficiency of vitamin D absorption.

Vitamin D_2 is utilized poorly by poultry (NRC, 1984a). Thus, vitamin D requirements for avian species generally are expressed as International Chick Units (ICU) where 1 ICU = .025 μg of vitamin D_3. Other species appear capable of utilizing D_2 as well as D_3, although at least one report has suggested that D_3 is more bioactive than D_2 for swine also (Horst *et al.*, 1982). Studies in grazing sheep confirm that ultraviolet irradiation is as effective as vitamin D_3 addition to the diet insofar as effecting significant increases in plasma D_3 and 25-hydroxy D_3 concentrations. In fact, shorn sheep exposed for 10 hr daily to uv sunlight (provided by sunlamps) had higher levels of both D_3 and 25-OH D_3 in their plasma than those not exposed to uv sunlight but instead fed 50 mg µg/day of vitamin D_3 (Hidiroglou and Karpinski, 1989). This suggests that utilization of oral D_3 by sheep is not 100% efficient relative to that synthesized in the skin from 7-dehydrocholesterol. This is probably due to ruminal degradation of vitamin D (Sommerfeldt *et al.*, 1983). Both synthetic D_2 and D_3 are quite stable when stored as the vitamin product itself at room temperature. In complete feeds and mineral-vitamin premixes, Schneider (1986) reported activity losses of 10 to 30% after either 4 or 6 months of storage at 22°C. Human foods, nonetheless, have been suggested as retaining most of their vitamin D potency after cooking, storage, or processing (Sauberlich, 1985).

C. Vitamin E

Vitamin E is the generic term for all tocol and tocotrienol derivatives having α-tocopherol biological activity. There are eight naturally occurring forms of vitamin E: α-, β-, γ-, and σ-tocopherols and α-, β-, γ-, and σ-tocotrienols. Among these, D-α-tocopherol possesses the greatest biological activity (Bieri and McKenna, 1981). One IU of vitamin E is the activity of 1 mg of DL-α-tocopheryl acetate. All-*rac* or DL-α-tocopherol has about 70% of the activity of pure D-α-tocopherol. Bieri and McKenna (1981) consider β-tocopherol and γ-tocopherol to have only 40 and 10% of the activity, respectively, of α-tocopherol (set at 100%). The only other natural form to possess activity is α-tocotrienol, which on the rating scale used above was listed by Bieri and McKenna (1981) as containing a biopotency of 25%. For purposes of diet supplementation, DL-α-tocopheryl acetate is the form commonly used.

Based principally on rat bioassay work (rat antisterility assay) and using DL-α-tocopheryl acetate as a standard (1 mg = 1 IU), 1 mg DL-α-tocopherol = 1.1 IU, 1 mg D-α-tocopheryl acetate = 1.36 IU, and 1 mg D-α-tocopherol = 1.49 IU. Recent work with beef cows involving blood and tissue increases in tocopherol upon feeding 1000 IU daily of various vitamin E supplements resulted in the following estimates of vitamin E potency: DL-α-tocopheryl acetate, 1 IU/mg; DL-α-tocopherol, 1.37 IU/mg; D-α-tocopheryl acetate, 2.58 IU/mg; D-α-tocopherol, 3.60 IU/mg (Hidiroglou *et al.*, 1988). These results are more in line with human results (Horwitt *et al.*, 1984) than with rodent values. This suggests that incomplete hydrolysis of the acetate may limit its complete utilization (Baker *et al.*, 1980). Also, it is apparent that D-α-tocopherol as well as D-α-tocopheryl acetate are considerably more bioactive as vitamin E supplements than the L-epimer. Astrup *et al.* (1974) have provided evidence that, unlike vitamins A and D, vitamin E is not metabolized to any great extent in the rumen.

Plant-source ingredients are richer in vitamin E bioactivity than animal-source feed ingredients. Plant oils are particularly rich in bioactive vitamin E, although corn and corn oil contain about six times more γ-tocol than α-tocol (Ullrey, 1981). Solvent-extracted soybean meal has very little vitamin E activity.

Vitamin E is subject to destruction by oxidation, and this process is accelerated by heat, moisture, unsaturated fat, and trace minerals. Losses of 50 to 70% occur in alfalfa hay stored at 32°C for 12 weeks; losses up to 30% have been known to occur during dehydration of alfalfa (Livingston *et al.*, 1968). Diets for cats, dogs and commercial fur-bearing animals that are rich in polyunsaturated fatty acids (e.g., fish or fish oil) generally are overfortified with vitamin E to guard against oxidative losses of vitamin E potency (NRC, 1986). In fermented grains, all vitamin E presumably is destroyed. Treatment of high-moisture grains with organic acids also greatly enhances vitamin E destruction (Young *et al.*, 1975; 1977; 1978). Even mildly alkaline conditions of vitamin E storage, however, are also very detrimental to vitamin E stability (Schneider, 1986). Thus, finely ground limestone or MgO coming in direct contact with vitamin E markedly reduces bioavailability.

D. Vitamin K

This fat-soluble vitamin exists in three series: phylloquinones (K_1) in plants, menaquinones (K_2) formed by microbial fermentation, and menadiones (K_3) which are synthetic. All three forms of vitamin K are biologically active. In metabolism, vitamin K functions in specific carboxylation reactions in which glutamyl residues of proteins are γ-carboxylated, thereby converting precursors of specific proteins to biologically active forms. Unlike the other fat-soluble vitamins, vitamin K has a rapid turnover rate in the body. As the γ-carboxylated proteins are degraded, γ-carboxyglutamic acid is released and quantitatively excreted in the urine. Liver stores of vitamin K can be depleted very rapidly during even short periods of vitamin K-deficient diet consumption (Kindberg and Suttie, 1989).

Water-soluble forms of menadione are used, primarily, to supplement animal diets. The commercially available forms of K_3 supplements are menadione sodium bisulfite (MSB), menadione sodium bisulfite complex (MSBC), and menadione dimethylpyridinol bisulfite (MPB). These contain 52, 33 and 45.5% menadione, respectively. Stability of these K_3 supplements in premixes and diets is impaired by moisture, choline chloride, trace elements, and alkaline conditions. Coelho (1991) suggests that either MSBC or MPB may lose almost 80% of bioactivity if stored for 3 months in a vitamin-trace mineral premix containing choline; losses in activity, however, are far less if stored in the same premix containing no choline. Coated K_3 supplements generally are more stable than uncoated supplements. Menadione pyridinol bisulfite is more bioactive than either MSB or MSBC for chicks (Griminger, 1965; Charles and Huston, 1972). Seerley *et al.* (1976) also found MPB effective for swine. Oduho *et al.* (1993) tested a new synthetic form of vitamin K: menadione nicotinamide bisulfite. It was found to be equal in potency to MPB for decreasing prothrombin time of chicks.

Although certain feed ingredients are known to be rich in vitamin K activity for swine, e.g., alfalfa meal (Fritschen, 1971), little quantitative information exists on the bioavailability of vitamin K in feedstuffs. Natural plant-source vitamin K_1 is virtually atoxic when ingested at high levels; also, menadione products are tolerated well when fed in excess, 1000 times the required level having no adverse effects (NRC, 1987).

Table I. Relative bioavailability of biotin in feedstuffs for poultry[a]

Source	RV	Standard	Response criterion	Meth cal	Type diet	Reference
Alfalfa meal	56	D–Biotin	Growth	SC	SP	Frigg (984)
Barley	20	D–Biotin	Growth	PL	SP	Frigg (1976)
Barley	53	D–Biotin	Growth	SC	AA	Anderson et al. (1978)
Barley	33	D–Biotin	Carbox	SC	AA	Anderson et al. (1978)
Barley	11	D–Biotin	Carbox	SC	N	Whitehead et al. (1982)
Barley	22	D–Biotin	Growth	SC	SP	Frigg (1984)
Barley	19	D–Biotin	Growth	SC	P	Misir and Blair (1988)
Canola meal	65	D–Biotin	Growth	SC	P	Misir and Blair (1988)
Canola meal	62	D–Biotin	Carbox	SC	N	Whitehead et al. (1982)
Corn	110	D–Biotin	Growth	SC	AA	Anderson et al. (1978)
Corn	97	D–Biotin	Carbox	SC	AA	Anderson et al. (1978)
Corn	133	D–Biotin	Carbox	SC	N	Whitehead et al. (1982)
Corn	107	D–Biotin	Growth	PL	SP	Frigg (1976)
Corn	75	D–Biotin	Yolk biotin	SC	SP	Buenrostro and Kratzer (1984)
Corn	125	D–Biotin	Pla biotin	SC	SP	Buenrostro and Kratzer (1984)
Corn	95	D–Biotin	Growth	SC	P	Misir and Blair (1988)
Grass meal	67	D–Biotin	Growth	SC	SP	Frigg (1984)
Milk, skim. dry	65	D–Biotin	Growth	SC	SP	Frigg (1984)
Milk, whey, dry	117	D–Biotin	Growth	SC	SP	Frigg (1984)

Table I. (continued)

Source	RV	Standard	Response criterion	Meth cal	Type diet	Reference
Molasses, beet	75	D-Biotin	Growth	SC	SP	Frigg (1984)
Oats	32	D-Biotin	Growth	PL	SP	Frigg (1984)
Oats	41	D-Biotin	Growth	SC	SP	Frigg (1984)
Peanut meal	53	D-Biotin	Growth	SC	SP	Frigg (1984)
Rice polishings	23	D-Biotin	Growth	SC	SP	Frigg (1984)
Rye	0	D-Biotin	Growth	SC	SP	Frigg (1984)
Safflower meal	32	D-Biotin	Carbox	SC	N	Whitehead et al. (1982)
Sorghum	20	D-Biotin	Growth	PL	SP	Frigg (1976)
Sorghum	38	D-Biotin	Growth	SC	AA	Anderson et al. (1978)
Sorghum	39	D-Biotin	Carbox	SC	AA	Anderson et al. (1978)
Sorghum	25	D-Biotin	Growth	SC	SP	Frigg (1984)
Sorghum	12	D-Biotin	Yolk biotin	SC	SP	Buenrostro and Kratzer (1984)
Sorghum	21	D-Biotin	Pla biotin	SC	SP	Buenrostro and Kratzer (1984)
Sorghum	30	D-Biotin	Growth	SC	P	Misir and Blair (1988)
Soybean meal	108	D-Biotin	Carbox	SC	N	Whitehead et al. (1982)
Soybean meal	100	D-Biotin	Yolk biotin	SC	SP	Buenrostro and Kratzer (1984)
Soybean meal	77	D-Biotin	Growth	SC	P	Misir and Blair (1988)
Sunflower meal	35	D-Biotin	Carbox	SC	N	Whitehead et al. (1982)
Sunflower meal	39	D-Biotin	Carbox	SC	SP	Frigg (1984)

Tapioca meal	6	D-Biotin	Growth	SC	SP	Frigg (1984)
Triticale	16	D-Biotin	Growth	SC	P	Misir and Blair (1988)
Wheat	0	D-Biotin	Growth	PL	SP	Frigg (1976)
Wheat	43	D-Biotin	Growth	SC	AA	Anderson *et al.* (1978)
Wheat	51	D-Biotin	Carbox	SC	AA	Anderson *et al.* (1978)
Wheat	5	D-Biotin	Carbox	SC	N	Whitehead *et al.* (1982)
Wheat	4	D-Biotin	Growth	SC	SP	Frigg (1984)
Wheat	0	D-Biotin	Yolk biotin	SC	SP	Buenrostro and Kratzer (1984)
Wheat	19	D-Biotin	Pla biotin	SC	SP	Buenrostro and Kratzer (1984)
Wheat	17	D-Biotin	Growth	SC	P	Misir and Blair (1988)
Wheat bran	18	D-Biotin	Growth	SC	SP	Frigg (1984)
Wheat germ	55	D-Biotin	Growth	SC	SP	Frigg (1984)
Wheat middlings	6	D-Biotin	Growth	SC	SP	Frigg (1984)

[a] Abbreviations can be found in Appendix 1.

REFERENCES

Abad, A. R. and J. F. Gregory. 1988. Assessment of folate bioavailability in the rat using extrinsic dietary enrichment with radiolabeled folates. *J. Agr. Food Chem.* **36**:97.

Adams, C. R. 1982. Vitamins--The life essentials. *In* "Proceedings of the NFIA Nutrition Institute." pp. 1-8.

Akiyama, T., J. Selhub and I. H. Rosenberg. 1982. FMN phosphatase and FAD pyrophosphatase in rat intestinal brush borders: Role in intestinal absorption of dietary riboflavin. *J. Nutr.* **112**:263.

Anderson, P. A., D. H. Baker and S. P. Mistry. 1978. Bioassay determination of the biotin content of corn, barley, sorghum and wheat. *J. Anim. Sci.* **47**:654.

Anderson, P. A., D. H. Baker, P. A. Sherry and J. E. Corbin. 1979. Choline-methionine interrelationship in feline nutrition. *J. Anim. Sci.* **49**:522.

Anderson, J. O. and R. E. Warnick. 1970. Studies of the need for supplemental biotin in chick rations. *Poult. Sci.* **49**:569.

Anonymous. 1979. Nomenclature Policy: Generic descriptors and trivial names for vitamins and related compounds. *J. Nutr.* **109**:8.

Anonymous. 1986. Pellagragenic effect of excess leucine. *Nutr. Rev.* **44**:26.

Anonymous. 1987. Dietary fiber reduces ß-carotene utilization. *Nutr. Rev.* **45**:350.

Arnich, L. and V. A. Arthur. 1980. Interactions of fat-soluble vitamins in hypervitaminoses. *Ann. N.Y. Acad. Sci.* **355**:109.

Astrup, H. M., S. C. Mills, L. G. Cook and T. W. Scott. 1974. Persistence of α-tocopherol in the post rumen. *Acta Vet. Scand.* **15**:454.

Axelson, J. E. and M. Gibaldi. 1972. Absorption and excretion of riboflavin in the rat - an unusual example of nonlinear pharmacokinetics. *J. Pharm. Sci.* **61**:404.

Bailey, L. B. 1988. Factors affecting folate bioavailability. *Food Technol.* **42**:206.

Baker, D. H. 1986a. Problems and pitfalls in animal experiments designed to establish dietary requirements for essential nutrients. *J. Nutr.* **116**:2339.

Baker, D. H. 1986b. Bioavailability of selected B-complex vitamins in feedstuffs. *In* "Proceedings of the BASF Technical Symposium." pp. 13-23.

Baker, D. H., N. K. Allen and A. J. Kleiss. 1973. Efficiency of tryptophan as a niacin precursor in the chick. *J. Anim. Sci.* **36**:299.

Baker, D. H., K. M. Halpin, G. L. Czarnecki and C. M. Parsons. 1983. The choline-methionine interrelationship for growth of the chick. *Poult. Sci.* **62**:133.

Baker, D. H., J. T. Yen, A. H. Jensen, R. G. Teeter, E. N. Michel and J. H. Burns. 1976. Niacin activity in niacinamide and coffee. *Nutr. Rep. Int.* **14**:115.

Baker, H. O., D. C. Angelis and S. Feingold. 1980. Plasma tocopherol in man at various times after ingesting free and acetylated tocopherol. *Nutr. Rep. Int.* **21**:531.

Bao-Ji, C. and G. F. Combs. 1986. Evaluation of biopotencies of nicotinamide and nicotinic acid for broiler chickens. *Poult. Sci.* **65**(Suppl. 1):24 [Abstract].

Bauchop, T. and L. King. 1968. Amprolium and thiamin pyrophospho-transferase. *Appl. Microbiol.* **16**:961.

Berry, E. P., C. W. Carrick, R. E. Roberts and S. M. Hauge. 1943. A deficiency of available choline in soybean oil and soybean oil meal. *Poult. Sci.* **22**:442.

Bieri, J. G. and M. C. McKenna. 1981. Expressing dietary values for fat-soluble vitamins: changes in concepts and terminology. *Am. J. Clin. Nutr.* **34**:289.

Braude, R., A. S. Foot, K. M. Henry, S. K. Kon, S. Y. Thompson and T. H. Mead. 1941. Vitamin A studies with rats and pigs. *Biochem. J.* **35**:693.

Brent, B. E. and E. E. Bartley. 1984. Thiamin and niacin in the rumen. *J. Anim. Sci.* **59**:813.

Bryant, K. L., E. T. Kornegay, J. W. Knight, H. P. Veit and D. R. Notter. 1985a. Supplemental biotin for swine. III. Influence of supplementation to corn-and-wheat-based diets on the incidence and severity of toe lesions, hair and skin characteristics and structural soundness of sows housed in confinement during four parities. *J. Anim. Sci.* **60**:154.

Bryant, K. L., E. T. Kornegay, J. W. Knight, K. E. Webb, Jr. and D. R. Notter, 1985b. Supplemental biotin for swine. I. Influence on feedlot performance, plasma biotin and toe lesions in developing gilts. *J. Anim. Sci.* **60**:136.

Buenrostro, J. L. and F. H. Kratzer. 1984. Use of plasma and egg yolk biotin of White Leghorn hens to assess biotin availability from feedstuffs. *Poult. Sci.* **63**:1563.

Carpenter, K. J., M. Schelstraete, V. C. Vilicich and J. S. Wall. 1988. Immature corn as a source of niacin. *J. Nutr.* **118**:165.

Carter, E. G. A. and K. J. Carpenter. 1982. The available niacin values of foods for rats and their relation to analytical values. *J. Nutr.* **112**:2091.

Charles, O. W. and T. M. Huston. 1972. The biological activity of vitamin K materials following storage and pelleting. *Poult. Sci.* **51**:1421.

Chung, T. K. and D. H. Baker. 1990. Riboflavin requirement of chicks fed purified amino acid and conventional corn-soybean meal diets. *Poult. Sci.* **69**:1357.

Chung, T. K., J. W. Erdman, Jr. and D. H. Baker. 1990. Hydrated sodium calcium aluminosilicate: effects on zinc, manganese, vitamin A and riboflavin utilization. *Poult. Sci.* **69**:1364.

Coelho, M. B. 1991. Vitamin stability. *Feed Management* **42**(10):24.

Cook, N. E. and K. J. Carpenter. 1987. Leucine excess and niacin status in rats. *J. Nutr.* **117**:519.

Czarnecki, G. L., K. M. Halpin and D. H. Baker. 1983. Precursor (amino acid):product (vitamin) interrelationship for growing chicks as illustrated by tryptophan-niacin and methionine-choline. *Poult. Sci.* **62**:371.

Darby, W. J., K. W. McNutt and N. E. Todhunter 1975. Niacin. *Nutr. Rev.* **33**:289.

Davies, M. K., M. E. Gregory and K. M. Henry. 1959. The effect of heat on the vitamin B_6 of milk. I. A Comparison of biological and microbiological tests of evaporated milk. *J. Dairy Res.* **26**:215.

DeRitter, E. 1976. Stability characteristics of vitamins in processed foods. *Food Technol.* **30**:48.

DuVigneaud, V., J. P. Chandler, M. Cohn and G. B. Brown. 1940. The transfer of the methyl group from methionine to choline and creatine. *J. Biol. Chem.* **134**:787.

Easter, R. A., P. A. Anderson, E. J. Michel and J. R. Corley. 1983. Response of gestating gilts and starter, grower and finisher swine to biotin, pyridoxine, folacin and thiamine additions to corn-soybean meal diets. *Nutr. Rept. Int.* **28**:945.

Ellenbogen, L. 1984. Vitamin B_{12}. *In* "Handbook of Vitamins" (L. J. Machlin, ed.). Marcel Dekker, New York.

Elliot, J. M. 1980. Propionate metabolism and vitamin B_{12}. *In* "Digestive Physiology and Metabolism in Ruminants" (Rukebuscin and Thioend, Eds.), pp. 485-530. AVI, Westport, CT.

Erdman, J. W. Jr., G. C. Fahey, Jr. and C. B. White. 1986. Effects of purified dietary fiber sources on ß-carotene utilization by the chick. *J. Nutr.* **116**:2415.

Erdman, J. W., C. L. Poor and J. M. Dietz. 1988. Processing and dietary effects on the bioavailability of vitamin A, carotenoids and vitamin E. *Food. Technol.* **42**:214.

Farrer, K. H. T. 1955. The thermal degradation of vitamin B-1 in foods. *Adv. Food. Res.* **6**:257.

Fox, H. M. 1984. Pantothenic acid. *In* "Handbook of Vitamins" (L. J. Machlin, Ed.), pp. 437-458. Marcel Dekker, New York.

Frank, G. R., J. M. Bahr and R. A. Easter. 1988. Riboflavin requirement of lactating swine. *J. Anim. Sci.* **66**:47.

Frigg, M. 1976. Bio-availability of biotin in cereals. *Poult. Sci.* **55**:2310.

Frigg, M. 1984. Available biotin content of various feed ingredients. *Poult. Sci.* **63**:750.

Fritschen, R. D., O. D. Grace and E. R. Peo. 1971. *In* "Nebraska Swine Report," Publ. 1 EC 71, **219**:22

Fritz, J. C., T. Roberts and J. W. Boehne. 1967. The chick's response to choline and its application to an assay for choline in feedstuffs. *Poult. Sci.* **46**:1447.

Gadient, M. 1986. Effect of pelleting on nutritional quality of feed. *In* "Proceedings of the Maryland Nutrition Conference." pp. 73-79.

Ghosh, H. P., P. K. Sarkar and B. C. Guha. 1963. Distribution of the bound form of nicotinic acid in natural materials. *J. Nutr.* **79**:451.

Goetsch, A. L. and F. N. Owens. 1987. Influence of supplemental sulfate (Dynamate) and thiamin HCl on passage of thiamin to the duodenum and site of digestion in steers. *Arch. Anim. Nutr.* **37**:1075.

Gregory, J. F. III and J. R. Kirk. 1981. The bioavailability of vitamin B_6 in foods. *Nutr. Rev.* **39**:1.

Griminger, P. 1965. Relative vitamin K potency of two water-soluble menadione analogues. *Poult. Sci.* **44**:210.

Hamilton, C. R. and T. L. Veum. 1984. Response of sows and litters to added dietary biotin in environmentally regulated facilities. *J. Anim. Sci.* **59**:151.

Hamilton, P. B., H. T. Tung, R. D. Wyatt and W. E. Donaldson. 1974. Interaction of dietary aflatoxin with some vitamin deficiences. *Poult. Sci.* **53**:871-877.

Harper, J. M. 1988. Effect of extrusion processing on nutrients. *In* "Nutritional Evaluation of Food Processing " (E. Karmas and R. S. Harris, Eds.), 3rd ed. Van Nostrand-Reinhold, New York.

Hawkins, D. R. 1968. Treatment of schizophrenia based on the medical model. *J. Schiz.* **2**:3.

Henderson, L. M. and C. J. Gross. 1979. Metabolism of niacin and niacinamide in perfused rat intestine. *J. Nutr.* **109**:654.

Hidiroglou, M. and K. Karpinski. 1989. Providing vitamin D to confined sheep by oral supplementation vs. ultraviolet irradiation. *J. Anim. Sci.* **67**:794.

Hidiroglou, N., L. F. Laflamme and L. R. McDowell. 1988. Blood plasma and tissue concentrations of vitamin E in beef cattle as influenced by supplementation of various tocopherol compounds. *J. Anim. Sci.* **66**:3227.

Hilker, D. M. and J. C. Somogy. 1982. Antithiamins of plant origin: their chemical nature and mode of action. *Ann. N. Y. Acad. Sci.* **378**:137.

Hilton, J. W., C. Y. Cho and S. J. Slinger. 1977. Factors affecting the stability of supplemental ascorbic acid in practical trout diets. *J. Fish Res. Board. Can.* **34**:683.

Hodson, A. Z. 1956. Vitamin B_6 in sterilized milk and other milk products. *J. Agric. Food Chem.* **4**:876.

Hoffman-LaRoche. 1989. "Vitamin Nutrition of Poultry," pp. 1-118.

Hornig, D., F. Weber and O. Wiss. 1973. Site of intestinal absorption of ascorbic acid in guinea pigs and rats. *Biochem. Biophys. Res. Commun.* **52**:168.

Horst, R. L., J. L. Napoli and E. T. Littledike. 1982. Discrimination in the metabolism of orally dosed ergocalciferol and cholecalciferol by the pig, rat, and chick. *Biochem. J.* **204**:185.

Howard, L., C. Wagne, and S. Schenker. 1974. Malabsorption of thiamin in folate-deficient rats. *J. Nutr.* **104**:1024.

Horwit, M., W. H. Elliot, P. Kanjananggulpan and C. D. Fetch. 1984. Serum concentration of α-tocopherol after ingestion of various vitamin E preparations. *Am. J. Clin. Nutr.* **40**:240.

Hudson, C. A., A. A. Betschart and S. M. Oace. 1988. Bioavailability of vitamin B_6 from rat diets containing wheat bran or cellulose. *J. Nutr.* **118**:65.

Huff, W. E. and P. B. Hamilton. 1975. Decreased plasma carotenoids during ochratoxicosis. *Poult. Sci.* **54**:1308.

Hungate, R. E. 1966. "The Rumen and Its Microbes." Academic Press, New York.

Jaster, E. H. 1988. Nicotinic acid or nicotinamide for lactating dairy cows. *In* "Proceedings of the Degussa Technical Symposium," pp. 3-15. Atlanta, GA.

Jaster, E. H., D. F. Bell and T. A. McPherron. 1983a. Nicotinic acid and serum metabolite concentrations of lactating dairy cows fed supplemental niacin. *J. Dairy Sci.* **66**:1039.

Jaster, E. H., G. F. Hartnell and M. F. Hutjens. 1983b. Feeding supplemental niacin for milk production in six dairy herds. *J. Dairy Sci.* **66**:1046.

Jukes, T. H., J. J. Oleson and A. Dornbush. 1945. Observations on monomethylaminoethanol and dimethylaminoethanol in the diet of chicks. *J.Nutr.* **30**:219.

Jusko, W. J. and G. Levy. 1975. *In* "Riboflavin" (R. S. Rivilin, Ed.), pp. 99-152. Plenum Press,New York.

Kabir, H., J. E. Leklem and L. T. Miller. 1983. Relationship of the glycosylated vitamin B-6 content of foods to vitamin B-6 bioavailability in humans. *Nutr. Rep. Int.* **28**:709.

Keltz, F. R., C. Kies and H. M. Fox. 1978. Urinary ascorbic acid excretion in the human as affected by dietary fiber and zinc. *Am. J. Clin. Nutr.* **31**:1167.

Ketola, H. G. and M. C. Nesheim. 1974. Influence of dietary protein and methionine levels on the requirement for choline by chickens. *J. Nutr.* **104**:1484.

Kindberg, C. G. and J. W. Suttie. 1989. Effect of various intakes of phylloquinone on signs of vitamin K deficiency and serum and liver phylloquinone concentrations in the rat. *J. Nutr.* **119**:175.

Kodicek, E. and P. W. Wilson. 1960. The isolation of niacytin, the bound form of nicotinic acid. *Biochem. J.* **76**:27.

Kratzer, F. H., K. Knollman, L. Earl and J. L. Buenrostro. 1988. Availability to chicks of biotin from dried egg products. *J. Nutr.* **118**:604.

Krumdieck, C. L., A. J. Newman and C. E. Butterworth Jr. 1973. A naturally occurring inhibitor of folic acid conjugase (petroylpolyglutamyl hydrolase) in beans and other pulses. *Am. J. Clin. Nutr.* **26**:460. [Abstract].

Leklem, J. E. 1988. Vitamin B₆ bioavailability and its application to human nutrition. *Food Technol.* **42**:194.

Lewis, A. J., G. L. Cromwell and J. E. Pettigrew. 1989. Effect of supplemental biotin on the reproductive performance of sows. *J. Anim. Sci.* **67**(Suppl. 2): 114 [Abstract].

Lindemann, M. D. and E. T. Kornegay. 1989. Folic acid supplementation to diets of gestating-lactating swine over multiple parities. *J. Anim. Sci.* **67**:459.

Livingston, A. L., J. W. Nelson and G. O. Kohler. 1968. Stability of α-tocopherol during alfalfa dehydration and storage. *J. Agric. Food Chem.* **16**:492.

Lott, D. G. 1951. The use of thiamin in mare's tail poisoning of horses. *Can. J. Comp. Med. Vet Sci.* **15**:274.

Lovell, T. 1989. "Nutrition and Feeding of Fish." Van Nostrand-Reinhold, New York .

Lowry, K. R. and D. H. Baker. 1987. Amelioration of ethionine toxicity in the chick. *Poult. Sci.* **66**:1028.

Lowry, K. R. and D. H. Baker. 1989. Effect of excess leucine on niacin provided by either tryptophan or niacin. *FASEB J.* **3**:A666 [Abstract].

Lowry, K. R., O. A. Izquierdo and D. H. Baker. 1987. Efficacy of betaine relative to choline as a dietary methyl donor. *Poult. Sci.* **66** (Suppl.1):120 [Abstract].

Luce, W. G., E. R. Peo and D. B. Hudman. 1966. Availability of niacin in wheat for swine. *J. Nutr.* **88**:39.

Luce, W. G., E. R. Peo and D. B. Hudman. 1967. Availability of niacin in corn and milo for swine. *J. Anim. Sci.* **26**:76.

March, B. E. and C. MacMillan. 1980. Choline concentration and availability in rapeseed meal. *Poult. Sci.* **59**:611.

Martin, A. A. 1975. Nigro pallidal encephalomalacia in horses caused by chronic poisoning with yellow star thistle. *Nutr. Abstr. Rev.* **45**:85.

Matte, J. J., C. L. Girard, and G. C. Brisson. 1984. Folic acid and reproductive performance of sows. *J. Anim. Sci.* **59**:1020.

McGinnis, C. H. 1986. Vitamin stability, and activity of water-soluble vitamins as influenced by manufacturing processes and recommendations for the water-soluble vitamins. In "Proceediings of the NFIA Nutrition Institute". pp. 1-44.

Menon, I. A. and E. Sognen. 1971. Amprolium and transport of thiamine in suspensions of intestinal cells. *Acta. Vet. Scand.* **12**:111.

Miller, B. L., S. D. Plegge, R. D. Goodrich and J. C. Meiske. 1983a. Influence of monensin on B-vitamin synthesis and absorption in beef steers. Minnesota Beef Report B-301.

Miller, B. L., S. D. Plegge, R. D. Goodrich and J. C. Meiske. 1983b. Influence of dietary grain level on production and absorption of B-vitamins in beef steers. Minnesota Beef Report B-300.

Misir, R. and R. Blair. 1988a. Biotin bioavailability of protein supplements and cereal grains for starting turkey poults. *Poult. Sci.* **67**:1274.

Misir, R. and R. Blair. 1988b. Biotin bioavailability from protein supplements and cereal grains for weanling pigs. *Can. J. Anim. Sci.* **68**:523.

Molitoris, B. A. and D. H. Baker. 1976a. Choline utilization in the chick as influenced by levels of dietary protein and methionine. *J. Nutr.* **106**:412.

Molitoris, B. A. and D. H. Baker. 1976b. Assessment of the quantity of biologically available choline in soybean meal. *J. Anim. Sci.* **47**:481.

Murata, K. 1982. Actions of two types of thiaminase on thiamin and its analogues. *Ann. N. Y. Acad. Sci.* **378**:146.

National Research Council (NRC). 1982. "Nutrient Requirements of DomesticAnimals. Nutrient Requirements of Mink," 2nd revised ed. National Academy of Sciences, Washington, DC.

National Research Council (NRC). 1984a. "Nutrient Requirements of Domestic Animals. Nutrient requirements of Poultry," 8th revised ed. National Academy of Sciences, Washington, DC.

National Research Council (NRC). 1984b. "Nutrient Requirements of Domestic Animals. Nutrient Requirements of Beef Cattle," 6th revised ed. National Academy of Sciences, Washington, DC.

National Research Council (NRC). 1985. "Nutrient Requirements of Domestic Animals. Nutrient requirements of Dogs," 2nd revised ed. National Academy of Sciences, Washington, DC.

National Research Council (NRC). 1986. "Nutrient Requirements of Domestic Animals. Nutrient Requirements of Cats," 2nd revised ed. National Academy of Sciences, Washington, DC.

National Research Council (NRC). 1987. "Vitamin Tolerence of Animals." National Academy of Sciences, Washington, DC.

National Research Council (NRC). 1988. "Nutrient Requirements of Domestic Animals. Nutrient Requirements of Swine," 9th revised ed. National Academy of Sciences, Washington, DC.

National Research Council (NRC). 1989a. " Nutrient Rrequirements of Domestic Animals. Nutrient Requirements of Dairy Cattle," 6th revised ed. National Academy of Sciences, Washington, DC.

National Research Council (NRC). 1989b. "Nutrient Requirements of Domestic Animals. Nutrient Requirements of Horses," 5th revised ed. National Academy of Sciences, Washington, DC.

NCR-42 Committee on Swine Nutrition. 1976. Effect of supplemental choline on reproductive performance of sows: A cooperative regional study. *J. Anim. Sci.* **42**:1211.

NCR-42 Committee on Swine Nutrition. 1980. Effect of supplemental choline on performance of starting, growing and finishing pigs: A cooperative regional study. *J. Anim. Sci.* **50**:99.

Oduho, G. and D. H. Baker. 1993. Quantitative efficacy of niacin sources for the chick: nicotinic acid, nicotinamide, NAD and tryptophan. *J. Nutr.* **123**:2201.

Oduho, G. W., T. K. Chung and D. H. Baker. 1993. Menadione nicotinamide bisulfite is a bioactive source of vitamin K and niacin activity for chicks. *J. Nutr.* **123**:737.

Oduho, G. W., Y. Han and D. H. Baker. 1994. Iron deficiency reduces the efficacy of tryptophan as a niacin precursor for chicks. *J. Nutr.* **124**:444.

Olson, J. A. 1984. "Vitamin A. In Handbook of Vitamins" (L. J. Machlin, Ed.). Marcel Dekker, New York.

Partridge, I. G. and M. S. McDonald. 1990. A note on the response of growing pigs to supplemental biotin. *Anim. Prod.* **50**:195.

Patsch, J. R., D. Yeshurm, R. L. Jackson and A. M. Gotto. 1977. Effects of clofibrate, nicotinic acid and diet on the properties of the plasma lipoproteins in a subject with type III hyperlipoproteinemia. *Am. J. Med.* **63**:1001.

Pharazyn, A. and F. X. Aherne. 1987. Folacin requirement of the lactating sow. *In* "66th Annual Feeders Day Report," pp. 16-17. University of Alberta.

Poston, H. A. and R. N. DiLorenzo. 1973. Tryptophan conversion to niacin in brook trout (Solvenlinus fontalis). *Proc. Soc. Exp. Biol. Med.* **144**:1103.

Rao, N. and B. S. N. Rao. 1970. Absorption of dietary carotenes in human subjects. *Am. J. Clin. Nutr.* **23**:105.

Reiners, R. A. and C. M. Gooding. 1975. " In Culture, Processing Products" (G. E. Inglett, Ed.).

Riddell, D. O., E. E. Bartley and A. D. Dayton. 1980. Effect of nicotinic acid on rumen fermentation in vitro and in vivo. *J. Dairy Sci.* **63**:1429.

Riddell, D. O., E. E. Bartley and A. D. Dayton. 1981. Effect of nicotinic acid on microbial protein synthesis in vitro, on dairy cattle growth and milk production. *J. Dairy Sci.* **64**:782.

Roberts, H. E., E. T. Evans and W. C. Evans. 1949. The production of bracken staggers in the horse and its treatment by vitamin B$_1$ therapy. *Vet. Rec.* **61**:549.

Rodriquez, M. S. and M. I. Irwin. 1972. A conspectus of research on vitamin A requirements of man. *J. Nutr.* **102**:909.

Rosenberg, H. R. 1942. *In* "Chemistry and Physiology of the Vitamins." Interscience, New York.

Rudnick, R. C. and G. L. Czarnecki-Maulden. 1988. Development of a zinc-deficient diet for dogs: effect of processing on feeding value of spray-dried egg white. *FASEB J.* **2**:A868 [Abstract].

Ruiz, N. and R. H. Harms. 1988. Comparison of biopotencies of nicotinic acid and nicotinamide for broiler chickens. *Br. Poult. Sci.* **29**:491.

Sauerlich, H. 1985. Bioavailability of vitamins. *Prog. Food Nutr. Sci.* **9**:1.

Sauer, W. C., R. Mosenthin and L. Ozimek. 1988. The digestibility of biotin in protein supplements and cereal grains for growing pigs. *J. Anim. Sci.* **66**:2583.

Schneider, J. 1986. Vitamin stability and activity of fat-soluble vitamins as influenced by manufacturing processes. *In* "Proceedings of the NFIA Nutrition Institute." pp. 1-6.

Schroeder, H. H. 1971. Losses of vitamins and trace minerals resulting from processing and preservation of foods. *Am. J. Clin. Nutr.* **24**:562.

Seerley, R. W., O. W. Charles, H. C. McCampbell and S. P. Bertsch. 1976. Efficacy of menadione dimethylpyrimidinol bisulfite as a source of vitamin K in swine diets. *J. Anim. Sci.* **42**:599.

Seetharam, B. and D. H. Alpers. 1982. Absorption and transport of cobalamin (vitamin B$_{12}$). *Annu. Rev. Nutr.* **2**:343.

Sharma, B. K. and R. A. Erdman. 1989. Effects of dietary and abomasally infused choline on milk production responses of lactating dairy cows. *J. Nutr.* **119**:248.

Smith, J. C. 1980. The vitamin A-zinc connection: A review. *In* "Micronutrient Interactions: Vitamins, Minerals and Hazardous Elements" (O. A. Levander and L. Cheng, Eds.), p. 62. New York Academy of Science.

Solomons, N. W. and R. M. Russell. 1980. The interaction of vitamin A and zinc: Implications for human nutrition. *Am. J. Clin. Nutr.* **33**:2031.

Solomons, N. W. and F. E. Viteri. 1982. Biological interaction of ascorbic acid and mineral nutrients. *In* "Ascorbic Acid: Chemistry, Metabolism, and Uses" (P. A. Seib and B. H. Tolbert, Eds.), pp. 551-569. American Chemical Society, Washington, DC.

Sommerfeldt, J. L., J. L. Napoli and E. T. Littledike. 1983. Metabolism of orally administered [^{3}H]-ergocalciferol and [^{3}H]-cholecalciferol by dairy cows. *J. Nutr.* **113**:2595.

Southern, L. L. and D. H. Baker. 1981. Bioavailable pantothenic acid in cereal grains and soybean meal. *J. Anim. Sci.* **53**:403.

Spenser, R. P., S. Purdy, R. Hoeldeke, T. M. Bow and A. Markulus. 1963. Studies on intestinal absorption of L-ascorbic acid 1-^{14}C. *Gastroenterology* **44**:768.

Staten, F. E., P. A. Anderson, D. H. Baker and P. C. Harrison. 1980. The efficacy of DL-pantothenic acid relative to D-pantothenic acid in chicks. *Poult. Sci.* **59**:1664 [Abstract].

Stockland, W. L. and L. G. Blaylock. 1974. Choline requirement of pregnant sows and gilts under restricted feeding conditions. *J. Anim. Sci.* **39**:1113.

Tamura, T., and E. L. R. Stokstad. 1973. The availability of food folate in man. *Br. J. Haematol* **25**:513.

Tarr, J. B., T. Tamura and E. L. R. Stokstad. 1981. Availability of vitamin B$_6$ and pantothenate in an average American diet in man. *Am. J. Clin. Nutr.* **34**:1328.

Thaler, B. 1988. Study shows effects of folic acid addition on sows. *Feedstuffs* **60**(38):18.

Thompson, A. D., H. Baker and C. M. Leevy. 1971. Folate-induced malabsorption of thiamin. *Gastroenterology* **60**:756 [Abstract].

Tomarelli, R. M., E. R. Spence and F. W. Bernhart. 1955. Biological availability of vitamin B$_6$ in heated milk. *J. Agric. Food Chem.* **3**:338.

Trumbo, P. R., J. F. Gregory and D. B. Sartain. 1988. Incomplete utilization of pyridoxine-beta-glucoside as vitamin B$_6$ in the rat. *J. Nutr.* **118**:170.

Tucker, B. W. and J. E. Halver. 1984. Ascorbate-2 sulfate metabolism in fish. *Nutr. Rev.* **42**:173-179.

Tung, H. T. and P. B. Hamilton. 1973. Decreased plasma carotenoids during aflatoxicosis. *Poult. Sci.* **52**:80.

Ullrey, D. E. 1972. Biological availability of fat-soluble vitamins: vitamin A and carotene. *J. Anim. Sci.* **35**:648.

Ullrey, D. E. 1981. Vitamin E for swine. *J. Anim. Sci.* **53**:1039.

Verbeeck, J. 1975. Vitamin behavior in premixes. *Feedstuffs* **47**(36):45.

Warner, R. G., H. F. Travis, C. F. Bassett, B. McCarthy and R. P. Abernathy. 1968. Niacin requirement of growing mink. *J. Nutr.* **95**:563.

Waterman, R., J. W. Schwalm and L. H. Schultz. 1972. Nicotinic acid treatment of bovine ketosis. 1. Effects of circulatory metabolites and interrelationships. *J. Dairy Sci.* **55**:1447.

Weber, F. 1983. Absorption of fat-soluble vitamins. *Int. J. Vit. Nutr. Res. (Suppl.)* **25**:55.

White, H. B. and C. C. Whitehead. 1987. Role of avidin and other biotin-binding proteins in the deposition of biotin in chicken eggs. *Biochem. J.* **241**:677.

Whitehead, C. C., J. A. Armstrong and D. Waddington. 1982. The determination of the availability to chicks of biotin in feed ingredients by a bioassay based on the response of blood pyruvate carboxylase (EC 6.4.1.1) activity. *Br. J. Nutr.* **48**:81.

Wornick, R. C. 1968. The stability of micro-ingredients in animal feed products. *Feedstuffs* **40**(48):25.

Yen, J. T., A. H. Jensen and D. H. Baker. 1976. Assessment of the concentration of biologically available vitamin B_6 in corn and soybean meal. *J. Anim. Sci.* **42**:866.

Yen, J. T., A. H. Jensen and D. H. Baker. 1977. Assessment of the availability of niacin in corn, soybeans and soybean meal. *J. Anim. Sci.* **45**:269.

Young, L. G., A. Lun, J. Pos, R. P. Forshaw and D. E. Edmeades. 1975. Vitamin E stability in corn and mixed feed. *J. Anim. Sci.* **40**:495.

Young, L. G., R. B. Miller, D. E. Edmeades, A. Lun, G. C. Smith and G. J. King. 1977. Selenium and vitamin E supplementation of high moisture corn diets for swine reproduction. *J. Anim. Sci.* **45**:1051.

Young, L. G., R. B. Miller, D. E. Edmeades, A. Lun, G. C. Smith and G. J. King. 1978. Influence of method of corn storage and vitamin E and selenium supplementation on pig survival and reproduction. *J. Anim. Sci.* **47**:639.

Zhuge Q. and C. F. Klopfenstein. 1986. Factors affecting storage stability of vitamin A, riboflavin and niacin in a broiler diet premix. *Poult. Sci.* **65**:987.

Zinn, R. A., F. N. Owens, R. L. Stuart, J. R. Dunbar and B. B. Norman. 1987. B-vitamin supplementation of diets for feedlot calves. *J. Anim. Sci.* **64**:267.

APPENDIX I

Table I. Abbreviations

AA	Crystalline amino acid
Abs	Absorption
AD	Air-dried
Alb	Albumin
Alk	Alkaline
Anhyd	Anhydrous
Arg	Arginine
App	Apparent
BBP	Biotin binding protein
BBS	Bone breaking strength
BW	Body weight
Cal	Calculation
Carbox	Carboxylase activity
Cell	Cellulose
Cer	Ceruloplasmin
Co-A	Coenzyme A
Cryst	Crystalline
CSM	Cottonseed meal
Cys	Cystine
Dig	Digestion
DIS	Diiodosalicylic acid
DM	Dry matter
DNA	Deoxyribonucleic acid
ED	Exudative diathesis
EDDI	Ethylenediamine dihydriodide
EDTA	Ethylenediaminetetraacetate
EGR	Erythrocyte glutathione reductase
Exc	Excretion
Ext	Extrinsic

FAD	Flavin adenine dinucleotide
FDNB	1-Fluoro-2,4-dinitrobenzene
Fert	Fertilized
FG	Feed grade
FH_4	Tetrahydrofolate
Fib	Fibrosis
Fl	Fluid
FMN	Flavin mononucleotide
GSH-Px	Glutathione peroxidase
Hr	Hour
Hat	Hatchability
Hb	Hemoglobin
His	Histidine
Hyd	Hydrate
ICU	International chick unit
Ile	Isoleucine
Int	Intrinsic
IU	International units
K_1	Phylloquinone
K_2	Menaquinone
K_3	Menadione
Kid	Kidney
Lab	Label
Lcell	Lignocellulose
Leu	Leucine
Liv	Liver
Lys	Lysine
MB	Monobasic
MBM	Meat and bone meal
Met	Methionine
Meth	Method
Min	Minute
Mo	Month
MPB	Menadione pyridinol bisulfite

MR	Mean ratio
MSB	Menadione sodium bisulfite
MSBC	Menadione sodium bisulfite complex
N	Natural
n	Number
NAD	Nicotinamide adenine dinucleotide
NDF	Neutral detergent fiber
Nec	Necrosis
NG	Not given
OH-M	Methionine hydroxy analog
P	Purified
PA	Pantothenic acid
PABA	Para-aminobenzoic acid
Panc	Pancreatic
PCOP	Pentacalcium orthoperiodate
Phe	Phenylalanine
Phos	Phosphatase
PI	Perosis index
PL	Parallel lines
Pla	Plasma
PM	Purified medium
Prod	Production
Prot	Protein
Qual	Quality
RA	Radioactivity
RBC	Red blood cell
RBV	Relative bioavailability value
RE	Retinol equivalent
Reg	Regeneration
Ret	Retention
RG	Reagent grade
Rum	Rumen or ruminal
RV	Relative value
SAA	Sulfur amino acids

SC	Standard curve
Ser	Serum
SH	Sulfhydral
Sim	Simulated
SOD	Single oral dose
SOM	Single oral meal
SP	Semipurified
Spl	Spleen
SR	Slope ratio
Syn	Synthesis
Thr	Threonine
Thy	Thyroid
TNBS	2,4,6-Trinitrobenzene sulfonic acid
TP	Three point
Trp	Tryptophan
Tyr	Tyrosine
Upt	Uptake
Ur	Urinary
USP	United States pharmacopoeia
UV	Ultraviolet
Val	Valine
WB	Whole blood
Wk	Week
Wt	Weight
Yr	Year

Index

ISBN 0-12-056250-2

9 780120 562503

90293>

UNIVERSITY OF LINCOLN